THE WASHINGTON MANUAL™

Hematology and Oncology Subspecialty Consult

Second Edition

Editors

Amanda F. Cashen, MD
Assistant Professor of Medicine
Department of Internal Medicine
Division of Oncology
Section of Bone Marrow Transplantation
and Leukemia
Washington University School of Medicine
Barnes-Jewish Hospital
St. Louis, Missouri

Tanya M. Wildes, MD
Fellow, Hematology and Oncology
Department of Internal Medicine
Division of Hematology/Oncology
Washington University School of Medicine
Barnes-Jewish Hospital
St. Louis, Missouri

Series Editors

Katherine E. Henderson, MD
Instructor in Medicine
Department of Internal Medicine
Division of Medical Education
Washington University School of Medicine
Barnes-Jewish Hospital
St. Louis, Missouri

Thomas M. De Fer, MD
Associate Professor of Internal Medicine
Washington University School of Medicine
St. Louis, Missouri

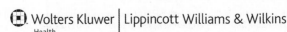
Wolters Kluwer | Lippincott Williams & Wilkins
Health
Philadelphia • Baltimore • New York • London
Buenos Aires • Hong Kong • Sydney • Tokyo

Acquisitions Editor: Ave McCracken
Managing Editor: Michelle LaPlante
Project Manager: Bridgett Dougherty
Marketing Manager: Kimberly Schonberger
Manufacturing Manager: Kathleen Brown
Design Coordinator: Stephen Druding
Cover Designer: Joseph DePinho
Production Service: Aptara, Inc.

Second Edition

© 2008 by Department of Medicine, Washington University School of Medicine

Printed in China

9 8 7 6 5 4

Library of Congress Cataloging-in-Publication Data

The Washington manual hematology and oncology subspecialty consult. —
2nd ed. / editors Amanda Cashen, Tanya Wildes,
    p. ; cm.
  Includes bibliographical references and index.
  ISBN 978-0-7817-9156-4 (pbk. : alk. paper)
  1. Cancer—Handbooks, manuals, etc.   2. Oncology—Handbooks, manuals, etc.   3. Hematology—Handbooks, manuals, etc.   4. Blood—Diseases— Handbooks, manuals, etc.   I. Cashen, Amanda.
II. Wildes, Tanya.   III. Title: Hematology and oncology subspecialty consult.
  [DNLM: 1. Hematologic Diseases—Handbooks.   2. Neoplasms—Handbooks.   3. Diagnosis, Differential—Handbooks.   4. Drug Therapy—methods—Handbooks. WH 120 W319 2008 /
WH 39 W319 2008]
  RC262.W265 2008
  616.99'4—dc22   2008001356

To purchase additional copies of this book, call our customer service department at **(800) 638-3030** or fax orders to **(301) 223-2320**. International customers should call **(301) 223-2300**.

Visit Lippincott Williams & Wilkins on the Internet: http://www.lww.com. Lippincott Williams & Wilkins customer service representatives are available from 8:30 am to 6:00 pm, EST.

Table of Contents

PART II. ONCOLOGY

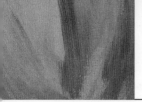

Contributing Authors

Nina Asrani, MD
Resident Physician
Department of Medicine
Washington University School of Medicine
St. Louis, Missouri

Kristan M. Augustin, PharmD, BCOP
Clinical Pharmacist
BMT/Leukemia
Department of Pharmacy
Barnes-Jewish Hospital
St. Louis, Missouri

Amanda F. Cashen, MD
Assistant Professor of Medicine
Department of Medicine, Division of Oncology
Washington University School of Medicine
St. Louis, Missouri

Walter W. Chan, MD
Clinical and Research Fellow in Medicine
Division of Gastroenterology, Hepatology and
Endoscopy
Brigham and Women's Hospital
Harvard Medical School
Boston, Massachusetts

Jinny E. Chang, MD
Resident Physician
Department of Medicine
Washington University School of Medicine
St. Louis, Missouri

Mariana Chavez-MacGregor, MD, MSc
Resident Physician
Department of Medicine
Washington University School of Medicine
St. Louis, Missouri

Yee Hong Chia, MD
Resident Physician
Department of Medicine
Washington University School of Medicine
St. Louis, Missouri

Lee Demertzis, MD
Instructor in Medicine
Chief Resident, Shatz-Strauss Firm
Washington University School of Medicine
St. Louis, Missouri

Bryan A. Faller, MD
Instructor in Medicine
Division of Hospital Medicine
Department of Medicine
Washington University School of Medicine
St. Louis, Missouri

Todd A. Fehniger, MD, PhD
Fellow
Department of Medicine
Division of Hematology/Oncology
Washington University School of Medicine
St. Louis, Missouri

Priya K. Gopalan, MD, PhD
Fellow
Department of Medicine
Division of Hematology/Oncology
Washington University School of Medicine
St. Louis, Missouri

Andrea R. Hagemann, MD
Resident Physician
Department of Obstetrics and Gynecology
Washington University School of Medicine
St. Louis, Missouri

Anna Margrét Halldórsdóttir, MD
Transfusion Medicine Fellow
Division of Laboratory and Genomic Medicine
Department of Pathology and Immunology
Washington University School of Medicine
St. Louis, Missouri

Coy Heldermon, MD, PhD
Fellow
Department of Medicine
Division of Hematology/Oncology
Washington University School of Medicine
St. Louis, Missouri

Lindsay M. Hladnik, PharmD
Clinical Pharmacist
Department of Pharmacy
Barnes-Jewish Hospital
St. Louis, Missouri

Chanda Ho, MD
Resident Physician
Department of Medicine
Washington University School of Medicine
St. Louis, Missouri

Nasreen Ilias, MD
Resident Physician
Department of Medicine
Washington University School of Medicine
St. Louis, Missouri

Meagan A. Jacoby, MD, PhD
Fellow
Department of Medicine
Division of Hematology/Oncology
Washington University School of Medicine
St. Louis, Missouri

Sakib K. Khalid, MD
Fellow, Section of Digestive Diseases
Department of Internal Medicine
Yale University School of Medicine
New Haven, Connecticut

David Kuperman, MD
Instructor
John Cochran VA Medical Center
Washington University School of Medicine
St. Louis, Missouri

Philip E. Lammers, MD
Resident Physician
Department of Medicine
Washington University School of Medicine
St. Louis, Missouri

Nathan Martin, MD
Resident Physician
Department of Medicine
Washington University School of Medicine
St. Louis, Missouri

Mike G. Martin, MD
Fellow
Department of Medicine
Division of Hematology/Oncology
Washington University School of Medicine
St. Louis, Missouri

James C. Mosley, III, MD
Fellow
Department of Medicine
Division of Hematology/Oncology
Washington University School of Medicine
St. Louis, Missouri

Mohsen Nasir, MD
Resident Physician
Department of Medicine
Washington University School of Medicine
St. Louis, Missouri

Parag J. Parikh, MD
Instructor
Radiation Oncology & Biomedical Engineering
Washington University School of Medicine
St. Louis, Missouri

Prapti Patel, MD
Resident Physician
Department of Medicine
Washington University School of Medicine
St. Louis, Missouri

Pablo Ramirez, MD
Fellow
Department of Medicine
Division of Hematology/Oncology
Washington University School of Medicine
St. Louis, Missouri

Giridharan Ramsingh, MD
Fellow
Department of Medicine
Division of Hematology/Oncology
Washington University School of Medicine
St. Louis, Missouri

Caron Rigden, MD
Assistant Professor of Medicine
Department of Medicine, Division of Oncology
Washington University School of Medicine
St. Louis, Missouri

Mark A. Schroeder, MD
Fellow
Department of Medicine
Division of Hematology/Oncology
Washington University School of Medicine
St. Louis, Missouri

Robert Schwartz, MD, PhD
Resident Physician
Department of Internal Medicine
Washington University School of Medicine
St. Louis, Missouri

Janakiraman Subramanian, MD, MPH
Fellow
Department of Medicine
Division of Hematology/Oncology
Washington University School of Medicine
St. Louis, Missouri

Brian A. Van Tine, MD, PhD
Fellow
Department of Medicine
Division of Hematology/Oncology
Washington University School of Medicine
St. Louis, Missouri

Vamsidhar Velcheti, MD
Resident Physician
Department of Internal Medicine
Ochsner Clinic Foundation
New Orleans, Louisiana

Saiama Waqar, MD
Resident Physician
Department of Internal Medicine
Washington University School of Medicine
St. Louis, Missouri

Lukas D. Wartman, MD
Fellow
Department of Medicine
Division of Hematology/Oncology
Washington University School of Medicine
St. Louis, Missouri

John S. Welch, MD, PhD
Fellow
Department of Medicine
Division of Hematology/Oncology
Washington University School of Medicine
St. Louis, Missouri

Tanya M. Wildes, MD
Fellow
Department of Medicine
Division of Hematology/Oncology
Washington University School of Medicine
St. Louis, Missouri

Israel Zighelboim, MD
Fellow
Department of Obstetrics and Gynecology
Division of Gynecologic Oncology
Washington University School of Medicine
St. Louis, Missouri

Imran Zoberi, MD
Associate Professor
Radiation Oncology
Washington University School of Medicine
St. Louis, Missouri

Chairman's Note

Medical knowledge is increasing at an exponential rate, and physicians are being bombarded with new facts at a pace that many find overwhelming. The Washington Manual™ Subspecialty Consult Series was developed in this context for interns, residents, medical students, and other practitioners in need of readily accessible practical clinical information. They, therefore, meet an important unmet need in an era of information overload.

I would like to acknowledge the authors who have contributed to these books. In particular, the series editors, Katherine E. Henderson, MD and Thomas M. De Fer, MD, for their oversight of the project. I'd also like to recognize Melvin Blanchard, MD, Chief of the Division of Medical Education in the Department of Medicine at Washington University for his guidance and advice. The efforts and outstanding skill of the lead authors are evident in the quality of the final product. I am confident that this series will meet its desired goal of providing practical knowledge that can be directly applied to improving patient care.

Kenneth S. Polonsky, MD
Adolphus Busch Professor
Chairman, Department of Medicine
Washington University School of Medicine
St. Louis, Missouri

Preface

S ignificant advances in the understanding and treatment of hematologic and oncologic diseases have occurred in recent years. New therapies move from the developmental phase to clinical practice at an ever-quickening pace. Antibody-based therapies and small molecules directed at the abnormal phenotype or aberrant signaling pathways in malignant cells provide effective new therapies that in many instances are less toxic than or synergistic with conventional chemotherapy. The discovery of new molecular biomarkers, including cytogenetic abnormalities and gene expression patterns, provides prognostic information that augments and complements traditional staging systems and clinical models.

At this time of rapid advances in the field, we take pride in introducing the second edition of *The Washington Manual™ Hematology and Oncology Subspecialty Consult*. This edition has been updated to include new standards in the treatment of malignancies, mechanisms of action of new therapeutic agents, and current use of molecular prognostic factors. Our goal is to provide a concise, practical reference for fellows, residents, and medical students rotating on hematology and oncology subspecialty services. Most of the authors are hematology-oncology fellows or internal medicine residents, the physicians who have recent experience with the issues and questions that arise in the course of training in these subspecialties. We hope that primary care practitioners and other health care professionals also will find this manual useful as a quick reference source in hematology and oncology.

As the practice of hematology and oncology continues to evolve, changes in dosing and indications for chemotherapy and targeted therapies will occur frequently. Likewise, staging systems are modified as our understanding of prognostic factors changes. Therefore, a handbook of chemotherapy regimens and an oncology staging manual will complement the information in this manual. And of course, clinical judgment is imperative when applying the principles presented herein to the care of individual patients.

We appreciate the effort and expertise of the many people who contributed to the second edition of the *Hematology and Oncology Subspecialty Consult*. We would like to thank Dr. Katherine Henderson for her thoughtful editorial comments and insights. We recognize the faculty in the divisions of hematology, medical oncology, and bone marrow transplantation for their mentorship and commitment to education. Finally, we thank the authors for working enthusiastically to distill volumes of new scientific literature into concise chapters.

—T.W. and A.C.

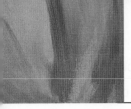

Introduction and Approach to Hematology

Pablo Ramirez

INTRODUCTION

Hematologic diseases are a heterogeneous group of diseases that can have multiple clinical and laboratory manifestations that mimic nonhematologic diseases. For that reason, a detailed clinical history and physical exam are essential. Frequently, laboratory tests will be necessary to confirm the clinical diagnosis.

The goal of this handbook is to provide an understanding of the basic mechanisms for hematologic disorders and the initial evaluation of them. The major clinical manifestations and the usual management options for these diseases are also discussed in each chapter.

APPROACH TO THE HEMATOLOGY PATIENT

Hematologic disorders can be approached by identifying the primary hematologic component that is affected: RBCs, WBCs, platelets, or the coagulation system. The major abnormalities in hematology are quantitative in nature, with either excessive or deficient production of one of the hematopoietic constituents (e.g., leukemias, anemias). Qualitative abnormalities also can be inherited (e.g., sickle cell disease) or acquired.

History

The medical history is the first step in hematology diagnostic assessment. With simple questions we can evaluate causes of a suspected anemia, the rapid onset of a hematological neoplasia, or a genetic hematological disease. Table 1-1 offers some general questions for evaluation of a hematological disorder.

Physical Exam

The physical exam is also an important part of the diagnostic process. Along with the history, it can suggest a diagnosis, guide lab testing, and aid in the differential diagnosis. Table 1-2 offers some general physical exam findings that are useful in the hematology patient.

Lab Evaluation

The clinician should be comfortable using the CBC and peripheral smear to evaluate patients for possible hematologic disorders. Patients may be referred to a hematologist based on a lab abnormality that is drawn for a reason other than the diagnosis of a primary hematologic disorder. There are certain limiting values in hematology that can help exclude or confirm the need for further testing or warn us of the possibility of potential physiological consequences (see Table 1-3).

TABLE 1-1	PERTINENT HISTORY IN THE HEMATOLOGY PATIENT
Pertinent Medical History	**Hematologic Differential Diagnosis**
History of present illness	
Recent infections	
Fever, chills, rigors	Leukemias, lymphomas, multiple myeloma
Antibiotic use	Hemolysis
Bleeding	
Hemorrhage, epistaxis, bleeding gums, petechiae, ecchymosis, menorrhagia	Thrombocytopenia, leukemias, coagulation disorder
Hemarthrosis	Clotting factor deficiency
Skin coloration	
Pallor	Anemia
Jaundice	Hemolysis
Dyspnea, chest pain, orthostasis	Anemia
Pica	Iron deficiency
Abdominal fullness, early satiety	Splenomegaly
Alcoholism, poor nutrition, vegetarianism	Megaloblastic anemia
Neurologic	
Headache, neurologic deficits	Leukostasis, thrombocytopenia, thrombosis, Waldenström macroglobulinemia
Pruritus	Polycythemia, Hodgkin lymphoma
Medical history	
Prior malignancies, chemotherapy	Secondary malignancies (leukemia), myelodysplasia
HIV risk factors	Anemia, thrombocytopenia
Previous hepatitis	Anemia, cryoglobulinemia
Pregnancy	Anemia, HELLP syndrome
Venous thrombosis	Thrombophilia
Family history	
Bleeding disorders	Hemophilias, von Willebrand disease
Anemia (African American, Mediterranean, Asian)	Hemoglobinopathies

HELLP, hemolysis, elevated liver enzymes, and low platelet count.

THE PERIPHERAL SMEAR

The visual study of peripheral blood is necessary to diagnose hematologic and nonhematologic diseases. The peripheral smear obtained allows the study of the different cellular components of the blood and the determination of anomalies in red blood cells, leukocytes, and platelets affected directly by a hematologic disease or as a manifestation of other nonhematologic diseases. Moreover, there are some cases where the suspected disease makes the smear obligatory, such as thrombotic thrombocytopenic purpura and malaria. In these cases, as in others, automated hematology analyzers are able to provide a large

TABLE 1-2	PHYSICAL EXAM IN THE HEMATOLOGY PATIENT
Pertinent Exam Findings	Hematologic Differential Diagnosis
HEENT	
Conjunctival or mucosal pallor	Anemia
Jaundice	Hemolysis, hyperbilirubinemia
Conjunctival or mucosal petechiae	Thrombocytopenia
Glossitis	Iron deficiency, vitamin B_{12} deficiency
Lymphadenopathy	Lymphoma
Skin/nails	
Pallor	Anemia
Jaundice	Hyperbilirubinemia
Bronze appearance	Hemochromatosis
Spoon nails (koilonychia)	Iron deficiency
Ecchymosis, petechiae	Thrombocytopenia
Erythematous, indurated plaques	Mycosis fungoides
Cardiovascular	
Tachycardia, S4, prominent post-MI	Severe anemia with high-output cardiac failure
Abdominal	
Splenomegaly	Hairy cell or other leukemias, polycythemia, lymphomas
Neurologic	Megaloblastic anemia
Loss of vibratory sense and proprioception (dorsal and lateral columns)	
Musculoskeletal	
Bone pain/tenderness	Multiple myeloma

HEENT, head, ears, eyes, nose, and throat.

number of data regarding all the blood cells but will not be able to detect subtle anomalies critical in the diagnosis.

Preparation
Slides for a peripheral smear are typically prepared either by automated methods or by qualified technicians in a specialized laboratory. This step is critical since poorly processed samples can lead to incorrect diagnoses.

Smears may be prepared on glass slides or coverslips. Ideally, blood smears should be prepared from uncoagulated blood and from a sample collected from a finger-stick. In practice, most slides are prepared from blood samples containing anticoagulants and are thus prone to the introduction of morphological artifacts. Blood smears are normally stained using Wright or May-Grünwald-Giemsa stain.

Examination
Examination of the smear should proceed systematically and begin under low power to identify a portion of the slide with optimal cellular distribution and staining, which normally corresponds to the thinner edge of the sample. As a general rule, the analysis starts with RBCs, continues with leukocytes, and finishes with platelets.

TABLE 1-3	DECISION LIMITING VALUES FOR COMMON HEMATOLOGIC TESTS	
Diagnostic Test	Limiting Value	Comment
Hgb	<5 g/dL	Transfusion indicated even in absence of symptoms
	<10 g/dL	Anemia workup indicated
Hct	>70%	Urgent phlebotomy indicated
Platelet count	<10,000/mm^3	Risk of spontaneous bleeding
	<50,000/mm^3	Risk of bleeding increased with surgery/trauma
	>500,000 to 1,000,000/mm^3	Risk of thrombosis
	>2,000,000/mm^3	Risk of bleeding
Neutrophil count	<500/mm^3	Greatest risk of infection
Blast count (acute myeloblastic leukemia)	>100,000/mm^3	Risk of leukostasis; urgent treatment indicated
Prothrombin time	<1.5× control	No increased bleeding risk
	>2.5× control	Risk of spontaneous bleeding
Partial prothrombin time	<1.5× control	No increased bleeding risk
	>2.5× control (>90 s)	Risk of spontaneous bleeding
Bleeding time	<20 min	Possible risk of spontaneous bleeding
Antithrombin III	<50% normal level	Risk of spontaneous thrombosis

Under *low power* (×10 to ×20) it is possible to analyze general characteristics of RBCs to discover, for example, the presence of Rouleaux associated with multiple myeloma, estimate the WBC and platelet counts, and determine the presence of abnormal populations of cells, such as blasts, by scanning over the entire smear.

Under *high power* (×100), each of the cell lineages is examined for any abnormalities in number or morphology.

Red Blood Cells

Quantitative analysis of RBCs is difficult on a peripheral smear. Automated analyzers are used to calculate:

MCHC, the mean cell Hgb concentration, expressed as grams per deciliter;
MCH, the mean corpuscular Hgb, expressed as picograms; and
MCV, the mean corpuscular volume, expressed as femtoliters (10^{-15} L).

Qualitative analysis of RBCs should demonstrate uniform round cells with smooth membranes and a pale central area with a round rim of red Hgb. Variations in size are called anisocytosis, and variations in shape, poikilocytosis.

RBC Abnormalities

- **Hypochromia:** Hypocromia corresponds to a very thin rim of Hgb and a larger central pale area. These red cells are often microcytic and are seen in iron deficiency, thalassemias, and sideroblastic anemia.
- **Microcytosis** (<6 μm): Differential diagnosis includes iron-deficiency anemia, anemia in chronic disease, thalassemias, and sideroblastic anemia. These cells are usually hypochromic and have prominent central pallor.
- **Macrocytosis** (>9 μm in diameter): Differential diagnosis includes liver disease, alcoholism, aplastic anemia, and myelodysplasia. Megaloblastic anemias (B_{12} and folate deficiencies) have macro-ovalocytes (large oval cells). *Reticulocytes* are large immature red cells with polychromatophilia.
- **Schistocytes** (fragmented cells): Schistocytes are caused by mechanical disruption of cells in the microvasculature by fibrin strands or by mechanical prosthetic heart valves. Differential diagnosis includes thrombotic thrombocytopenic purpura/hemolytic uremic syndrome, disseminated intravascular coagulation, hemolysis/elevated liver enzymes/low platelet count (HELLP) syndrome, and malignant hypertension.
- **Acanthocytes** (spiculated cells with irregular projections of varying length): These are seen in liver disease.
- **Crenated cells** (cells with short, evenly spaced cytoplasmic projections): Crenated cells may be an artifact of slide preparation or found in renal failure and uremia.
- **Bite cells** (cells with a smooth semicircle extracted): Bite cells are due to spleen phagocytes that have removed Heinz bodies consisting of denatured Hgb. They are found in hemolytic anemia due to glucose-6-phosphate dehydrogenase deficiency.
- **Spherocytes** (round, dense cells with absent central pallor): Spherocytes are seen in immune hemolytic anemia and hereditary spherocytosis.
- **Sickle cells** (sickle-shaped cells): Sickle cells are due to polymerization of Hgb S. They are found in sickle cell disease but not in sickle cell trait.
- **Target cells** (cells with extra Hgb in the center surrounded by a rim of pallor; bull's-eye appearance): Target cells are due to an increase in the ratio of cell membrane surface area to Hgb volume within the cell. These have a central spot of Hgb surrounded by a ring of pallor from the redundancy in cell membrane. They are found in liver disease, postsplenectomy, in hemoglobinopathies, and in thalassemia.
- **Teardrop cells/dacryocytes** (teardrop-shaped cells): These are found in myelofibrosis and myelophthisic states of marrow infiltration.
- **Ovalocytes** (elliptical cells). Ovalocytes are due to the abnormal membrane cytoskeleton found in hereditary elliptocytosis.
- **Polychromatophilia** (blue hue of cytoplasm): This is due to the presence of RNA and ribosomes in reticulocytes.
- **Howell-Jolly bodies** (small, single, purple cytoplasmic inclusions): These represent nuclear remnant DNA and are found after splenectomy or with functional asplenism.
- **Basophilic stippling** (dark-purple inclusions, usually multiple): Basophilic stippling arises from precipitated RNA found in lead poisoning and thalassemia.
- **Nucleated red cells:** These are not normally found in peripheral blood. They appear in hypoxemia and myelofibrosis or other myelophthisic conditions, as well as with severe hemolysis.

- **Heinz bodies** (inclusions seen only on staining with violet crystal): Heinz bodies represent denatured Hgb and are found in glucose-6-phosphate dehydrogenase after oxidative stress.
- **Parasites:** A variety of parasites, including malaria and babesiosis, may be seen within red cells.
- **Rouleaux** (red cell aggregates resembling a stack of coins): Rouleaux is due to the loss of normal electrostatic charge-repelling red cells due to coating with abnormal paraprotein, such as in multiple myeloma.
- **Leukoerythroblastic smear** (teardrop cells, nucleated red cells, and immature white cells): This is found in marrow infiltration or fibrosis (myelophthisic conditions).

White Blood Cells

WBCs normally seen on the peripheral smear include mature granulocytes (neutrophils, eosinophils, and basophils) and mature agranulocytes (lymphocytes and monocytes). Under normal conditions immature myeloid and lymphoid cells are not seen and their presence is related to conditions such as infections and hematologic neoplasias.

- **Neutrophils:** Neutrophils comprise 55% to 60% of total WBCs (1.8×10^9 to 7.7×10^9/L, or thousands per cubic millimeter). They have nuclei containing three or four lobes and granular cytoplasm. The normal size is 10 to 15 μm. Hypersegmented neutrophils contain more than five lobes and are found in megaloblastic anemias. The cytoplasmatic granules correspond to enzymes that are used during the acute phase of inflammation. Increased prominence of cytoplasmic granules is indicative of systemic infection or therapy with growth factors and is known as *toxic granulation*. Neutrophils develop from myeloblasts through promyelocyte, myelocyte, metamyelocyte, and band forms and progress to mature neutrophils. Only mature neutrophils and bands are normally found in peripheral blood. Metamyelocytes and myelocytes may be found in pregnancy, infections, and leukemoid reactions. The presence of less mature forms in the peripheral blood is indicative of hematologic malignancy or myelophthisis.
- **Lymphocytes:** Lymphocytes comprise 25% to 35% (1×10^9 to 4.8×10^9/L, or thousands per cubic millimeter) of total WBCs. They contain a dark, clumped nucleus and a scant rim of blue cytoplasm. The differentiation of T and B cells is very difficult using light microscopy. The normal size is 7 to 18 μm. Atypical (or reactive) lymphocytes seen in viral infections contain more extensive, malleable cytoplasm that may encompass surrounding red cells.
- **Eosinophils:** Eosinophils comprise 0.5% to 4% of total WBCs (0.2×10^9/L, or thousands per cubic millimeter). These are large cells containing prominent red/orange granules and a bilobed nucleus. The normal size is 10 to 15 μm. Increased numbers are found in parasitic infections and allergic disorders.
- **Monocytes:** Monocytes comprise 4% to 8% of total WBCs (0×10^9 to 0.3×10^9/L, or thousands per cubic millimeter). These are the bigger circulating cells with an eccentric U-shaped nucleus. They contain blue cytoplasm and are the precursors of the mononuclear phagocyte system (macrophages, osteoclasts, alveolar macrophages, Kupfer cells, and microglia). The usual size is 12 to 20 μm.
- **Basophils** comprise 0.01% to 0.3% of total WBCs (0 to 0.1×10^9/L, or thousands per cubic millimeter). Their cytoplasm contains large dark-blue granules and a

bilobed nucleus. They are involved in inflammation reactions and increased numbers are also seen in chronic myeloid leukemia. As for eosinophils, the normal size is 10 to 15 μm.

WBC Abnormalities

Quantitative anomalies result in leukopenia and leukocytosis. Main causes of leukopenia include bone marrow failure (aplastic anemia), myelophthisis (acute leukemia), drugs (immunosuppressive drugs, propylthiouracil), and hypersplenism (portal hypertension). Main causes of leukocytosis are infection, inflammation, malignancies, and allergic reactions.

- **Pelger-Huet anomaly** (neutrophils have a bilobed nucleus connected by a thin strand and decreased granulation): This anomaly is seen in myelodysplastic syndromes.
- **Hypersegmented neutrophils** (more than nuclear lobes): These are found in megaloblastic anemias (vitamin B_{12} and folate deficiency).
- **Blast cells** (myeloblasts or lymphoblasts; large cells with large nuclei and prominent nucleoli): Blast cells are seen in acute leukemia.
- **Auer rods** (rodlike granules in blast cytoplasm): Auer rods are pathognomonic for acute myelogenous leukemia, especially acute promyelocytic leukemia (M3).
- **Hairy cells** (lymphoid cells with ragged cytoplasm): These are seen in hairy cell leukemia.
- **Sézary cells** (atypical lymphoid cells with cerebriform nuclei): Sézary cells are seen in cutaneous T cell lymphoma.

Platelets

Platelets appear as small (1- to 2-μm-diameter), purplish cytoplasmic fragments without a nucleus, containing red/blue granules. Derived from bone marrow giant cells called megakaryocytes, they are involved in the cellular mechanisms of primary hemostasis leading to the formation of blood clots. Normal counts are 150,000 to 400,000 per cubic millimeter of peripheral blood (150×10^9 to 400×10^9/L). The number of platelets per high-power field multiplied by 20,000 usually estimates the platelet count per microliter. Alternatively, one should find 1 platelet for every 10 to 20 red cells.

Numbers of platelets can decrease due to bone marrow disease (myelophthisic bone marrow), consumption (disseminated intravascular coagulation), or drugs. An increase in numbers can be seen in bone marrow overproduction (myeloproliferative syndromes) or in a normal response to massive bleeding. Pseudo-thrombocytopenia represents clumping of platelets in blood samples collected in EDTA, resulting in spuriously low platelet counts. This phenomenon can be avoided by using citrate to anticoagulate blood samples sent for blood counts.

BONE MARROW EVALUATION

Introduction

For many hematologic diseases that affect the bone marrow, evaluation of the peripheral blood smear does not provide sufficient information, and a direct examination of the bone marrow is required to establish the diagnosis. The bone marrow biopsy can be done at the bedside under local anesthesia, although some patients may require low doses of anxiolytics or opioids for the procedure. Despite advances in the bone marrow biopsy and aspiration techniques, they are still commonly considered painful procedures by patients and some physicians, but with expertise, both can be performed safely and with minimal discomfort to the patient.

Indications and Contraindications

The most common indications for bone marrow evaluation are workup of bone marrow malignancies, staging of marrow involvement by metastatic tumors, assessment of infectious diseases that may involve the bone marrow (i.e., HIV, tuberculosis), determination of marrow damage in patients exposed to radiation, drugs, and chemicals, and workup of metabolic storage diseases. There are a few absolute contraindications for the procedure, including infection, previous radiation therapy at the site of biopsy, and poor patient cooperation. Thrombocytopenia is not a contraindication to bone marrow biopsy, although it may be associated with more procedure-related bleeding. Patients who have a coagulopathy require factor replacement or withholding of anticoagulation to minimize bleeding complications.

Technique

In adults, the most common places to do the procedure are the posterior and anterior iliac crests, which are accessible and safe locations of active hematopoiesis. Other potential biopsy sites are the sternum and tibia.

The posterior iliac crest is the preferred site, as it allows collection of both aspirate and biopsy specimens and is associated with minimal morbidity or complications. The procedure can be performed with little patient discomfort under local anesthesia, but anxious patients may be sedated. In most cases, a *Jamshidi* bone marrow aspiration and biopsy needle is used. Aspirate smears are often prepared at the bedside, the quality of which is assessed by observing bone marrow spicules. Additional aspirate is often obtained for further studies such as flow cytometry, cytogenetics, and cultures. In some instances, marrow cannot be aspirated and only a biopsy is obtained (a "dry tap"). This can be due to technique or may signal myelofibrosis or previous local radiotherapy. In such cases, touch preparations of the biopsy can be made to allow for a cytological exam. Finally, the biopsy specimen is embedded in a buffered formaldehyde-based fixation for further processing.

Complications

Bleeding at the site of puncture is the most common complication. It is easily controlled with compression, but some thrombocytopenic patients will require platelet transfusions. Other uncommon complications are infections, tumor seeding in the needle track, and needle breakage.

Bone Marrow Examination

- The examination of the bone marrow aspirate begins under **low power** to obtain an impression of overall cellularity, an initial scan for any abnormal populations of cells or clumps of cells, and an evaluation of the presence or absence of bone marrow spicules. Megakaryocytes are normally seen under low power as large multinucleated cells. The overall cellularity of the marrow is difficult to estimate from the aspirate because of contamination with peripheral blood.
- The **myeloid-to-erythroid** (M:E) **ratio** is also determined under low power and is normally 3:1 to 4:1. The ratio is increased in chronic myeloid leukemia due to an increase in granulocyte precursors and is increased in pure red cell aplasia due to a decrease in red cell precursors. The ratio is decreased in hemolytic disorders in which increased erythroid precursors are present or in agranulocytic conditions secondary to chemotherapeutic agents or other drugs.

- Under **high power**, the aspirate should contain a variety of cells representative of various stages in myeloid and erythroid maturation. Myeloid cells progress from myeloblasts to promyelocytes, myelocytes, metamyelocytes, band forms, and then mature neutrophils. As these cells mature, their nuclear chromatin condenses, with a resultant decrease in the nuclear:cytoplasmic ratio. Their cytoplasm gradually develops granules seen in mature neutrophils.
- **Erythroid precursors** progress from proerythroblasts through varying stages of normoblasts known as *basophilic, chromatophilic,* and *orthochromic.* Again, the nucleus gradually condenses, and the cytoplasm gradually takes on the pinkish hue of Hgb found in mature red cells.
- **Bone marrow core biopsies** are fixed in a buffered formaldehyde-based solution and then embedded in paraffin or plastic. Biopsies are used to assess the cellularity of the bone marrow and the presence of neoplasias, infections, or fibrosis. Cellularity is estimated by observing the ratio of hematopoietic cells to fat cells. Cellularity is usually 30% to 60% but typically declines with advancing age.

Abnormalities in the Bone Marrow Evaluation

Listed below are some of the more common abnormal findings of the bone marrow. This list is by no means exhaustive, nor does it list all abnormalities noted in each condition.

- **Acute leukemia:** The presence of >20% blasts in the bone marrow confirms the diagnosis of acute leukemia.
- **Myelodysplastic syndrome:** This syndrome is a heterogeneous group of diseases characterized by the presence of immature erythroid precursors with loss of synchrony between nuclear and cytoplasmic maturation. Mature myeloid cells have decreased lobes (Pelger-Huet cells). Iron staining may reveal ring sideroblasts with iron granules surrounding the nucleus.
- **Chronic myeloid leukemia:** Findings include a hypercellular marrow with an increased M:E ratio. Myeloblasts represent <5% of cells, with the marrow containing predominantly myelocytes, metamyelocytes, and mature neutrophils.
- **Chronic lymphocytic leukemia** is marked by hypercellular marrow with small, round, mature lymphocytes with a thin rim of blue cytoplasm.
- **Myelofibrosis:** This is often the cause of a "dry tap." Bone marrow biopsy will reveal marrow infiltration with collagen and fibrous tissue.
- **Essential thrombocytosis:** Megakaryocyte hyperplasia is a common finding.
- **Polycythemia vera:** This is characterized by a hypercellular marrow.
- **Multiple myeloma:** The marrow is replaced by large numbers of abnormal, often immature plasma cells with eccentric nuclei containing a cartwheel pattern of nuclear chromatin. Flame cells contain pink, flamelike cytoplasm and are said to be associated with an IgA paraprotein.
- **Megaloblastic anemia:** Findings include hypercellular marrow with abnormalities in myeloid and erythroid precursors. Megaloblasts are erythroid cells that are larger than normal, with more nuclear chromatin. There is loss of synchrony between nuclear and cytoplasmic maturation.
- **Hodgkin lymphoma:** One may find the characteristic Reed-Sternberg cells infiltrating the bone marrow in conjunction with lymphoid elements.
- **Storage diseases:** Macrophages with striated cytoplasm due to accumulation of cerebrosides may be seen in patients with Gaucher disease. Individuals with Niemann-Pick disease may have macrophages with a foamy cytoplasm secondary to contained sphingomyelin.

KEY POINTS TO REMEMBER

- Hematologists are involved in the evaluation and treatment of bleeding and clotting disorders, blood cell count abnormalities, and abnormalities of blood cell morphology.
- The role of the history and physical exam is important when assessing a patient suspected to have a hematological disorder. They suggest differential diagnoses and appropriate lab tests to establish the definitive diagnosis.
- The peripheral blood smear is a key tool in hematology diagnosis and cannot be replaced by automated hematology counters.
- The peripheral slide should be reviewed systematically every time, looking at every cell line. Failure to do so may result in a missed diagnosis.
- RBCs are usually monotonous, with one third of their area demonstrating a central pallor.
- WBCs must be assessed in numbers and morphological characteristics. The most common leukocytes are neutrophils.
- A quick estimation of platelet number is: 1 platelet per high-power field equals 20,000 platelets per microliter in an automated count.
- A bone marrow aspirate and biopsy should both be attempted in the bone marrow exam.
- Inability to aspirate bone marrow—a "dry tap"—may be due to technique or may signal myelofibrosis.

REFERENCES AND SUGGESTED READINGS

Aster J, Kumar V. Myelodysplastic syndromes. In: Cotran R, Kumar V, Collins T, eds. *Robbins Pathologic Basis of Disease*. 6th ed. Philadelphia, PA: W. B. Saunders; 1999:678–679.

Bain BJ. Diagnosis from the blood smear. *N Engl J Med*. 2005;353:498–507.

Greer JP, Foester J, Lukens JN. *Wintrobe's Clinical Hematology*. 11th ed. Philadelphia, PA: Lippincott Williams & Wilkins; 2004.

Riley RS, Ben-Ezra JM, Pavot DR, et al. *An Illustrated Guide to Performing Bone Marrow Aspiration and Biopsy*. Richmond: Medical College of Virginia, Virginia Commonwealth University.

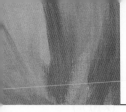

White Blood Cell Disorders: Leukopenia and Leukocytosis

2

Mark A. Schroeder

INTRODUCTION

The normal white blood cell count (WBC) varies between genders and ethnic groups but in general ranges from 4×10^9 cells to 11×10^9 cells/L (Table 2-1) and is composed of those cells committed to the leukocyte lineage: granulocytes (neutrophils, eosinophils, and basophils), monocytes, and lymphocytes. Neutrophils make up about 60% of the peripheral blood nucleated cells. When the total WBC count is elevated above the normal range, this is termed **leukocytosis,** and when it falls below this range, this is termed **leukopenia.** A person's gender and ethnic background should be taken into consideration when determining normal ranges. The specific white cell lineage affected helps to guide the differential diagnosis and treatment decisions. This chapter focuses on evaluation, etiology, and management of the abnormal WBC count, with specific etiologies discussed in detail elsewhere in this book.

LEUKOPENIA

Leukopenia is defined as a white blood cell count $<3.8 \times 10^9$ cells/L. This lower limit of normal varies with age (infants have lower absolute neutrophil counts [ANCs] than adults) and race (lower ANCs in persons of African ancestry and Yemenite Jews), and 5% of the normal population may fall outside of the normal reference range. It is best to divide the leukopenias according to clinically relevant cell lineages: neutrophils and lymphocytes.

Neutropenia

Definition
The ANC is obtained by taking the percentage of neutrophils identified on a 100-cell differential or by Coulter counter and multiplying by the total WBC count. **Neutropenia** is classified as mild (ANC, $<1.5 \times 10^9$ to 1×10^9/L), moderate (ANC, 1 to 0.5×10^9/L), or severe (ANC, $<0.5 \times 10^9$/L). **Agranulocytosis** is the total absence of granulocytes.

Epidemiology
Neutropenia is five times more prevalent in African Americans compared to Caucasians.

Causes
Differential Diagnosis. Causes of neutropenia in adults are reported in Table 2-2. Severe neutropenia can be congenital or acquired. Congenital causes include Kostmann syndrome or congenital agranulocytosis, Shwachman-Diamond-Oski syndrome, Chediak-Higashi syndrome, and cyclic neutropenia. Congenital causes are usually suggested by family history. Most cases of neutropenia are acquired and related to decreased granulocyte production and, less often, increased destruction. Acquired causes include drug toxicity,

TABLE 2-1	AVERAGE ADULT WBC COUNT	
Cell	Percentage	Absolute Count ($\times 10^9$/L)
Leukocytes		3.8–9.8
Neutrophils	40–75	1.8–6.6
Monocytes	4–13	0.2–1.2
Eosinophils	0–6	<0.5
Basophils	0–3	<0.2
Lymphocytes	20–54	1.2–3.3

Adapted from Barnes-Jewish Hospital Laboratory References, Barnes-Jewish Hospital, St. Louis, MO.

infection (viral and sepsis), autoimmune (rheumatoid, Felty syndrome, systemic lupus, and isoimmune neonatal neutropenia), hematologic malignancies, aplastic anemia, myelodysplastic syndrome, and hypersplenism. In addition, pseudo-neutropenia may be obtained by analyzing blood several hours old. Lower ANCs occur in African Americans as a result of either defective release of neutrophils from the marrow, a poor marrow reserve, or an increased marginated pool of neutrophils.

Pathophysiology. Neutropenia results from decreased production, ineffective granulopoiesis, increased margination to peripheral pools, or increased peripheral destruction. Acquired neutropenias are usually a result of infection, toxins/drugs, or immune disorders. Viral, parasitic, or bacterial infections may cause neutropenia, and this is usually short-lived. The underlying mechanism involves increased margination, sequestration, and increased destruction by circulating antibodies. Drug and toxin exposure usually follows a temporal course, with neutropenia developing after continued drug exposure of days to months. The mechanism of drug-induced neutropenia is either antibody-mediated or direct toxic effects on the marrow. Certain drugs at higher risk of causing neutropenia are highlighted in Table 2-3. Primary immune disorders mediate neutropenia through antibody-mediated neutrophil destruction.

Presentation. Neutropenia is often incidentally discovered on a CBC but may present with fever or infection. Signs of infection, such as purulence, may be less evident given the low neutrophil count. The risk of infection is directly related to the degree and duration of neutropenia. The risk of infection increases at an ANC $<1 \times 10^9$/L, but clinical symptoms usually do not become manifest until the ANC falls below 0.5×10^9/L.

Management

Workup. The initial evaluation should include a complete history and physical exam. The history should focus on systemic symptoms of infection, recent exposures or new medications, history of neutropenia, and family history of neutropenia. The physical exam may suggest the cause of neutropenia, and attention should be paid to vital signs that would suggest sepsis or infection, oral cavity exam for gingivitis or tooth abscess, macroglossia to suggest vitamin deficiency, lymphadenopathy to suggest malignancy or infection, skin and joint changes suggesting a rheumatologic disorder, and splenomegaly (sequestration and Felty's syndrome).

Lab Analysis. Initial laboratory evaluation starts with the CBC with complete differential and review of the peripheral blood smear. Additional testing to consider includes nutritional studies of vitamin B_{12}, folate, and possibly copper. If a clonal process is suspected, lymphocyte immunophenotyping by flow cytometry and T cell-receptor gene

TABLE 2-2　CAUSE OF NEUTROPENIA

Primary hematological disorders	Congenital/Inherited
	Severe congenital neutropenia (Kostmann syndrome)
	Cyclic neutropenia
	Familial benign neutropenia
	Diamond-Blackfan syndrome
	Schwachman-Diamond syndrome
	Chédiak-Higashi syndrome
	Glycogen storage disease type Ib
	Fanconi anemia
	Acquired
	Acute leukemia
	Myelodysplastic syndromes
	Chronic lymphocytic leukemia
	Hodgkin lymphoma
	Non-Hodgkin lymphoma
	Aplastic anemia and pure white cell aplasia
	Chronic idiopathic neutropenia
	Nutritional: copper, vitamin B_{12}, and folate
Secondary disorders	Immune neutropenias
	Isoimmune neutropenia of the neonate (transplacental IgG specific for paternal neutrophil antigens)
	Autoimmune neutropenia
	Neutropenia with autoimmune diseases
	Systemic lupus erythematosus
	Rheumatoid arthritis
	Felty syndrome
	Sjögren syndrome
	Neutropenia with clonal large granular lymphocytosis
	Marrow infiltrative process
	Drug induced (see Table 2-3)
	Neutropenia with infectious diseases
	Sepsis
	Viral: EBV, parvovirus, and HIV
	Hypersplenism

rearrangement studies may be useful. Antinuclear antibody and antineutrophil antibody testing can be sent to evaluate for autoimmune neutropenia. HIV and EBV serologies start the initial infectious workup. If anemia or thrombocytopenia occurs in combination with neutropenia, direct examination of the bone marrow via bone marrow biopsy is usually warranted unless a cause is obvious. In cases of asymptomatic mild neutropenia serial CBC examination to rule out cyclic neutropenia may be considered. In mild cases of neutropenia that do not improve in a couple of months with observation, a bone marrow biopsy should be considered.

Treatment. Treatment is guided by the underlying etiology and severity of neutropenia. This can range from close observation in patients with benign neutropenia to growth factor support and antibiotics in patients with neutropenic fevers. Growth factors can be used to speed count recovery in drug-induced neutropenia. The major complication associated with

TABLE 2-3	DRUGS CAUSING NEUTROPENIA

Drug Class	Common Example
Analgesics and anti-inflammatory agents	Indomethacin Para-aminophenol derivatives, e.g., acetaminophen Pyrazolon derivatives, e.g., phenylbutazone
Antibiotics	Cephalosporins Chloramphenicol Penicillins Sulfonamides Trimethoprim-sulfamethoxazole Vancomycin
Anticonvulsants	Phenytonin Carbamazepine
Antidepressants	Amitriptyline Imipramine
Antihistamines, H2-blockers	Cimetidine Ranitidine
Antimalarials	Dapsone Quinine Chloroquine
Antithyroid drugs	Carbimazole Methimazole Propylthiouracil
Cardiovascular drugs	Captopril Hydralazine Propranolol
Diuretics	Hydrochlorothiazide Acetazolamide
Hypnotics and sedatives	Chlordiazepoxide Benzodiazepines
Atypical antipsychotics	Chlorpromazine Olanzapine Clozapine
Other drugs	Allopurinol Colchicine Penicillamine Ticlopidine

neutropenia is infection. Supportive care with broad-spectrum antibiotics in the ill or febrile patient is an essential part of initial care while the workup for a cause of neutropenia is under way. Common sites of infection include mucous membranes, skin, perirectal and genital areas, disseminated intravascular coagulation bloodstream, and lungs. Most commonly, endogenous bacterial flora is the pathogen (*Staphylococcus* from skin or gram-negative organisms from the gut). Antibiotics should be continued until the ANC is >500 for 2 days and the fever subsides. If fever and neutropenia persist, empiric antifungal coverage should be considered.

Cases caused by drug toxicity should improve, with removal of the drug within 1 to 3 weeks. Drug-related neutropenia can be confirmed by testing antineutrophil-associated drug antibodies. Infectious etiologies resolve with treatment of the infection or shortly after a viral infection has subsided. Autoimmune diseases can be treated by immunosuppression with corticosteroids and can be confirmed by testing antineutrophil antibodies. Congenital etiologies are often supported with growth factors such as granulocyte colony-stimulating factor (G-CSF) but have a high risk of progression to leukemia. The involvement of other blood cell lineages (RBCs and platelets) suggests aplastic anemia, leukemia, myelodysplastic syndromes, or megaloblastic anemia.

Lymphopenia

Definition

Lymphopenia is defined as an absolute lymphocyte count $<1.2 \times 10^9/L$. The absolute lymphocyte count is 80% T cells and 20% B cells. Sixty-six percent of the T cell population is CD4+ cells and the remaining is mainly CD8+ cells.

Etiology

Lymphopenia is most often acquired but congenital causes should also be considered. Etiologies of lymphopenia are listed in Table 2-4 and are mainly acquired. Acquired causes include immunosuppressive drugs, viral and bacterial infections, critical illness, autoimmune

TABLE 2-4	CAUSES OF LYMPHOPENIA
Congenital	Severe combined immunodeficiency Common variable immune deficiency Congenital thymic aplasia (DiGeorge syndrome) X-Linked agammaglobulinemia (Brutun agammaglobulinemia) Wiskott-Aldrich syndrome Purine nucleoside phosphorylase deficiency Ataxia-telangiectasia

Acquired	Aplastic anemia
	Infectious diseases
	  Viral: HIV/AIDS, severe acute respiratory syndrome (SARS), hepatitis, influenza, Herpes simplex virus
	  Bacterial diseases
	    Tuberculosis, pneumonia, richettsiosis, ehrlichiosis, sepsis malaria—acute phase
	  Immunosuppressive agents
	    Antilymphocyte globulin, alemtuzumab, glucocorticoids
	  Chemotherapy
	  Radiation
	  Renal or hematopeitic stem cell transplantation
	  Hemodialysis

Systemic diseases	Autoimmune diseases: systemic lupus erythematosus, periarteritis Hodgkin lymphoma Carcinoma Sarcoidosis
Nutritional	Ethanol abuse Zinc deficiency

and connective tissue diseases, chronic renal insufficiency, excess alcohol, older age, and thymoma. Congenital causes include common variable immune deficiency, severe combined immunodeficiency, congenital thymic aplasia (DiGeorge syndrome), and X-linked agammaglobulinemia (Brutun agammaglobulinemia).

Management
Most causes of lymphocytopenia are acquired and the management focuses on treating the underlying illness. The most common infectious cause is acquired immunodeficiency syndrome (AIDS). Other viral and bacterial diseases also cause lymphocytopenia, which usually resolves a couple of weeks after antimicrobial therapy. Zinc deficiency responds to repletion of zinc and should be part of the initial screen, along with examination of the peripheral blood smear. Inherited causes predispose to recurrent and opportunistic infections and detailed discussion of management is beyond the scope of this text. In general, prophylactic antibiotics can be used, as well as best supportive care.

LEUKOCYTOSIS

Definition
Leukocytosis is defined as a WBC $>10 \times 10^9$/L.

Etiology
An elevated WBC most commonly reflects a normal bone marrow response to inflammation or infection. Occasionally leukemia or myeloproliferative disorders are to blame. The maturation of WBCs is influenced by colony-stimulating factors, interleukins, tumor necrosis factor, and complement components.

Classification
Leukocytosis should be divided into granulocytosis, monocytosis, and lymphocytosis to guide the workup and differential diagnosis.

Causes
Most cases of leukocytosis are a result of the bone marrow reacting to inflammation or infection. A **leukemoid reaction** is an excessive WBC response (usually >50,000) associated with a cause outside of the bone marrow (growth factors, infection, or differentiating agents such as all-trans retinoic acid [ATRA]). Leukocytosis may also be caused by physical and emotional stress and usually resolves in hours once the stress is eliminated. In postsplenectomy patients, a transient leukocytosis can be seen, lasting for weeks to months secondary to the demargination of leukocytes typically stored in the spleen. Other etiologies include medications, but leukocytes should not rise above 20,000 to 30,000 in this case. The leukocytosis seen in hemolytic anemias (sickle cell and autoimmune types) is related to the nonspecific effects of increased erythropoiesis and inflammation. Nonhematopoietic malignancy can also cause a leukocytosis that is multifactorial in etiology. Finally, acute and chronic leukemias and myeloproliferative disorders usually present with a leukocytosis.

Pathophysiology
The pathophysiology of leukocytosis stems from the production, maturation, and survival of leukocytes. Stem cells give rise to erythroblasts, myeloblasts, and megakaryoblasts. Seventy-five percent of nucleated cells in the bone marrow are committed to production of leukocytes. At any given time, 90% of WBCs remain in storage in the bone marrow, with 7% to 8% in the tissue compartment and the remainder in circulation. This large storage pool allows for a rapid increase in WBCs (mostly neutrophils). In addition, a percentage

TABLE 2-5   CAUSES OF LEUKOCYTOSIS

Normally responding bone marrow

Infection

Inflammation
  Tissue necrosis, infarction, burns, arthritis

Stress
  Overexertion, seizures, anxiety, anesthesia

Drugs
  Corticosteroids, lithium, beta-agonists

Trauma
  Splenectomy
  Hemolytic anemia
  Leukemoid malignancy
  Leukocytosis of pregnancy

Abnormal bone marrow
  Acute leukemias
  Chronic leukemias
  Myeloproliferative disorders

of circulating WBCs is marginated along blood vessel walls and is mobilized by inflammatory stimuli. The two basic causes of leukocytosis are a normal bone marrow response to external stimuli or primary bone marrow disorder.

Differential Diagnosis

The differential diagnosis of leukocytosis is extensive, and common causes are listed in Table 2-5. Increases in the absolute numbers of lymphocytes, eosinophils, monocytes, or basophils are less common than neutrophilia and help to direct the differential diagnosis.

Neutrophilia

Background

Neutrophilia is defined as an ANC $>6.6 \times 10^9$ cells/L. The neutrophil count is influenced by shifts in neutrophils among four major compartments: the bone marrow, the circulation, the marginated pool, and the tissues. Only about 5% of neutrophils are in circulation at any given time, with a half-life of 6 to 10 hours. Most neutrophils and their precursors are contained in storage pools in the bone marrow at 10 to 20 times their circulating numbers. About 50% of peripheral blood neutrophils are circulating, and the other 50% marginated along vessel walls and in the spleen. This pool can be rapidly increased, within hours from the bone marrow stores or within minutes from demarginating neutrophils along blood vessel walls. Neutrophils move to sites of inflammation and infection and act as phagocytes. Their trafficking depends on chemotaxins and surface molecules such as selectins to mediate rolling and integrins to mediate adhesion and transmigration of blood vessels.

Causes

  Pathophysiology. The pathophysiology of **primary neutrophilia** may be related to inherited deficiencies in adhesion molecules or, in the case of myeloproliferative disorders, constitutive expression and activation of a growth-promoting receptor tyrosine kinase such as *bcr/abl* or Jak2. **Secondary neutrophilia**, seen in infection and inflammation, is related to demargination from storage pools in the bone marrow and peripheral blood signaled by

TABLE 2-6	CAUSES OF NEUTROPHILIA
Spurious causes	Cryoglobulinemia Platelet clumping
Primary causes	Hereditary neutrophilia Chronic idiopathic neutrophilia Chronic myelogenous leukemia Myeloproliferative disorders (polycythemia vera and myelofibrosis) Leukocyte adhesion deficiency Down syndrome

Secondary
  causes
	Infection
	Smoking
	Medications: glucocoticoids, beta-agonists, lithium,
	    granulocyte colony-stimulating factor (G-CSF)/
	    granulocyte-macrophage CSF (GM-CSF), all-trans
	    retinoic acid (ATRA)
	Nonhematologic malignancy: large cell lung cancer
	Stress
	Exercise
	Hemolytic anemia/sickle cell disease
	Leukoerythroblastic reaction: marrow invasion by tumor,
	    fibrosis, and granulomatous reaction
	Asplenia

endotoxin and proinflammatory cytokines such as tumor necrosis factor-alpha, interleukin (IL)-6, IL-1B, IL-8, G-CSF, and granulocyte/macrophage colony-stimulating factor (GM-CSF).

Differential Diagnosis. Neutrophilia can be spurious, of primary hematologic origin, or related to secondary causes. Etiologies of neutrophilia are listed in Table 2-6. Spurious leukocytosis can be a result of the automated cell counter (Coulter counter) counting clumps of platelets as leukocytes and is usually associated with pseudo-thrombocytopenia. In addition, cryoglobulins can agglutinate and be counted as leukocytes at temperatures lower than body temperature. Primary causes of neutrophilia may be hereditary (usually resulting in splenomegaly and leukocyte counts of 20×10^9 to 100×10^9/L) or associated with familial syndromes. Other primary causes include myeloproliferative disorders (e.g., chronic myeloid leukemia [CML]) and leukocyte adhesion deficiency. Secondary causes are by far the most common cause of neutrophilia. Common secondary causes include infection, smoking (25% increase), chronic inflammation (e.g., rheumatoid arthritis and inflammatory bowel disease), stress, medications, chronic marrow stimulation (hemolytic anemia and idiopathic thrombocytopenic purpura), asplenia, marrow invasion, and nonhematologic malignancy.

Management

Workup. Initial laboratory evaluation starts with review of the peripheral blood smear to confirm automated counts and rule out spurious leukocytosis. The smear may suggest a secondary cause such as infection or inflammation with increased bands, vacuolization, Döhle bodies, and toxic granulations in neutrophils. A marrow infiltrating process is suggested by a leukoerythroblastic reaction that shows a "left shift" (increased myelocytes and metamyelocytes in the marrow and bands in the peripheral blood) and nucleated RBCs. Acute leukemia is suggested by circulating blasts, which may be incorrectly counted as monocytes or neutrophils by the Coulter counter. If no secondary causes of neutrophilia can be identified, peripheral blood analysis for *bcr/abl* by fluorescence in situ hybridization (FISH) or cytogenetics may be helpful to exclude CML. A leukocyte alkaline phosphatase (LAP) score is of historical importance but is no longer commonly used because of intra-operator variability and the evolution of cytogenetic testing. A low LAP score can be seen in CML, and a high LAP score may suggest inflammation or infection.

Treatment. Treatment depends on the underlying etiology. Treatment of primary etiolgies such as CML and myeloproliferative disorders are discussed elsewhere in this book. Treatment of neutrophilia related to a secondary cause revolves around treating the underlying cause.

Eosinophilia

Background
Eosinophilia is defined as an absolute eosinophil count $>0.5 \times 10^9/L$. Eosinophilia is most commonly due to secondary causes. Table 2-7 reviews causes of eosinophilia. Secondary causes of eosinophilia include parasites, drugs (IL-2), allergy and asthma, vasculitides, lymphoma, and metastatic cancer. Absolute eosinophil counts $>4 \times 10^9/L$ suggest primary eosinophilia as a result of either clonal expansion (chronic leukemia variant or acute leukemia variant) or hypereosinophilic syndrome.

Management
Workup. Initial evaluation of eosinophilia should include review of the peripheral smear, stool examination for ova and parasites, and serum tryptase, IgE, and IL-5 levels. If no secondary source can be identified, T cell immunophenotyping and T cell-receptor gene rearrangement analysis and bone marrow biopsy with cytogenetic analysis and FISH for the platelet-derived growth factor-receptor rearrangement (FIP1L1-PDGFRA) should be performed to evaluate for a clonal disorder.

TABLE 2-7	CAUSES OF EOSINOPHILIA

Allergic

Parasites

Dermatologic

Infections
    Scarlet fever, chorea, leprosy, genitourinary infections

Immunologic disorders
    Rheumatoid arthritis, periarteritis, lupus erythematosus, eosinophilia-myalgia syndrome

Pleural and pulmonary conditions
    Loffler syndrome, pulmonary infiltrates, and eosinophilia

Malignancies
    Non-Hodgkin lymphoma, Hodgkin lymphoma

Myeloproliferative disorders
    Chronic myelogenous leukemia, polycythemia vera, myelofibrosis

Adrenal insufficiency: Addison disease

Sarcoidosis

Treatment. Hypereosinophilic syndrome can cause end organ damage, including cardiac involvement causing conduction defects and cardiomyopathy, as well as pulmonary involvement. In patients with evidence of end organ damage, treatment with corticosteroids and hydroxyurea may be needed to decrease the eosinophil count rapidly. Leukopheresis may be used as well to lower the eosinophil count rapidly. Recent evidence suggests that patients with idiopathic hypereosinophilic syndrome and chronic eosinophilic leukemia with the FIP1L1-PDGFRA rearrangement may be effectively treated with the tyrosine kinase inhibitor imatinib. See Chapter 9 for further discussion.

Basophilia

Background

Basophilia is defined as an absolute basophil count $>0.2 \times 10^9$/L. Basophils are inflammatory mediators and their granules contain histamine, glycosaminoglycans, major basic protein, proteases, and other inflammatory and vasoactive substances. They primarily function to activate the type 1 hypersensitivity reaction mediated through surface receptors for IgE.

Etiology

Basophilia can be associated with hypersensitivity reactions to drugs and food. Basophilia may also be seen in chronic inflammatory states such as tuberculosis and ulcerative colitis. However, these reactions are rare, and the most common setting of basophilia is in myeloproliferative disorders such as CML.

Management

Workup. Review of the peripheral smear confirms basophilia and management focuses on the underlying etiology. Peripheral blood can be sent for Jak2 and *bcr/abl* to evaluate for a myeloproliferative disorder. If suspicion of a myeloproliferative disorder is high, a bone marrow biopsy is necessary. Myeloproliferative disorders are reviewed in Chapter 9.

Monocytosis

Background

Monocytosis is defined as an absolute monocyte count $>0.8 \times 10^9$/L. Monocytes are cells in transit to the tissues and are capable of transformation to macrophages in the tissues. Monocytes play a role in acute and chronic inflammatory reactions.

Etiology

Monocytosis usually represents a myeloproliferative disorder such as CML or acute monocytic leukemia. Secondary causes include infection (bacterial or tuberculosis) and relative monocytosis as seen with initial count recovery after chemotherapy and drug-induced neutropenia.

Management

Workup. Review of the peripheral smear confirms monocytosis, and treatment is focused on the underlying etiology. Peripheral blood can be sent for Jak2 and *bcr/abl* to evaluate for a myeloproliferative disorder. If suspicion of a myeloproliferative disorder is high, a bone marrow biopsy is necessary. A detailed discussion of the management of myeloproliferative disorders can be found in Chapter 9.

Lymphocytosis

Introduction

Lymphocytosis is defined as an absolute lymphocyte count $>3.3 \times 10^9$/L. Lymphocytosis may be of primary or secondary origin. Table 2-8 reviews causes of lymphocytosis. Primary

TABLE 2-8	CAUSES OF LYMPHOCYTOSIS
Primary lymphocytosis	Malignancy Acute lymphocytic leukemia Chronic lymphocytic leukemia Prolymphocytic leukemia Hairy cell leukemia Adult T cell leukemia Large granular lymphocytic leukemia Essential monoclonal B cell lymphocytosis Persistent polyclonal B cell lymphocytosis

Secondary or reactive lymphocytosis	Mononucleosis syndromes
	EBV
	CMV
	Herpes simplex virus
	HIV
	Rubella
	Toxoplasma
	Adenovirus
	Hepatitis virus
	Varicella zoster
	Human herpesvirus (HHV)-6 and HHV-8
	  Bordetella pertussis
	Stress lymphocytosis
	  Surgery, myocardial infarction, septic shock, sickle cell crisis
	Hypersensitivity reactions
	  Insect bite and drugs
	Cancer: Thymoma
	Smoking
	Hyposplenism
	Chronic infection

etiologies include hematologic malignancy, particularly chronic lymphocytic leukemia (CLL), and secondary causes include infection, stress, hypersensitivity reactions, smoking, and hyposplenism. Cell surface markers are important in determining primary from secondary lymphocytosis.

Management

Workup. The blood smear should be reviewed to look for evidence of reactive lymphocytes associated with infection, large granular lymphocytes associated with large granular lymphocytic leukemia, smudge cells associated with CLL, or blasts associated with acute leukemia. Peripheral blood flow cytometry immunophenotyping allows identification of clonal disorders. Immunoglobulin or T cell-receptor gene rearrangements support a clonal disorder.

Treatment. Management of hematological malignancies including CLL is discussed in Chapter 29. Resolution of infectious etiologies results in resolution of the lymphocytosis. Finally, removal of allergens such as drugs or venom results in resolution of the lymphocytosis associated with hypersensitivity reactions.

KEY POINTS TO REMEMBER

- The "normal range" for WBCs varies among ethnic groups, age groups, and genders.
- Review of the peripheral smear is essential in the initial evaluation of the abnormal WBC count to confirm the findings of the Coulter counter and to rule out machine error.
- The subtype of the affected white cell guides the differential diagnosis and evaluation.
- Secondary causes of leukopenia and leukocytosis are the most common etiology.
- The risk of infection is inversely proportional to the ANC.
- Imatinib is a targeted therapy for idiopathic hypereosinophilic syndrome and chronic eosinophilic leukemia.

REFERENCES AND SUGGESTED READINGS

Abramson N, Melton B. Leukocytosis: basics of clinical assessment. *Am Fam Phys.* 2000;62(9):2053–2060.

Andersohn F, Konzen C, Garbe E. Systematic review: agranulocytosis induced by nonchemotherapy drugs. *Ann Intern Med.* 2007;146(9):657–665.

Bokoch GM. Chemoattractant signaling and leukocyte activation. *Blood.* 1995;86(5): 1649–1660.

Darko DF, et al. Neutrophilia and lymphopenia in major mood disorders. *Psychiatry Res.* 1988;25(3):243–251.

Jovanovic JV, et al. Low-dose imatinib mesylate leads to rapid induction of major molecular responses and achievement of complete molecular remission in FIP1L1-PDGFRA-positive chronic eosinophilic leukemia. *Blood.* 2007;109(11):4635–4640.

Lakshman R, Finn A. Neutrophil disorders and their management. *J Clin Pathol.* 2001;54(1):7–19.

Lichtman MA, Kipps TJ, Seligsohn U, et al. *Williams Hematology.* 7th ed. ed BE. New York: McGraw-Hill; 2006:2189.

McCarthy DA, et al. Leucocytosis induced by exercise. *Br Med J (Clin Res Ed).* 1987;295(6599):636.

Pardanani A, et al. Imatinib therapy for hypereosinophilic syndrome and other eosinophilic disorders. *Blood.* 2003;101(9):3391–3397.

Shastri KA, Logue GL. Autoimmune neutropenia. *Blood.* 1993;81(8):984–995.

Tefferi A, Hanson CA, Inwards DJ. How to interpret and pursue an abnormal complete blood cell count in adults. *Mayo Clin Proc.* 2005;80(7):923–936.

Tefferi A, Patnaik MM, Pardanani A. Eosinophilia: secondary, clonal and idiopathic. *Br J Haematol.* 2006;133(5):468–492.

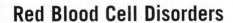

Red Blood Cell Disorders

3

Walter W. Chan and Jinny E. Chang

he disorders of RBCs fall into two main categories: anemia and polycythemia. *Anemia* is broadly defined as a decrease in the red cell mass characterized by a Hgb below the normal range, whereas *polycythemia* is defined as a red cell mass above the normal range.

ANEMIA

Introduction

Anemia is defined as a decrease in circulating RBC mass, the usual criteria being a Hgb <12 g/dL or Hct <36% for women and a Hgb <14 g/dL or Hct <41% in men. Anemia is commonly encountered in inpatient medicine and thus a frequent reason for hematology consults. A systematic approach to anemia is best at narrowing down the diagnosis and guiding the subsequent diagnostic workup.

Clinical Presentation

As with any other medical condition, the history and physical exam play key roles in approaching anemia. Based on symptomatology, one can discern the time line (acute, subacute, or chronic), the severity, and even the underlying etiology. Patients can be asymptomatic, but those patients with a Hgb <7 g/dL will usually have symptoms. Acute clinical manifestations include those typical of hypovolemia (pallor, visual impairment, syncope, hypotension, and tachycardia) and require immediate attention. Chronic symptoms will reflect tissue hypoxia (fatigue, headache, dyspnea, lightheadedness, and angina). A careful history of the clinical manifestations including initial presentation, time of onset, potential source of blood loss, family history, and medication history must be evaluated carefully. On exam, one can note pallor, alopecia, atrophic glossitis, angular cheilosis, congestive heart failure (with severe and chronic anemia), koilonychias (spoon nails), and brittle nails, as well as hypotension and tachycardia.

Causes

While there can be some overlap, anemia can be divided into three broad categories: **blood loss (acute or chronic)**, **increased destruction of RBCs (hemolysis)**, and **decreased production of RBCs**. Blood loss can be evaluated by a careful evaluation of the patient, including volume status. The reticulocyte count will usually help differentiate between states with decreased production (reticulocyte index [RI] <2%; see below for description of RI) and those associated with increased destruction (implied when the RI is >2%).

Diagnostic Approach

Lab Analysis

- The **complete blood count** (CBC) measures WBCs, Hgb, Hct, platelets, as well as measures of the *red cell indices*. The Hgb is a measurement of mass of Hgb in blood as reflected by grams per deciliter, whereas the Hct is the physical amount of space that the Hgb occupies as a percentage of the whole that the red cells occupy. Remember that the Hgb and Hct are unreliable indicators of red cell volume in the setting of rapid shifts of intravascular volume (i.e., an acute bleed).

- The most useful red cell indices include the **mean corpuscular volume** (MCV), **red cell distribution width** (RDW), and **mean cell Hgb concentration** (MCHC). MCV is the mean size of the red cells and the normal range is 80 to 100 fL. RBCs can be classified as microcytic when the MCV is <80 fL and macrocytic when it is >100 fL. RDW is a measure of variability in the size of the red cells and is calculated as: RDW = (standard deviation of red cell volume ÷ mean cell volume) ×100. An elevated RDW indicates increased variability in RBC size. The MCHC describes the concentration of Hgb in each cell.

- The **reticulocyte count** measures the immature red cells in the blood as a percentage of the whole and reflects the bone marrow's (BM's) response to anemia (i.e., a normal BM response is to increase the production of red cells in anemia so that the observed reticulocyte count goes up). A nascent RBC lives on average for 120 days, and the BM is constantly replenishing the bloodstream with new RBCs, with the normal reticulocyte count being ~1%. In the setting of anemia or blood loss, the BM should increase its production of RBC in proportion to loss of RBC, and thus a 1% reticulocyte count in the setting of anemia is inappropriate. The RI is calculated as percentage reticulocytes × (actual Hct/normal Hct) and is important in determining if a patient's BM is responding appropriately to the level of anemia. In normal individuals, an RI of 1.0 to 2.0 is acceptable, however, an RI of <2 with anemia indicates decreased production of RBCs. An RI of >2 with anemia may indicate hemolysis or loss of RBC leading to increased compensatory production of reticulocytes.

- The **peripheral smear** is a required part of the initial hematologic evaluation. Shapes, size, and orientation of cells in relation to each other are important factors to look for in a smear. RBCs can appear in many abnormal forms, such as acanthocytes, schistocytes, spherocytes, and teardrop cells, and abnormal orientations such as rouleaux formation.

- A **BM biopsy** may be indicated in cases of normocytic anemias with a low RI without an identifiable cause or anemia associated with other cytopenias. The biopsy may confirm myelophthisic process (i.e., presence of teardrop or fragmented cells, normoblasts, or immature WBCs on peripheral blood smear) in the setting of pancytopenias.

ANEMIAS ASSOCIATED WITH DECREASED PRODUCTION

The approach to an anemia associated with decreased production of red cells is to divide them into categories based on red cell size with the MCV. Depending on the MCV, *microcytic* (<80 fL), *normocytic* (80 to 100 fL), and *macrocytic* (>100 fL) anemias have distinct differential diagnoses.

Microcytic Anemias
Causes
Iron-deficiency anemia, sideroblastic anemia, and anemia of chronic disease make up the bulk of the microcytic anemias. The degree of microcytosis may give a clue to the possible underlying diagnoses. A very low MCV typically does not represent anemia of chronic disease or sideroblastic anemia (Table 3-1).

Iron-Deficiency Anemia
Etiologies
- **Dietary deficiency** is usually seen in infants who are milk-fed. In early childhood, it can be seen in meat-deficient diets. It can also occur in the setting of increased requirements, such as pregnancy and early childhood.

| TABLE 3-1 | CAUSES OF MICROCYTIC ANEMIAS BY MEAN CORPUSCULAR VOLUME (MCV) |

MCV, 70–80	MCV, <70
Iron deficiency	Thalassemia
Anemia of chronic disease	Iron deficiency
Thalassemia	
Sideroblastic anemia	

- **Malabsorption** can occur in the setting of partial gastrectomy, as hypochlorhydria/achlorhydria impairs iron absorption. Iron is most actively absorbed in the duodenum. Decreased transit time through duodenum, as seen in chronic diarrhea, may result in iron deficiency. Celiac sprue will result in iron deficiency that is refractory to oral iron therapy.
- **Chronic blood loss** is the most common cause of iron deficiency in adults. It is usually lost via the GI tract by ulcerative disease, gastritis, cancer, hemorrhoids, or arteriovenous malformation, with ulcers and colon malignancies being the most common. Menorrhagia/menstruation, hematuria due to genitourinary cancer, frequent blood donation, and frequent phlebotomy in hospitalized patients are additional causes of chronic blood loss.
- In addition to the usual symptoms of anemia, iron deficiency is often associated with **pica** (consumption of nonfood substances such as corn starch or ice).
- It should be noted that the diagnosis of iron deficiency in an adult mandates evaluation for GI malignancy.

Diagnosis

- Diagnosis involves serum testing of iron via an iron panel and ferritin level. The iron panel includes **serum iron level**, **total iron binding capacity** (TIBC), **unsaturated iron binding capacity** (UIBC), and **transferrin saturation** (Tsat). Serum iron levels reflect the level of iron immediately available for blood production. TIBC is an indirect method of determining the transferrin level in serum. Transferrin is an iron-transporting protein that is capable of associating reversibly with up to 1.254 g of iron per 1 g of protein. Serum **ferritin** (intracellular iron storage protein) should also be checked and, when low, almost always signifies iron deficiency. However, it is an acute phase reactant and can be falsely elevated in inflammatory states. Typically, in iron-deficiency anemia, the iron level is low, the TIBC is in the normal to high range, and ferritin is depleted. The Tsat, the percentage of transferrin that is bound to iron, can be a somewhat less reliable measure of iron. Low transferrin saturation is associated with iron-deficiency states, while high saturation is associated with excess iron. The gold standard for diagnosis of an iron deficiency anemia is a BM biopsy with iron staining; however, this is rarely necessary.
- Of note, patients can have microcytic normochromic (concentration of Hgb in the erythrocytes is within the normal range of 32% to 36%) anemia that eventually progresses to microcytic hypochromic as the anemia progresses. With worsening iron-deficiency anemia, there is a gradual increase in anisocytosis and poikilocytosis (abnormally shaped cells).

Treatment

- In addition to diagnosing the patient with iron-deficiency anemia, it is important to discover and treat the underlying cause of the iron deficiency, if possible. **Iron**

replacement may be given by oral iron salts, which should be given between meals because food or antacids may decrease absorption. Ascorbic acid given with iron sulfate may increase absorption. One replacement regimen is ferrous sulfate, 325 mg PO tid (equivalent of 65 mg elemental iron tid). Enteric-coated forms are not well absorbed and should not be used.

- **Parenteral iron** is given when the patient is intolerant of oral iron, when iron losses exceed the capacity to replete orally, or in the setting of malabsorption. There is an ~1 in 300 risk of a serious reaction including anaphylaxis.
- The amount of Fe needed can be calculated as the amount of Fe needed to replace the missing Hgb added to the amount necessary to replete the total body Fe stores (usually estimated as approximately 1000 mg) by the formula:

$$\text{Total dose(mg)} = \{[\text{normal Hgb(g/dL)} - \text{patient Hgb(g/dL)}] \times \text{body weight [kg]} \times 2.2)\} + 1000 \text{ mg}$$

However, in practice, iron is often infused at a dose of 1 to 1.2 g without formal calculation of iron repletion.

- **Follow-up.** One can expect an increase in the reticulocyte count within 7 to 10 days, and correction of anemia usually occurs within 6 to 8 weeks if ongoing blood loss is stopped. Treatment should continue for approximately 6 months (on PO iron) to fully restore tissue stores.

Sideroblastic Anemias

Sideroblastic anemias are characterized by ineffective erythropoiesis and the presence of ringed sideroblasts in the BM. The term *ringed* refers to the accumulation of iron in the mitochondria that surround the periphery of the nucleus. There are hereditary and idiopathic forms, as well as forms associated with drugs or toxins such as alcohol, lead, isoniazid (INH), and chloramphenicol. There is no cure for hereditary sideroblastic anemia, and treatment is aimed at preventing end-organ damage from iron overload (chelation therapy). Drug-induced sideroblastic anemias are commonly reversible when the offending agent is discontinued. For sideroblastic anemia caused by isoniazid treatment, high-dose pyridoxine supplementation (up to 200 mg/day PO) often reverses the anemia and allows for continuation of the drug.

Lead Poisoning

An additional diagnosis to consider in cases of microcytic, hypochromic anemias is **lead poisoning**. This is a rare but treatable form of microcytic anemia in adults and usually results from a work or an environmental exposure. The diagnosis is suggested by finding basophilic stippling on the peripheral smear.

Anemia of Chronic Disease

Anemia of chronic disease usually presents as a normocytic anemia, however, it can be microcytic (usually mild) in a minority of cases. It is a disease state usually associated with malignancy, infection, and inflammatory states and is covered in detail under Normocytic Anemia, below.

Thalassemias

In general, thalassemia results from a number of genetic defects that lead to decreased or absent synthesis of alpha- or beta-globin chains. *Beta-thalassemia* is more common in Mediterranean, African, and Southeast Asian populations and is thought to offer resistance to falciparum malaria. Beta-thalassemia major results from a total lack of production of beta-globin chain. It causes lack of adequate Hgb A formation, leading to microcytic, hypochromic cells. Complications of severe beta-thalassemia include skeletal deformities resulting from erythropoietin-stimulated expansion of BM, hepatosplenomegaly from extramedullary hematopoiesis, and secondary hemochromatosis from repeat blood transfusions and increased dietary absorption of iron. Beta-thalassemia minor is loss of only one of the two alleles coding for the beta-globulin gene. It is usually an asymptomatic condition manifested by microcytosis and a normal red cell distribution width. It is accompanied by a mild anemia (if any). *Alpha-thalassemia* results from decreased production of alpha-globin chains, of which there are four in total. The severity of anemia depends on the number of defective alpha genes. Diagnosis is by Hgb electrophoresis for beta-thalassemia and severe alpha-thalassemia. Mild alpha-thalassemia may be detected by alpha:beta ratio or by molecular testing, although neither is widely available.

The treatment of thalassemias usually depends on the severity of the genetic defect and resultant clinical sequelae. The minor thalassemias are commonly asymptomatic and require no therapy. The major thalassemias may be treated by chronic transfusions, chelation therapy to avoid iron overload (due to transfusions), and splenectomy. For ferritin concentrations >1000 ng/mL, chelation therapy may reduce the long-term complications of iron overload. Options for chelation include the intramuscular or subcutaneous iron chelator deferoxamine and the recently approved oral iron chelator deferasirox.

Normocytic Anemias

Normocytic anemias can be associated with an elevated reticulocyte count, which represents hemolytic anemia (HA) or bleeding (see following sections), whereas a decreased reticulocyte count typically represents hypoproliferative disorder (Table 3-2). Normocytic anemia may be an early finding in BM failure. Aplastic anemia is actually a BM failure syndrome and is discussed in Chapter 8. Pure RBC aplasia involves a selective destruction of RBC precursors and can be congenital or acquired. It is often associated with viral infections (e.g., parvovirus). Symptoms are related to the anemia. Diagnosis is via BM biopsy showing absence of erythroid elements but with preservation of other cell lines. Treatment includes supportive measures with transfusions as needed.

TABLE 3-2	CAUSES OF NORMOCYTIC ANEMIA ASSOCIATED WITH A DECREASED RETICULOCYTE COUNT

Malignancies and other marrow infiltrative diseases
   Leukemia and lymphoma
   Metastatic cancer
   Plasma cell disorders
   Granulomatous disease
Stem cell disorders
   Myelofibrosis
   Aplastic anemia
   Pure red cell plasma
   Myelodysplasia
Due to other medical conditions
   Anemia of renal disease
   Anemia of chronic disease
   Endocrine disorders

Anemia of Chronic Disease (Anemia of Chronic Inflammation)
This condition is often associated with malignancy, infection, and inflammatory states. It may occur in patients with chronic infections (e.g., osteomyelitis), HIV, or inflammatory diseases (e.g., lupus or rheumatoid arthritis). These disorders have in common the inhibition of normal RBC synthesis due to the underlying disorder. They may act by inadequate release of or insensitivity to erythropoietin. Other etiologies include deficiency in mobilization of iron from the reticuloendothelial system. The anemia is most often a normocytic, normochromic anemia with a decreased reticulocyte count but may also present as a mild microcytic anemia. The serum iron concentration and total iron-binding capacity are usually both low, often giving a normal transferrin saturation (although this may be low or low-normal range). Serum ferritin, however, is an acute phase reactant and is often elevated in inflammatory diseases and infections. BM exam, if done, typically shows present iron stores. Symptoms and physical exam of the anemia of chronic disease patient are dependent on the patient's underlying condition. The anemia is typically mild and does not require blood transfusion. The more appropriate treatment is to treat the underlying condition.

Myelophthisic Anemias
Myelophthisic anemias refer to those with evidence of hematopoiesis outside the BM or infiltration of the BM by nonhematologic cells. The most common cause is metastatic carcinoma to the BM (e.g., breast, lung, prostate, and kidney). Other causes include myeloproliferative disorders, multiple myeloma, leukemias, and lymphoma. These are often suspected by a typical appearance of the peripheral smear (nucleated RBC, teardrop-shaped RBCs, and immature WBCs) and a "dry tap" on BM aspiration. BM biopsy results are dependent on the underlying disease. Treatment is directed toward the underlying disorder.

Anemia of Chronic Renal Failure
Anemia of chronic renal failure is due to erythropoietin deficiency. The anemia generally starts when CrCl <45 mL/min and worsens with declining renal function. When possible, treatment involves first treating the underlying renal dysfunction. Erythropoietin can be given at 50 to 100 U/kg IV or SC 3×/week, with readjustments based on response. In follow-up, expect an increase in Hct in 8 to 12 weeks.

Endocrine Disorders
Anemia due to endocrine disorders is seen in hypothyroidism, adrenal insufficiency, and gonadal dysfunction. Estrogens tend to inhibit red cell synthesis, and testosterone tends to stimulate it. Correction of the underlying endocrine disorder may improve the anemia.

Macrocytic Anemias

Anemias that have a MCV of more than ~100 fL are macrocytic anemias. These may be separated into two categories based on features seen on peripheral smear: megaloblastic and nonmegaloblastic. *Megaloblastic* features include the presence of oval macrocytes and hypersegmentation of the PMNs. They are a consequence of abnormal maturation of these cells and nuclear/cellular asynchrony. Examples of megaloblastic anemia include vitamin B_{12} deficiency, folate deficiency, and drug-induced megaloblastic anemia. *Nonmegaloblastic* features include the presence of round macrocytes without hypersegmentation of the PMNs. Causes of nonmegaloblastic macrocytic anemia include liver disease, hypothyroidism, alcohol-induced reticulocytosis and reticulocytosis secondary to HA, and myelodysplastic syndrome (see Chap. 8 for further discussion).

Vitamin B_{12} Deficiency
The daily requirement of vitamin B_{12} is 2 µg/day, and a typical diet provides 5 to 15 µg/day, with the liver capable of storing ~2000 to 5000 µg. Thus, it takes up to 3 to 6 years for deficiency to develop once absorption completely ceases.

Etiologies. Etiologies include pernicious anemia (the most common cause), gastrectomy or gastric bypass surgery, ileal disorders (sprue, inflammatory bowel disease, and lymphoma), bacterial overgrowth in the small intestine, fish tapeworms, and inadequate intake (this is very rare and only occurs in the strict vegetarian).

History and Physical Exam. Symptoms include burning sensation of the tongue, vague abdominal pain, diarrhea, numbness, paresthesia, and mental clouding. On exam, one can note glossitis, smooth tongue, dorsal column findings (decreased vibration and proprioception), and corticospinal tract findings (motor weakness, spasticity, positive Babinski sign). *Of note, patients can present with neurologic signs without overt anemia.*

Diagnosis. In cases of borderline-low B_{12} values, one can measure serum methylmalonic acid and homocysteine levels, which are elevated in vitamin B_{12} deficiency. Once deficiency is established, an attempt should be made to identify the etiology. The presence of anti-intrinsic factor antibodies or anti-parietal cell antibodies lends support to the diagnosis of pernicious anemia. Surgical history can reveal postsurgical etiologies. Suspicion of ileal disorder can be evaluated by endoscopy. Stool ova and parasites should be performed if suspicious for parasitic infection. A therapeutic trial of antibiotics may be given if bacterial overgrowth is suspected. The Schilling test is rarely used today but may delineate the underlying pathology.

Treatment. Treatment usually includes vitamin B_{12}, 1 mg IM or SC daily for 7 days, then weekly for 1 month, followed by monthly doses thereafter. There are data suggesting that oral vitamin B_{12} at doses of 1 to 2 mg daily is just as effective as IM administration. Failure to correct or identify the underlying mechanism of deficiency may result in lifelong therapy.

Follow-up. Reticulocytosis should occur in 5 to 7 days, with resolution of hematologic abnormalities in ~2 months. Resolution of neurologic abnormalities depends on their duration before treatment and may take up to 18 months but can also be permanent.

Folate Deficiency

The daily requirement of folate is 50 to 100 μg/day, with body stores of ~5 to 10 mg. Depletion can occur after ~2 to 4 months of persistent negative balance. Etiologies include inadequate intake (e.g., alcoholics), decreased absorption (e.g., sprue, bacterial overgrowth, certain drugs such as phenytoin and oral contraceptives), or states of increased requirements (HA, pregnancy, chronic dialysis, exfoliative dermatitis). Folate deficiency can also be iatrogenic, such as treatment with folic acid antagonists (e.g., methotrexate, trimethoprim). Symptoms and physical exam are similar to vitamin B_{12} deficiency except that *neurologic features are not present.* Both serum and RBC folate levels must be measured. Serum folate is more labile and subject to acute rise after a folate-rich meal; RBC folate is a better indicator of tissue stores. It is important to *rule out vitamin B_{12} deficiency* before repletion with folate, because folate may improve the hematologic abnormalities in vitamin B_{12} deficiency but will not correct the neurologic manifestations. Treatment is with oral folate (1 mg/day), with resolution of hematologic abnormalities in ~2 months.

Drug-Induced Disorders

Several drugs can cause a macrocytic anemia by affecting DNA synthesis. Offenders include purine analogues (e.g., 6-mercaptopurine, azathioprine), pyrimidine analogues (5-fluorouracil, cytarabine), hydroxyurea, and anticonvulsants (phenytoin, phenobarbital). Reverse transcriptase inhibitors (AZT, etc.) may cause macrocytosis without anemia. Therapy is cessation of the offending agent or toleration of a mild anemia if the drug is therapeutically needed.

Nonmegaloblastic Anemia

Nonmegaloblastic anemias typically have round macrocytes without hypersegmentation of PMNs on peripheral smear. MCV of nonmegaloblastic anemias is rarely >110 to 115. A value higher than this would tend to support a megaloblastic etiology. When the reticulo-cyte count is elevated, it suggests an etiology such as alcohol, hypothyroidism, or liver disease. HA can produce a macrocytosis via increased production of reticulocytes. Nonmega-loblastic anemias are usually treated by identifying and treating the underlying etiology, such as discontinuation of alcohol use and thyroid hormone replacement.

ANEMIAS ASSOCIATED WITH INCREASED DESTRUCTION

Table 3-3 lists causes of anemia associated with increased RBC destruction. The following discussion is based on the acquired vs. hereditary classification.

Classification of Hemolytic Anemias
Location of Hemolysis
- **Extravascular:** Cell destruction occurs in the reticuloendothelial system, usually in the spleen.
- **Intravascular:** RBC destruction takes place within the circulation.

Mechanism of Hemolysis
- **Intrinsic:** Hemolysis is caused by a defect in the RBC membrane or contents.
- **Extrinsic:** Factors outside the RBC, such as serum antibody, trauma within circulation, infection, etc., lead to RBC damage
- In general, most intrinsic causes are hereditary, and most extrinsic causes are acquired.

Hemolytic Anemias
HAs are disorders in which the destruction of RBCs leads to a decrease in circulating RBC mass. Acute hemolysis may be accompanied by a wide variety of signs and symptoms, many of which may point to the underlying etiology. Patients may present with fever, chills, jaundice, back and abdominal pain, splenomegaly, and brown or red urine. Peripheral blood smear remains a useful tool both to confirm the diagnosis of hemolysis and to aid in discerning the underlying etiology. Some signs commonly found on peripheral smears include spherocytes (autoimmune HA, hereditary spherocytosis), helmet cells or schistocytes (microangiopathic HA), sickle cells and Howell-Jolly bodies (sickle cell anemia), spur cells (in liver diseases), bite cells or Heinz bodies (glucose-6-phosphate dehydrogenase [G-6-PD] deficiency), and agglutination (cold agglutinin). Laboratory abnor-

TABLE 3-3	CAUSES OF INCREASED RBC DESTRUCTION
Hereditary	**Acquired**
RBC membrane disorders	Immune related
Spherocytosis	Warm antibody
Elliptocytosis	Cold agglutinin
RBC enzyme disorders	Transfusion reaction
Pyruvate kinase deficiency	Nonimmune
Hexokinase deficiency	Microangiopathic hemolytic anemia
G-6-PD deficiency	Infection
Disordered Hgb synthesis	Hypersplenism
Hemoglobinopathy (i.e., sickle cell)	Paroxysmal nocturnal hemoglobinuria
Thalassemias	

malities suggestive of hemolysis, though not specific, include increased lactate dehydrogenase, decreased haptoglobin, and increased unconjugated bilirubin. In addition, signs of compensatory increased RBC production such as an increase in reticulocyte count are typically present. Other useful lab tests include the **direct Coombs test**, which is a direct antiglobulin test that detects antibodies (usually IgG) or complement (usually C3) bound to the surface of circulating RBCs by mixing *patient RBCs* with *anti-IgG*. Positive results occur when allo- or autoantibodies to RBC antigens are present, or when there is nonspecific adherence of other Ig or immune complexes to the RBC surface. The **indirect Coombs** test, which mixes the *patient's serum* with *normal RBCs*, is used to detect the presence of any anti-RBC antibody in the serum.

Sickle Cell Anemia

Sickle cell anemia is caused by a defect in the beta-globin chain, resulting in sickling of RBC under oxidative stress. See Chapter 11 for further details.

Glucose-6-Phosphate Dehydrogenase Deficiency

G-6-PD deficiency is an X-linked disorder that is fully expressed in males and homozygous females and variably expressed in heterozygous females. G-6-PD is the rate-limiting enzyme in the pentose phosphate pathway that helps maintain intracellular levels of glutathione, which serves to protect RBC against oxidative damage. In patients with G-6-PD deficiency, the presence of oxidative stress results in an inability to maintain Hgb in a reduced state, which, in turn, leads to Hgb precipitation within RBCs (Heinz body formation) and intravascular hemolysis. Two main variants of G-6-PD lead to clinically significant hemolysis: *G-6-PD A⁻* and *G-6-PD Mediterranean*. G-6-PD A⁻, which occurs in 10% of black individuals, has normal enzyme activity in young RBCs but a marked deficiency of enzyme activity in older cells. Therefore, when oxidatively challenged, only the older cells lyse. This form is typically milder and self-limited. The G-6-PD Mediterranean variant occurs in people of Middle Eastern and Mediterranean descent, and is characterized by a nearly complete lack of G-6-PD. Hemolysis in this form tends to be more severe compared to the A⁻ variant.

The diagnosis of G-6-PD deficiency is suspected when hemolysis occurs after any form of oxidative stress, most commonly from starting on drugs known to precipitate hemolysis in a G-6-PD-deficient patient (Table 3-4). Other triggers of hemolytic crises include certain foods, most notably fava beans, illnesses such as severe infections, and diabetic ketoacidosis. Findings on the peripheral blood smear suggestive of the diagnosis

TABLE 3-4	PRECIPITANTS OF HEMOLYSIS IN GLUCOSE-6-PHOSPHATE DEHYDROGENASE DEFICIENCY

Infection: *E. coli*, salmonella, *S. pneumoniae*, viral hepatitis

Drug-induced

    Antimalarials: primaquine and chloroquine

    Antibiotics: sulfonamides, dapsone (dapsone USP, DDS), nitrofurantoin (Macrodantin)

    Phenazopyridine (Pyridium)

    Analgesics: in some cases, salicylates

Fava beans (in the Mediterranean variant only)

Naphthalene

include Heinz bodies and "bite" cells. Heinz bodies are Hgb precipitants in the RBC, while bite cells are deformed RBCs that result from attempts by macrophages in the spleen to remove the Heinz bodies. Definitive diagnosis is made by measuring G-6-PD enzyme activity level. **In suspected G-6-PD A⁻ variant, enzyme levels should not be measured during acute hemolysis.** In these patients, older RBCs containing the defective enzymes have mostly been lysed during acute hemolysis, and the normal enzyme activities in the remaining younger RBCs and reticulocytes will provide a false-negative result. It is, therefore, advisable to *wait 3 to 4 weeks after the acute episode* to get a true representation of the enzyme activity level. The same does not apply to the Mediterranean variant, as both younger and older red cells are affected. Treatment is supportive, with transfusions as needed, and preventive, with avoidance of oxidative precipitant.

Hereditary Spherocytosis (Membrane Defect)

Hereditary spherocytosis is an autosomal dominant disorder most common in patients of Northern European descent. In these patients, a defect in a membrane cytoskeletal protein leads to loss of surface area on the RBCs, resulting in spherocyte formation. Hemolysis of the spherocytic RBCs occurs primarily in the spleen. Clinical presentation may vary from asymptomatic to profound anemia and jaundice, depending on the severity of spherocytosis. Some patients may present with cholelithiasis. Splenomegaly is detected in most patients due to extravascular hemolysis. Peripheral blood smears reveal spherocytes. The *osmotic fragility test*, which measures the RBC resistance to hemolysis when incubated in hypotonic saline, will show increased hemolysis. Treatment is largely supportive, with transfusions as needed and folate supplement to support increased erythropoiesis. Splenectomy, which corrects the anemia but not the underlying defect, can be curative and may be considered in patients with severe anemia.

Acquired Immune Hemolytic Anemia

Warm Antibody. Warm antibody is the most common form of autoimmune HA. The most common antibodies involved are IgG and they are most active at 37°C. Sixty percent of cases are *idiopathic* (or *primary*), whereas 40% are *secondary*. Secondary causes include chronic lymphocytic leukemia, non-Hodgkin lymphoma, Hodgkin lymphoma, autoimmune disorders (such as systemic lupus erythematosus), and drugs. **Drug-related antibodies** can occur by three main mechanisms.

- **Autoantibody:** Antibody against Rhesus (e.g., methyldopa) is produced.
- **Hapten:** Drug binds to the RBC membrane, acting as hapten, which serves as a target for antibodies. Hemolysis typically occurs 1 to 2 weeks after treatment (e.g., penicillin, cephalosporins).
- **Immune complex:** Drug binds to plasma protein, evoking an antibody response. The drug-protein-antibody complex then nonspecifically coats RBCs, resulting in complement-mediated lysis (e.g., quinidine, INH, sulfonamides).

Warm antibodies usually cause extravascular hemolysis by the spleen, leading to splenomegaly. Almost all are panagglutinins (i.e., react with most donor RBCs), thus making crossmatching difficult. Treatment for drug-induced hemolysis is withdrawal of the offending agent, as hemolysis will stop with clearance of the drug. **Steroids (prednisone) and immunoglobulins remain the most commonly used initial therapies.** Prednisone up to 1 mg/kg/day may be used for severe hemolysis in idiopathic forms, until Hgb reaches normal levels over a few weeks, and then tapered. Intravenous immunoglobulins may be effective in controlling hemolysis, though its benefits tend to be short-lived. **Splenectomy** is an option for patients who fail or relapse after steroid taper. If steroids and splenectomy both fail, other immunosuppressives such as cyclosporine, azathioprine, and rituximab should be considered. **Transfusions should be avoided**, if possible, as they may result in more hemolysis.

Cold Antibody. Most cold antibodies are IgM and active at <30°C. Acute onset is often associated with infectious causes such as mycoplasma pneumonia and infectious mononucleosis, whereas chronic forms occur with lymphoproliferative disorders or are idiopathic. The two main manifestations are acrocyanosis (ears, nose, and distal extremities) and hemolysis (complement mediated). Symptoms mainly occur in distal body parts, where the temperature often drops below 30°C. In these cold temperatures, IgM will bind to the RBCs, leading to complement fixation and hemolysis. The antibody dissociates from the RBCs as the temperature rises above 30°C. Treatment mainly involves avoidance of cold exposure and treatment of the underlying disorder. While certain immunosuppressive agents may be effective, splenectomy and steroids are of limited therapeutic value.

Acquired Nonimmune Hemolytic Anemia
Acquired causes of nonimmune HA are often secondary to physical damages from the environment, chemical changes, or infections. Microangiopathic and macroangiopathic HAs represent the most common causes of environmental damages. In these cases, changes in the vasculature result in the destruction of RBCs due to physical stress. Conditions associated with these forms of HAs include disseminated intravascular coagulation (DIC), thrombotic thrombocytopenic purpura (TTP), hemolytic-uremic syndrome (HUS), prosthetic heart valves, and severe aortic stenosis. DIC, TTP, and HUS are discussed in Chapter 4. Osmotic changes and certain snake and spider venom are examples of chemical damages to RBC's. HA is a characteristic feature of malarial infections. Table 3-5 lists the causes of acquired nonimmune HA.

TABLE 3-5	TYPES OF ACQUIRED NONIMMUNE HEMOLYTIC ANEMIAS

1. Microangiopathic hemolytic anemia
   a. Thrombotic thrombocytopenic purpura
   b. Disseminated intravascular coagulation
   c. Hemolytic-uremic syndrome
   d. Eclampsia
   e. Malignant hypertension
   f. Metastatic adenocarcinoma
2. Macroangiopathic hemolytic anemia
   a. Prosthetic valve
   b. Severe aortic stenosis
3. Physical and chemical
   a. Snake and spider venom
   b. Osmotic hemolysis from freshwater drowning
   c. Damage to RBC membranes from third-degree burns
4. Infection
   a. Malaria
   b. *Clostridium difficile*
   c. Babesiosis
5. Hypersplenism
6. Paroxysmal nocturnal hemoglobinuria

SECONDARY POLYCYTHEMIA

Secondary polycythemia refers to erythrocytosis, which is defined as increased RBC mass. Chronic generalized or local hypoxia causes the body to respond by producing RBC mass to compensate. Chronic hypoxia from congenital heart disease, lung diseases including chronic obstructive lung disease and smoking with increased carboxyhemoglobin levels, or even local hypoxia to kidneys may increase erythropoietin levels from the kidneys (appropriate or inappropriate), resulting in increased production of RBCs. On physical exam, a ruddy complexion can be seen in patients with secondary polycythemia. In patients who are suffering from chronic hypoxia at severe levels, clubbing or even cyanosis may be found. Usually, no therapy is indicated in patients with erythrocytosis, as it is a physiological response to hypoxia and is a compensatory mechanism. **Secondary polycythemia can be distinguished from primary polycythemia (polycythemia vera) by the erythropoietin level**, which is elevated in secondary polycythemia and low or normal in polycythemia vera. Polycythemia vera is a stem cell disorder leading to increased RBC mass, which is discussed further discussed in Chapter 9.

KEY POINTS TO REMEMBER

- Always consider active bleeding as a source of anemia.
- The initial workup of anemia includes a thorough history and physical, assessment of cell counts and red cell indexes, tests of the coagulation system, and viewing of the peripheral slide.
- The Hgb and Hct are often inaccurate in the setting of acute bleeding.
- Patients with iron deficiency can have microcytic normochromic indexes initially that eventually progress to microcytic hypochromic. Worsening iron-deficiency anemia is also associated with a gradual increase in anisocytosis and poikilocytosis (abnormally shaped cells).
- Patients with vitamin B_{12} deficiency can present with neurologic signs without overt anemia.
- It is important to rule out vitamin B_{12} deficiency before instituting folate repletion. While folate can improve the hematologic abnormalities in vitamin B_{12} deficiency, it has no effect on the neurologic manifestations.
- In G-6-PD A⁻, enzyme levels should not be measured during an acute hemolytic attack. It is best to wait 3 to 4 weeks, because it is the older RBCs that have the marked deficiency in enzyme activity, which are the cells that have been lysed. Testing during an acute attack can render false-negative results.
- While steroids are effective initial therapy in warm antibody HA, they are of limited value in the cold antibody-mediated form.

REFERENCES AND SUGGESTED READINGS

Berkow R, ed. Anemias. In: *The Merck Manual*. 16th ed. Rahway, NJ: Merck Research Laboratories; 1992:1136–1174.

Blinder M. Anemia and transfusion therapy. In: Ahya SN, Flood K, Paranjothi S, eds. *The Washington Manual of Medical Therapeutics*. 30th ed. Philadelphia: Lippincott Williams & Wilkins; 2001:413–428.

Burd R. Hematology/oncology. In: Ferri FF, ed. *Practical Guide to the Care of the Medical Patient*. 3rd ed. St. Louis: Mosby; 1995:376–387.

Davenport J. Macrocytic anemia. *Am Fam Phys*. 1996;53(1):155–162.

Dubois RW, Goodnough LT, Ershler WB, et al. Identification, diagnosis, and management of anemia in adult ambulatory patients treated by primary care physicians: evidence-based and consensus recommendations. *Curr Med Res Opin*. 2006;22(2):385–395.

Eckman JR. Orderly approach to the evaluation and treatment of anemia. *Emory Univ J Med*. 1991;5(2):80–90.

Goroll AH. Evaluation of anemia. In: Goroll AH, May LA, Mulley AG, eds. *Primary care Medicine: Office Evaluation and Management of the Adult Patient*. 3rd ed. Philadelphia: J. B. Lippincott; 1995:447–455.

Kuzminski AM, Del Giacco EJ, Allen RH, et al. Effective treatment of cobalamin deficiency with oral cobalamin. *Blood*. 1998;92(4):1191–1198.

Massey A. Microcytic anemia, differential diagnosis and management of iron deficiency anemia. *Med Clin North Am*. 1992;76(3):549–566.

Robbins SL, Cotran RS, Kumar V. Diseases of red cells and bleeding disorders. In: Cotran RS, Robbins SL, Kumar V, et al., eds. *Pathologic Basis of Disease*. 5th ed. Philadelphia: W. B. Saunders; 1994:583–616.

Rosse W, Bunn HF. Hemolytic anemias. In: Isselbacher KJ, Braunwald E, Wilson JD, et al., eds. *Harrison's Principles of Internal Medicine*. 13th ed. New York: McGraw-Hill; 1994:1743–1754.

Sandstad J, McKenna RW, Keffer JH, eds. Erythrocyte disorders. In: Keffer JH, ed. *Handbook of Clinical Pathology*. Chicago: ASCP Press; 1992:193–211.

Steensma DP, Hoyer JD, Fairbanks VF. Hereditary red blood cell disorders in Middle Eastern patients. *Mayo Clin Proc*. 2001;76(3):285–293.

Vichinsky E, Styles L. Pulmonary complications. *Hematol Oncol Clin North Am*. 1996;10(6):1275–1287.

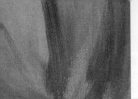

Platelets: Thrombocytopenia and Thrombocytosis

4

Sakib K. Khalid and Chanda Ho

THROMBOCYTOPENIA

Introduction
Platelets are essential for primary hemostasis—the process in which a platelet plug forms to initiate clotting. When the platelet number is too low (thrombocytopenia) or the platelets are not functioning properly, bleeding may result.

Causes
Pathophysiology
Thrombocytopenia results from decreased platelet production, platelet destruction/sequestration, or a combination thereof.

Differential Diagnosis
Decreased Platelet Production
- Infection: HIV, hepatitis C, parvovirus, varicella, rubella, mumps
- Chemotherapy
- Radiation
- Congenital or acquired primary bone marrow failure: Fanconi anemia, megakaryocytic thrombocytopenia, paroxysmal nocturnal hemoglobinuria
- Vitamin deficiencies: folate, B_{12}
- Alcohol

Increased Platelet Destruction
- Drugs: heparin, valproic acid, quinine
- Autoimmune platelet destruction: idiopathic thrombocytopenic purpura (ITP), thrombotic thrombocytopenic purpura (TTP)/hemolytic-uremic syndrome (HUS)
- HELLP (hemolysis, elevated liver enzymes, and low platelets) syndrome
- Disseminated intravascular coagulation (DIC)
- Pseudothrombocytopenia
- Splenic sequestration
- Platelet clumping

Inherited Abnormalities of Platelets
Although inherited abnormalities of platelets are quite rare, they deserve brief mention because of their historical significance and importance in understanding platelet function. **Glanzmann thrombasthenia** is an autosomal recessive disorder caused by a defect in GpIIb-IIIa, an important glycoprotein involved in binding fibrinogen, forming the primary hemostatic plug and activating platelets. A defect in GpIIb-IIIa due to any number

of possible mutations leads to the typical mucosal bleeding pattern seen in acquired platelet disorders. Mild to severe bleeding may be seen. Platelet count is normal in this disorder. **Bernard-Soulier syndrome** is an autosomal recessive disorder due to a defect in GpIb-IX. GpIb-IX acts as the receptor for von Willebrand factor (vWF), and its absence leads to improper platelet-vWF binding. The disorder is characterized by giant platelet forms (up to 20 μm) and thrombocytopenia. **Pseudo-vWD,** or "platelet-type vWD," is due to an abnormality in GpIb, which has an increased affinity for vWF. Abnormal platelet binding leads to increased clearance of vWF from the plasma. The **May-Hegglin** anomaly is an autosomal dominant disorder characterized by giant platelets and thrombocytopenia-like Bernard-Soulier syndrome. There are a number of other inherited disorders associated with platelet defects, and these should be distinguished from acquired platelet abnormalities. A key distinguishing feature is giant platelets seen on peripheral blood smear. Many of these disorders are treated with platelet transfusions.

Thrombotic Thrombocytopenic Purpura and Hemolytic-Uremic Syndrome
Background
TTP and HUS are clinically similar disorders that are often grouped together as *TTP-HUS*. Although pathophysiology distinguishes the two disorders, both involve microvascular damage and platelet destruction and have significant clinical similarities. They are classically defined by **thrombocytopenia** and **microangiopathic hemolytic anemia** (MAHA) in the absence of another apparent cause. Neurologic and renal impairments are also characteristic. When neurologic impairment is present, the patient is said to have TTP, whereas acute renal failure is considered to be the hallmark for HUS. In some cases, there is a significant overlap and patients can have both renal and neurological impairment.

Epidemiology
TTP has an incidence of ~3.7 cases/100,000 persons. HUS is an uncommon disorder with two forms—a sporadic form more typical of adults and a childhood form that is associated with verotoxin and *Escherichia coli* O157:H7. Both cause thrombocytopenia with MAHA but are distinct entities. TTP-HUS once had a 90% mortality rate until the development of plasma exchange. Now its mortality is <30% with treatment. Therefore, treatment should be initiated in anyone with thrombocytopenia and MAHA without other cause.

Etiology
Although it is idiopathic in most cases, certain conditions have been associated with TTP-HUS (Table 4-1). Microvascular damage and platelet aggregation appear to be key in the development of these disorders. High shear stress and damage to endothelial cells are also noted as causative factors. Platelet thrombi subsequently form in the vasculature.

Causes
Pathophysiology
   Thrombotic Thrombocytopenic Purpura. Over the past few years, there has been significant advancement in the understanding of the pathophysiology of TTP. Endothelial cells produce ultralarge vWF (ULvWF) molecules that are cleaved by ADAMTS 13 (a metalloprotease) into their typical-length multimers in normal circumstances (Fig. 4-1A) In a significant number of TTP patients, there is either a marked deficiency (<5% of normal activity) or an inhibitor of ADAMTS 13. This protease deficiency may be recessively inherited. Antibodies (Abs; IgG) to this protease that act as inhibitors are also associated with TTP and may be induced by some drugs. When these ULvWF molecules persist, they induce abnormal platelet aggregation in the microcirculation in areas of high shear stress. This leads to platelet consumption and fragmenting and destruction of RBCs. These ULvWF molecules also disappear in acute episodes of TTP, suggesting their consumption

TABLE 4-1	ETIOLOGY OF TTP-HUS

1. Idiopathic (most common)
2. Estrogen use
3. Pregnancy
4. Infections (EHEC 0157:H7 in HUS, pneumococcal infection, HIV)
5. Stem cell transplantation
6. Autoimmune diseases (SLE, antiphospholipid syndrome)
7. Cardiac surgery
8. Drugs
   a. Quinine
   b. Ticlopidine
   c. Clopidogrel
   d. Cyclosporine
   e. Tacrolimus
9. Familial

in an abnormal proteolytic process (Fig. 4-1B). It should be noted that, at times, patients can have significant deficiency in ADAMTS 13 levels without developing TTP, implicating other unidentified factors.

Hemolytic-Uremic Syndrome. Although HUS has long been thought to be related to TTP, ADAMTS 13 inhibitors or deficiency does not appear to be the etiology of HUS. HUS is associated with selective endothelial damage in kidneys and, occasionally, in brain as well. CD36 is thought to play a role. Heredity has been identified as the cause in <5% of cases of HUS, and a familial form with recurrent episodes of HUS has been described. Factor H is a complement regulatory protease that appears to be involved. Factor H mutations have been linked to familial forms of the disease, although it is not clear how these mutations predispose patients to HUS. As mentioned earlier, the childhood HUS variant is associated with Shiga verotoxin and is frequently seen after an episode of hemorrhagic

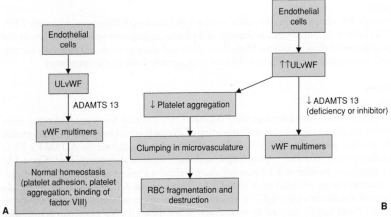

FIGURE 4-1. A: Role of ADAMTS 13 in a normal subject. **B:** Role of ADAMTS 13 deficiency in thrombotic thrombocytopenic purpura. vWF, von Willebrand factor; ULvWF, ultralarge vWF.

TABLE 4-2	THROMBOTIC THROMBOCYTOPENIC PURPURA/HEMOLYTIC-UREMIC SYNDROME (HUS): THE CLASSIC PENTAD OF FINDINGS

1. Thrombocytopenia
2. Microangiopathic hemolytic anemia
3. Neurologic changes
4. Renal dysfunction (predominates in HUS)
5. Fever

diarrhea. Outbreaks have been documented in children secondary to *E. coli* O157:H7, but it is also seen in adults.

Presentation

Clinical Presentation

The **classic findings** of TTP-HUS include a pentad of physical exam and lab findings as reported in Table 4-2. The complete pentad does not have to be present for the diagnosis, and HUS often presents without fever or neurologic dysfunction. Renal failure in HUS may be oliguric or nonoliguric. TTP may be preceded by a few weeks of malaise, but neurologic symptoms (including headache, confusion, vision changes, tinnitus, and seizures) are frequently the first symptoms that bring a patient to medical attention. These symptoms may wax and wane over minutes. Some patients may progress to coma. Bleeding problems are commonly seen (90%). Pancreatitis has also been associated with TTP, and patients can have abdominal pain, nausea, and vomiting. At times diarrhea may also be present. Urine output can drop off dramatically.

Differential Diagnosis

Differential diagnosis includes other etiologies of MAHA (DIC, prosthetic valve hemolysis, malignant hypertension, adenocarcinoma, vasculitis). Although fever is part of the pentad, it should also prompt workup of sources of infection. Evan syndrome (autoimmune thrombocytopenia and autoimmune hemolytic anemia) should be distinguished by the presence of spherocytes and absence of schistocytes in the peripheral smear.

Management

Diagnostic Evaluation

Anemia and thrombocytopenia are universal. The thrombocytopenia tends to be worse in TTP than in HUS. The WBC count is frequently normal, but significant neutrophilia may occur. An elevated **lactate dehydrogenase (LDH)**, elevated **indirect bilirubin,** and decreased **haptoglobin** will help identify hemolysis associated with the disorder, but a **peripheral blood smear** is mandatory for diagnosis by identifying schistocytes consistent with MAHA. A **direct Coombs** test is negative. The reticulocyte count should be elevated, but coagulation studies (PT/INR, PTT) are usually within normal limits. A DIC panel, including fibrinogen, fibrinogen degradation products (FDPs), and D-dimer, is useful to evaluate DIC as an alternate diagnosis. ADAMTS 13 activity levels may be undetectable; however, treatment should not be delayed waiting for this test. If the patient's **creatinine** is significantly elevated, HUS is suggested. The urinalysis may be unimpressive, with only mild findings, but proteinuria and red cells are typical when there are abnormalities. With fever, blood cultures should be drawn to evaluate for sepsis. In unclear cases, some have suggested a renal biopsy, but this is problematic in patients with thrombocytopenia.

Treatment

The primary treatment for TTP-HUS is **plasma exchange** (plasmapheresis), with one estimated plasma volume being exchanged daily. Some patients require plasma exchange twice daily, in severe cases or in cases that progress despite daily treatments. Because of the high mortality of untreated TTP-HUS, thrombocytopenia and MAHA are all that is required to initiate plasma exchange if no other cause can be identified. ADAMTS 13 levels should not be used in management decisions. Plasma exchange has also shown benefits in other thrombotic microangiopathies, so it should not be withheld in urgent cases. Plasma exchange carries a high complication rate, so a specialist in hematology should be involved in the decision to initiate it. The goal of daily plasma exchange should be to reverse the thrombocytopenia and hemolysis. This can be monitored with LDH and CBC measurements and typically requires 1 to 2 weeks of plasma exchange, but can take considerably longer. The frequency of plasma exchange is typically decreased to taper the treatment after the LDH and platelets are within normal limits. Some patients require dialysis, if the renal failure is severe. Platelet transfusions are relatively contraindicated, except in cases of life-threatening bleeding. After remission, exacerbations due to discontinuing plasma exchange (<30 days) should lead to immediate retreatment with plasma exchange. With remission, neurologic symptoms often improve dramatically, but renal problems frequently persist. The childhood variant associated with verotoxin is not typically treated with plasmapheresis, and supportive treatment is often all that is necessary.

In patients who appear **resistant to plasma exchange** at a frequency that has increased to twice a day, attempts with the cryosupernatant portion of plasma may be attempted. Methylprednisolone, 125 mg IV bid, or prednisone, 1 mg/kg/day, should also be added. Splenectomy is controversial. Drug-induced forms caused by agents like mitomycin C and cyclosporine often will not respond well and have a poor prognosis.

Follow-up

After **remission,** approximately one third of patients will relapse in 10 yrs, and routine follow-up is required. LDH levels should be monitored. Chronic renal insufficiency is a frequent problem, but if the disease is quickly identified, mortality and this long-term complication may be avoided.

Disseminated Intravascular Coagulation

Introduction

Although DIC is usually considered a malfunction in coagulation or secondary hemostasis, it is discussed here because it may have findings similar to those of disorders mentioned previously, especially the TTP-HUS spectrum. Rapid onset of thrombocytopenia or a significant drop in platelet count can be a clue that a patient with certain predisposing conditions (Table 4-3) is developing DIC.

Pathophysiology

DIC is an acquired disorder of hemostasis that involves inappropriate thrombosis systemically but is most notable in small and medium-sized vessels. DIC evolves from a condition in which the patient is **hypercoagulable,** to end-organ damage by **thrombosis and ischemia,** to one in which the clotting factors are depleted, and culminates in the development of **bleeding problems** and **life-threatening hemorrhage**. There are many associated conditions, but the unifying cause appears to be widespread endothelial damage and/or extensive release of inflammatory cytokines, most notably interleukin-6, tumor necrosis factor-alpha, and interleukin-1. This exposes tissue factor, which interacts with factor VII, initiating the coagulation cascade. Subsequent to this is the generation of thrombin molecules and, therefore, the *consumption of the coagulation factors*, specifically factor V, factor VIII, and fibrinogen. The increased thrombin generation leads to release

TABLE 4-3	CONDITIONS ASSOCIATED WITH DISSEMINATED INTRAVASCULAR COAGULATION

Systemic infection
    Gram-negative sepsis related to endotoxin
    Gram-positive organisms that may also cause sepsis and DIC

Cancer
    Solid tumors, including pancreatic, prostate, breast, and others
    Hematologic malignancy, most notably acute promyelocytic leukemia (AML-M3)

Trauma
    Head injury: usually life-threatening
    Serious burns involving large parts of the body
    Serious crushing injuries with substantial tissue damage
    Serious fractures, most notably a femur fracture with fat embolism

Obstetric complications
    Amniotic fluid embolism
    Placental abruption

Vascular disorders
    Aortic aneurysm
    Hemangiomas: usually giant

Immune-mediated reactions
    Anaphylaxis: mediated by cytokine release
    Transfusion reactions
    Transplant rejection

Toxins
    Snake venom
    IV drugs: possibly related to a drug affect, but IV drug abuse–associated systemic
      infections should be considered

of tissue plasminogen activator from endothelial cells, which results in the proteolysis of plasminogen to plasmin. Plasmin then leads to secondary fibrinolysis (degradation of fibrin to fibrin degradation products, which, in turn, further inhibits factors V and VIII). Antithrombin III (ATIII), proteins C and S, and tissue factor pathway inhibitor are also affected by DIC. These factors become depleted or are inhibited in various ways. ATIII may be the most important of these; low levels of ATIII due to consumption and degradation by elastase from neutrophils are associated with increased mortality. The net result of all these processes is systemic thrombosis and hemorrhage.

Presentation
Although minimal symptoms can be present in mild cases and early in the disease course, widespread bleeding, in the form of petechiae and oozing from venipuncture sites or wounds, is the most common presenting feature. In some patients, thrombosis, in the form of digit gangrene or systemic thrombosis (in kidneys, adrenal glands, liver, lungs, and central nervous system), is also present. As noted previously, these patients are usually gravely ill, and the history should be focused on assessing the patient for a condition or disease that is associated with DIC.

Management
    Diagnosis. There are a number of useful lab tests to assist in the diagnosis of DIC. A **CBC** to follow the platelet count and **PT/INR** and **PTT** are usually the first tests that indicate DIC is a potential problem. The platelets will usually show a substantial drop or a

count of <100,000/μL. The coagulation studies are typically abnormal, with prolongation of PT being universal and prolonged PTT in most of the patients. The CBC may also be useful to identify a high WBC count, often seen in sepsis. "DIC panels" often measure **fibrinogen, FDP, and D-dimer.** Fibrinogen levels are low as a result of consumption. The FDP and D-dimers are markers of clot dissolution and are usually elevated at the time of diagnosis, but because fibrinogen is an acute phase reactant and may be elevated at baseline, the levels may remain normal for some time. In such situations, a declining fibrinogen level over the course of days (half-life of fibrinogen is 4 days) provides a clue to the diagnosis of DIC. A **peripheral smear** may be useful in determining the diagnosis and will show schistocytes from destruction of red cells.

It is important to distinguish DIC from liver disease (low platelets and prolonged PT and PTT but normal fibrinogen—except in severe liver disease, which may show low fibrinogen), vitamin K deficiency (prolonged PT/PTT but normal platelets and fibrinogen), and TTP (MAHA and thrombocytopenia but normal PT, PTT, and fibrinogen).

Treatment. Management revolves around treatment of the underlying condition, replacement therapy, and treatment focused on thrombosis or bleeding (whichever is the predominant manifestation of DIC). Of these, the overriding and most important treatment for DIC is **treatment of the initiating condition.** Antibiotics in sepsis, for example, are more important than any direct intervention related to coagulation. Critical-care support should be tailored to the patient. In patients with high bleeding risk or active bleeding, fresh-frozen plasma and platelet **transfusions** are recommended. Platelet counts >50,000 are preferable. Cryoprecipitate to replace fibrinogen (in patients with a fibrinogen level ≤50 mg/dL) is also used to raise the fibrinogen level above 100 mg/dL. In patients predominantly in the thrombotic phase of DIC, **heparin** has been suggested, but this is controversial. The dose is typically a 300 to 500 U/h infusion. Low molecular weight heparin (LMWH) may have less risk for bleeding, and some consider it an alternative. In cases in which the patient has low ATIII levels and severe DIC, some consider ATIII replacement (with FFP or ATIII concentrates) a reasonable option. The goal of this therapy should be to achieve normal or supranormal levels. In patients with predominant bleeding, replacement therapy is the cornerstone of treatment. However, if this fails to control bleeding, aminocaproic acid (contraindicated with concurrent heparin administration) can be used. The role of activated protein C in DIC (outside sepsis) remains to be better defined.

Heparin-Induced Thrombocytopenia (HIT)

Classification

There are two forms of heparin-induced thrombocytopenia: HIT I and HIT II. HIT I is nonimmune-mediated and characterized by a transient fall in platelet count. This form of HIT is not an indication for discontinuing heparin. The remainder of this chapter focuses on HIT II.

Background

HIT is a complication of heparin therapy that is crucial to recognize given the potential life-threatening consequences. This phenomenon usually occurs 4 to 10 days after the initiation of heparin. This chapter focuses on HIT II, an immune-mediated disorder caused by IgG Abs that bind to platelet factor 4 (PF4). It has been noted in up to 3% of people treated with typical intravenous doses. Thrombosis has been noted in 30% of those who develop HIT, with 25% of these thromboses being arterial. As a result, these patients are at increased risk for pulmonary embolus, stroke, and myocardial infarction, making it essential to consider HIT in any patient having even a moderate reduction in platelets (50,000 to 100,000) with a history of heparin treatment within the previous 5 days.

Pathophysiology

PF4 binds to the Fc portion of the IgG Ab, leading to platelet activation, which explains the tendency of HIT patients to develop thrombosis rather than bleeding.

As with many primary specific immune responses, it has a delayed onset of at least 5 days after administration of heparin or LMWH. If the patient has been exposed previously, however, the thrombocytopenia can develop in hours. HIT is not usually seen after a patient has been on heparin for more than 2 weeks. The HIT-IgG Ab (HIT Ab) can activate platelets, generate platelet-derived microparticles, and promote tissue factor expression, leading to significant thrombosis, which can threaten limb circulation and potentially cause DIC. Although LMWH is associated with HIT, the incidence appears to be less than that for unfractionated heparin.

Management

Diagnosis. Thrombocytopenia, a fall in >50% of the platelet count, occurs in ~95% of patients diagnosed with HIT. The average platelet count is 50,000 to 60,000. It is important to take into account the patient's overall clinical picture before making a diagnosis of HIT. The presence of both thrombocytopenia and heparin administration does not necessarily mean that a patient has HIT. The differential diagnosis includes DIC and sepsis.

There are three time courses of HIT described in the literature: typical, rapid, and delayed-onset HIT. In typical-onset HIT (70%), thrombocytopenia develops ~5 to 10 days after initiation of heparin therapy, approximately the amount of time necessary to generate a humoral immune response. Twenty-five to thirty percent of patients experience rapid-onset HIT, where thrombocytopenia occurs within 24 hours, indicating a recent exposure to heparin during the preceding weeks. Delayed-onset HIT occurs days after heparin has been stopped. This form of HIT is not well understood. These patients typically have high-titer platelet-activating HIT Ab. It is uncommon for HIT to occur if heparin has been discontinued for more than 2 weeks.

Most patients with HIT experience thrombosis rather than bleeding complications given that the platelet count does not usually fall below 20,000. The most common manifestation is venous thromboembolism (deep venous thrombosis and pulmonary embolism) in the postoperative setting. Though less common, arterial thrombosis can occur and is manifested as stroke, myocardial infarction, or limb ischemia.

Lab Evaluation. The gold standard laboratory test for diagnosing HIT is the ^{14}C-serotonin release assay. This method was reported in 1986 by Sheridan et al. In this functional assay, donor platelets are first radiolabeled with ^{14}C-serotonin, then washed and added to patient serum at varying heparin concentrations (low, 0.1 U/mL; high, 100 U/mL). The test is considered positive when serotonin is released at a low concentration of heparin. This test has >95% sensitivity.

The platelet aggregation assay, another functional assay, has a 90% specificity but a much lower sensitivity. In this assay, normal platelet-rich plasma or washed donor platelets are added to patient platelet-poor plasma. A positive test is determined by platelet aggregation with varying concentrations of heparin.

There is also an antigenic assay. The solid phase ELISA measures Ab binding to heparin-PF4 complexes. The sensitivity of this test is >90% but its specificity is 74% to 86%.

Treatment. The first step in treating HIT is the discontinuation of heparin. Return of laboratory assay results often takes several days, therefore if HIT is suspected, all heparin products, including heparin flushes and heparin-coated catheters, should be discontinued immediately. Because of 90% cross-reactivity to the HIT Ab, LMWH should not be substituted. Patients with persistent thrombocytopenia after discontinuation of heparin, patients with thrombosis, and patients who were receiving heparin for significant anticoagulation needs should be treated with an alternative anticoagulant agent. One retrospective study of 62 patients reported that patients diagnosed with HIT had a 53% risk of thrombosis at 30 days. This finding stresses that patients with HIT may need to be treated with alternative agents even in the absence of thrombosis, given their underlying risk for developing complications.

There are a number of alternative agents that can be used to manage patients with HIT requiring anticoagulation for either treatment or prophylaxis. These agents can be used in HIT because they do not generate or cross-react with the HIT Ab. Warkentin and Greinacher classified HIT patients into three categories. This grouping creates a helpful framework for managing patients with HIT or with a history of HIT.

- **Active HIT.** Direct thrombin inhibitors such as lepirudin and argatroban are often used in the treatment of HIT. Lepirudin is a recombinant hirudin, a natural anticoagulant (found in the salivary glands of medicinal leeches *Hirudo medicinalis*). This drug has been approved by the FDA for patients with HIT for the prevention and treatment of thrombosis. **Lepirudin** is renally cleared and should therefore be dose-adjusted in patients with chronic kidney disease. If the CrCl is $\geq$60 mL/min, a 0.4 mg/kg bolus over 20 seconds, followed by 0.15 mg/kg/h, should be given. The PTT should be checked 4 hours after initiation of therapy and after dose changes—the goal PTT is 1.3 to 2$\times$ the control. Increased doses of this drug have been associated with bleeding.

  Argatroban has also been approved by the FDA for the prevention and treatment of thrombosis associated with HIT. This drug is hepatically cleared and should be used with caution in patients with impaired hepatic function. The starting dose is 0.5 to 1 μg/kg/min (start at 0.5 for those with hepatic insufficiency). The PTT should be checked 2 hours after initiation of therapy and after each dose change; the goal PTT is 1.5 to 3$\times$ the control. Argatroban has also been approved specifically for patients with HIT undergoing percutaneous coronary intervention. **Bivalirudin** is another direct thrombin inhibitor specifically approved for patients undergoing percutaneous coronary intervention.

  Danaparoid is a heparinoid factor Xa inhibitor that is no longer marketed in the United States. It had previously been approved by the FDA for prophylaxis in HIT patients undergoing hip replacement surgery. **Fondaparinux** is a synthetic pentasaccharide that will likely play a future role in the treatment of HIT.

  Warfarin should not be used to treat a patient with HIT in the acute setting given the risk of venous limb gangrene. Once the patient has been anticoagulated on one of the above agents and the platelet count has reached 100,000, warfarin can be started if long-term anticoagulation is clinically indicated.

- **Subacute HIT.** Subacute HIT refers to a state where the platelet count has returned to normal in the presence of +HIT Ab. The normalization of the platelet count is thought to reflect decreased HIT activity; however, IgG HIT Ab persists in the circulation for $\geq$100 days. Even after the platelet count recovers, patients are at risk for systemic complications as long as their HIT Ab is still positive. Therefore, it is safest to avoid heparin until the Ab is no longer detectable.

- **History of HIT where antibodies are no longer detectable.** There is no consensus regarding the treatment of patients with a history of HIT Ab without detectable Ab. There is some evidence that re-exposure to heparin has been successful in patients requiring short-term heparin while undergoing cardiopulmonary bypass. Otherwise, the use of other methods of anticoagulation would be a safer option.

Idiopathic Thrombocytopenic Purpura

Background

ITP (immune thrombocytopenic purpura) is a diagnosis of exclusion. It is often defined as an isolated thrombocytopenia where all other possible causes of thrombocytopenia have been excluded.

Epidemiology. The incidence of ITP has not been well defined but is thought to be 100 cases/1 million persons per year, of which 50% are in children. ITP occurs most commonly in the age range of 18 to 40, and women are two to three times more likely to be affected than men.

Pathophysiology

Abs to platelet surface GpIIb/IIIa, Gp-Ib/IX, Gp-Ia/IIa, and others have been identified as the likely causes of ITP. It is unclear why the immune system develops Abs to these markers, but the process appears to be related to antigen-presenting cell processing of the platelet glycoproteins and stimulation of T cells similar to foreign antigen processing. It also appears to be a polyclonal process, but the number of B cell clones may be limited. These Abs bind to intact platelet surface glycoproteins, which in turn bind to Fc-gamma receptors on macrophages, leading to clearance by the reticuloendothelial system, especially in the spleen. The body does try to compensate, and the platelets subsequently produced tend to be somewhat larger and more effective than typical platelets of the average population. The disease has been noted after viral infection, especially in children, which may initiate the malfunction in the immune system. There also appears to be a possible genetic predisposition, although more work is needed to assess the full role of genetics.

Presentation

The clinical spectrum of ITP is broad but is most often characterized by mucocutaneous bleeding. Petechiae, purpura, bruising, epistaxis, and gingival bleeding are commonly seen. These clinical signs can help the clinician distinguish from other disorders such as coagulopathies, often characterized by hemarthroses/deep hematomas, or vasculitides, evidenced by palpable purpura.

Management

Diagnosis. ITP is often diagnosed incidentally when thrombocytopenia is noted on routine lab work/CBC. After a thorough history and physical and exclusion of other causes of thrombocytopenia, a diagnosis of ITP can be made. It is important to rule out other etiologies of thrombocytopenia including TTP-HUS, DIC, hypersplenism, drugs, and infection. Falsely reported thrombocytopenia secondary to platelet clumping (induced by EDTA) should also be excluded. This occurs in 0.1% to 0.3% of the population. It is sometimes helpful to send a CBC in a citrate tube (blue top) rather than the traditional lavender-top tube containing EDTA. Bone marrow biopsy is recommended in patients >60 years old to rule out myelodysplastic syndrome. HIV/hepatitis C virus testing should be performed in at-risk populations. ITP can occur in pregnancy, but gestational thrombocytopenia and thrombocytopenia associated with pre-eclampsia and HELLP syndrome should be ruled out.

Treatment. The primary goal of treatment is to prevent bleeding complications in patients with ITP. There is no target therapeutic platelet count. The literature shows that patients with asymptomatic thrombocytopenia at platelet counts >30,000 to 50,000/μL often do fine without treatment. Major bleeding occurs when the platelet count is <10,000/μL. Therefore, treatment of ITP should be focused on the patient who is symptomatic or at risk for bleeding. The American Society of Hematology has established general guidelines.

- Patients with platelet counts >20,000/μL without bleeding should not be hospitalized.
- Patients with platelet counts >50,000/μL without bleeding do not need to be treated.

- Patients with platelet counts <50,000/μL with mucosal bleeding or counts <30,000/μL should be treated.
- Patients with platelet counts <50,000/μL and risk factors for bleeding are also appropriate to treat.

Initial Therapy. First-line therapy for management of ITP is glucocorticoids, typically prednisone at 1 mg/kg/day. Prednisone is usually given until there is a normalization of the platelet count, at which point the prednisone is tapered. Approximately 50% to 75% of patients have a response within the first 3 weeks. Once the prednisone is tapered, the majority of patients experience a relapse. Long-term use of glucocorticoids, however, is not recommended, given the risks associated with chronic use. If oral prednisone fails to boost the platelet count or decrease bleeding, other options include intravenous immune globulin (IVIG), high-dose methylprednisolone, and anti-D immune globulin (for Rh-positive patients). IVIG is given at 1 g/kg for 2 to 3 days. Anti-D is dosed at 50 to 75 μg/kg/day IV. Anti-D can only be given in Rh+ patients who have not undergone splenectomy. Both can cause a mild alloimmune hemolysis.

Second-Line Treatment. Splenectomy is the treatment of choice for those who have failed first-line therapy. It is recommended if the platelet count is <30,000/μL after 4 to 6 weeks of initial therapy. Approximately two thirds of patients who undergo surgery have a response. Two weeks prior to surgery, patients should be immunized against *Streptococcus pneumoniae, Haemophilus influenzae b,* and *Neisseria meningitidis*. If the patient's platelet count is <50,000/μL before surgery, platelet transfusion or therapy with steroids, IVIG, etc., should be given.

Chronic Refractory Idiopathic Thrombocytopenic Purpura

Approximately 30% to 40% of patients meet the criteria for chronic refractory ITP, which is defined by the following: platelet count <50,000/μL, presence of ITP for >3 months, and lack of response to splenectomy. Once a patient has chronic refractory ITP, there is no defined algorithm for treatment. Therapy should be individualized based on the patient's clinical presentation and severity of symptoms. Treatment is recommended for those with platelet counts <30,000/μL and bleeding. Often, steroids can be used in an acute setting; however, long-term steroid treatment is not recommended. Immunosuppression with azathioprine, cyclophosphamide, and rituximab has been used to treat patients with platelet counts <20,000/μL. Twenty to forty percent of patients have a response to azathioprine or cyclophosphamide. Cyclophosphamide can be given daily or monthly, and side effects include hemorrhagic cystitis and neutropenia. There are some data on rituximab, an anti-CD20 monoclonal Ab, in response to which patients have had an increase in their platelet counts to >50,000/μL. Other treatment modalities include dapsone, danazol, and vinca alkaloids; however, the efficacy of these agents is limited. There are some preliminary data on autologous stem cell transplant as a form of treatment, but more studies are needed at this time. Accessory splenectomy is another treatment consideration. Accessory spleens are suspected if Howell-Jolly bodies are not seen on peripheral smear after splenectomy and can be confirmed by radionuclide imaging.

Emergent Situations

In rare cases, ITP can lead to fatal bleeding, most commonly from intracranial hemorrhage. Patients can also have severe GI bleeding. Patients should be managed in an intensive care unit setting and supported via platelet transfusions, IVIG (1 g/kg/day for 2 to 3 days), and methylprednisolone. In catastrophic cases, one can also consider recombinant human factor VIIa and aminocaproic acid.

THROMBOCYTOSIS

A platelet count exceeding the reference range is called **thrombocytosis**. Thrombocytosis may be reactive or due to autonomous production of platelets by clonal megakaryocytes (essential thrombocythemia or other myeloproliferative disorders).

- **Essential thrombocytosis** is discussed in Chapter 9.
- **Reactive thrombocytosis** is thrombocytosis in the absence of a chronic myeloproliferative disorder. It can be seen in the setting of infection, surgery, malignancy, blood loss, and iron deficiency or postsplenectomy. The platelet count is expected to normalize when the underlying process is corrected.

KEY POINTS TO REMEMBER

- TTP-HUS is a disease that can be identified by MAHA and thrombocytopenia without other cause.
- TTP-HUS should be treated with plasma exchange.
- DIC is a condition of abnormal coagulation due to another underlying condition.
- The primary treatment for DIC is treatment of the underlying condition.
- HIT typically occurs 5 to 14 days after commencement of heparin and has only been seen prior to 5 days in cases in which heparin had been used before.
- LMWHs (e.g., enoxaparin [Lovenox]) should not be used in patients with HIT.
- Lepirudin and argatroban are effective treatment options for HIT.
- ITP is a diagnosis of exclusion.
- ITP is generally treated with steroids, and IV Ig is added in serious cases.

REFERENCES AND SUGGESTED READINGS

American Society of Hematology ITP Practice Guideline Panel. Diagnosis and treatment of idiopathic thrombocytopenic purpura: recommendations of the American Society of Hematology. *Ann Intern Med.* 1997;126:319–326.

Arepaly, GM, Ortel, TL. Clinical practice. Heparin-induced thrombocytopenia. *N Engl J Med.* 2006; 355:809.

Cines DB, Blanchette VS. Immune thrombocytopenic purpura. *N Engl J Med.* 2002;346: 995–1008.

de Jonge E, Levi M, Stoutenbeek CP, et al. Current drug treatment strategies for disseminated intravascular coagulation. *Drugs.* 1998;55:767–777.

Favaloro EJ. Laboratory assessment as a critical component of the appropriate diagnosis and sub-classification of von Willebrand's disease. *Blood Rev.* 1999;13:185–201.

George JN. How I treat patients with thrombotic thrombocytopenic purpura-hemolytic uremic syndrome. *Blood.* 2000;96:1223–1229.

George JN. Platelets. *Lancet.* 2000;355:1531–1539.

George JN, Shattil S. The clinical importance of acquired abnormalities of platelet function. *N Engl J Med.* 1991;32:27–39.

George JN, Woolf SH, Raskob GE, et al. Idiopathic thrombocytopenic purpura: a practice guideline developed by explicit methods for the American Society of Hematology. *Blood.* 1996;88:3–40.

George JN, Raskob GE, Shah SR, et al. Drug induced thrombocytopenia: a systematic review of the published case reports. *Ann Intern Med.* 1998;129:886–890.

Greinacher A, Volpel H, Janssens U, et al. Recombinant hirudin (lepirudin) provides safe and effective anticoagulation in patients with heparin-induced thrombocytopenia. *Circulation.* 1999;99:73–80.

Harrington WJ, et al. Demonstration of a thrombocytopenic factor in the blood of patients with thrombocytopenic purpura. *J Lab Clin Med.* 1951;38:1–10.

Hassell, K. The management of patients with heparin-induced thrombocytopenia who require anticoagulant therapy. *Chest.* 2005;127: 1–8.

Hatem CJ, Kettyle WM (Co-editors in Chief) with contributions by: Williams ME, Epstein PE, Kickler TS, et al. (Multiple Titles) MKSAP 12 (American College of Physicians–American Society of Internal Medicine). *Hematology.* 2001:32–82.

Lämmle B, Furlan M. New insights into the pathogenesis of thrombocytopenic purpura. *Hematology.* 1999:243–248.

Levi M, Ten Cate H. Disseminated intravascular coagulation. *N Engl J Med.* 1999;341: 586–592.

Lewis BE, Walenga JM, Wallis DE. Anticoagulation with Novastan (argatroban) in patients with heparin-induced thrombocytopenia and heparin-induced thrombocytopenia and thrombosis syndrome. *Semin Thromb Hemost.* 1997;23:197–202.

Mannucci PM. How I treat patients with von Willebrand disease. *Blood.* 2001;97: 1915–1919.

Nurden AT. Inherited abnormalities of platelets. *Thromb Haemost.* 1999;82:468–480.

Rock GA, Shumak KH, Buskard NA, et al. Comparison of plasma exchange with plasma infusion in the treatment of thrombotic thrombocytopenic purpura. *N Engl J Med.* 1991;325:393–397.

Sheridan, D, Carter, C, Leton, JG. A diagnostic test for heparin-induced thrombocytopenia. *Blood.* 1986;67:27.

Warkentin TE. Heparin-induced thrombocytopenia: a ten-year retrospective. *Annu Rev Med.* 1999;50:129–147.

Warkentin TE. New approaches to the diagnosis of heparin-induced thrombocytopenia. *Chest.* 2005;127:35–45.

Warkentin TE, Chong BH, Greinacher A. Heparin-induced thrombocytopenia: towards consensus. *Thromb Haemost.* 1998;79:1–7.

Warkentin TE, Greinacher A. Heparin-induced thrombocytopenia: recognition, treatment, and prevention: the Seventh ACCP Conference on Antithrombotic and Thrombolytic Therapy. *Chest.* 2004;126:311S.

Warkentin TE, Leton JG. A 14-year study of heparin-induced thrombocytopenia. *Am J Med.* 1996;101:502.

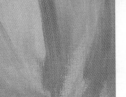

Introduction to Coagulation and Laboratory Evaluation of Coagulation

5

Anna Margrét Halldórsdóttir

INTRODUCTION

The hemostatic system is a complex, regulated, sequence of reactions involving interactions among platelets, endothelium, and coagulation factors. **Primary hemostasis**, which is comprised of platelet activation and platelet plug formation, is followed by **secondary hemostasis**, with activation of the coagulation cascade and formation of a stable fibrin complex. Fibrinolysis then limits the extent of thrombosis. Symptoms of mucosal bleeding, such as epistaxis, gum bleeding, hematochezia, melena, petechiae, and easy bruising, are often signs of defective primary hemostasis due to thrombocytopenia, platelet dysfunction, or abnormalities of von Willebrand factor (vWF). Hemarthroses, intramuscular hemorrhage, and bleeding into deeper structures are more commonly signs of secondary hemostasis disorders caused by coagulation factor deficiency or dysfunction. The laboratory evaluation of a patient with a suspected coagulation disorder is performed in a systematic fashion and begins with a complete blood count (CBC), prothrombin time (PT)/international normalized ratio (INR), and activated partial thromboplastin time (aPTT). Further workup depends on these results.

INITIAL LABORATORY TESTS IN THE WORKUP OF SUSPECTED HEMOSTASIS DISORDERS

Complete Blood Count

The CBC reveals thrombocytopenia if present and assesses whether the patient has developed clinically significant anemia. Leukocytosis or leukopenia may implicate a hematologic malignancy as the cause of a patient's coagulopathy or thrombocytopenia. Examination of the peripheral smear yields information regarding the presence of microangiopathy, platelet clumping, and white blood cell morphology.

Coagulation Tests

Prothrombin Time and International Normalized Ratio
PT is a measure of the extrinsic (tissue factor) and common pathways (Fig. 5-1). In this assay clotting is initiated by a commercial reagent called thromboplastin, which consists of tissue factor and phospholipid derived from human placenta, rabbit or oxen brain, or recombinant human tissue factor. Plasma, thromboplastin, and calcium are mixed and the clotting time is determined. The PT depends on the activities of prothrombin, factors V, X, and VII, and fibrinogen. Gamma-carboxylation of factors II, VII, and X is dependent on reduced vitamin K and therefore the PT is very sensitive to vitamin K antagonists (warfarin) or deficiencies of vitamin K (nutritional or malabsorption). As these clotting factors are synthesized in the liver, the PT is characteristically prolonged in liver disease. A prolonged PT

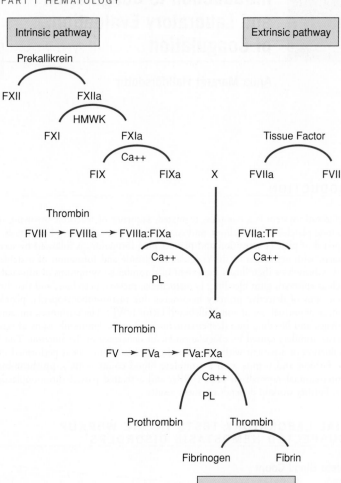

FIGURE 5-1. The normal coagulation cascade is split into the *intrinsic pathway* and the *extrinsic pathway*, either of which leads to activation of factor X to Xa. The factors after that point are referred to as the *common pathway*. Disorders of the intrinsic pathway are manifest as prolongation of the aPTT. Disorders of the extrinsic pathway are reflected by prolongation of the PT, whereas disorders of the common pathway will prolong both tests.

is rarely due to an acquired coagulation factor inhibitory autoantibody. Historically, PT values have varied from institution to institution due to differences in commercial thromboplastin sensitivities to factor deficiencies. The INR system has markedly reduced interlaboratory variability. This ratio standardizes all PT assays and is calculated as follows:

$$INR = [(PT \text{ patient})/(PT \text{ laboratory mean})]^{ISI}$$

ISI is the International Sensitivity Index for the thromboplastin reagent used.

Activated Partial Thromboplastin Time

The aPTT measures both intrinsic and common pathways. A phospholipid mixture and a surface activating agent (e.g., silica) are added to plasma. Calcium is then added and the clotting time recorded. The aPTT measures all factors except VII and XIII. Isolated factor deficiencies that prolong the aPTT and are associated with increased bleeding include factors IX, XI, and VIII. Deficiencies of factor XII, prekallikrein, and high molecular weight kininogen markedly prolong the aPTT but are not associated with increased bleeding. Deficiencies or inhibitors of common pathway factors can also prolong the aPTT. This test is also commonly used to screen for lupus anticoagulant (LA).

Thrombin Time (TT)

The TT is performed by adding purified bovine or human thrombin to plasma and monitoring the time for fibrin clot formation. This measures the final common step in the coagulation cascade. The TT may be prolonged in a variety of coagulation disorders, including hypo- and dysfibrinogenemia, high levels of fibrinogen degradation products, monoclonal gammopathies, the presence of heparin or heparinlike inhibitors, direct thrombin inhibitors such as lepirudin, argatroban, and bivalirudin, and thrombin antibodies. When the TT is prolonged, a heparin neutralizing substance is added to the patient's plasma, and the TT is repeated. If the TT corrects, then heparin or a heparin-like anticoagulant is present. If the TT does not correct, then one of the previously mentioned abnormalities may be the cause. If the plasma contains a direct thrombin inhibitor, it cannot be neutralized and a new specimen should be obtained when the patient is not receiving the drug.

GENERAL WORKUP OF ELEVATED PROTHROMBIN TIME OR ACTIVATED PARTIAL THROMBOBLASTIN TIME

Preanalytical variables that can prolong the PT and aPTT should be considered before embarking on additional testing, and if an artifact is suspected, screening tests should be repeated. Incomplete filling of blood collection tubes and heparin in intravenous lines are common causes of artificially prolonged clotting tests, but other potential confounding factors include a high hematocrit (>55%) and plasma turbidity (lipemic, hemolyzed or icteric specimens). An elevated PT or aPTT noted on lab evaluation involves first determining which pathway of the coagulation cascade is defective (or that both are). A *mixing study* is then typically performed to determine whether the abnormality is due to an inhibitor present in the patient's plasma or a factor deficiency. This will provide the differential diagnosis for further testing. Figures 5-2 through 5-4 detail the workup and differential diagnoses based on the coagulation abnormality present.

Mixing Studies

Mixing studies are performed to determine whether a prolonged PT or aPTT is more likely due to factor deficiencies or inhibitors. In this test, patient's plasma is mixed with normal plasma at a 1:1 ratio and the coagulation test in question, either the PT or the aPTT, is performed immediately and after incubation at 37°C for 1 hour. If a factor deficiency is the cause of the abnormal PT or aPTT, it should be corrected completely or within a few seconds of the upper limit of the reference range when mixed with normal plasma. If the prolonged PT or aPTT is not corrected, an inhibitor is present. Further workup is then required to determine the nature of the inhibitor (i.e., nonspecific vs. factor-specific LA). Typically, factor-specific inhibitory antibodies are time dependent, which means that the aPTT will be partially corrected immediately after mixing but prolonged again after 1 hour of incubation. LA inhibitors typically are not time dependent and will produce similar degrees of partial correction immediately and 1 hour after mixing.

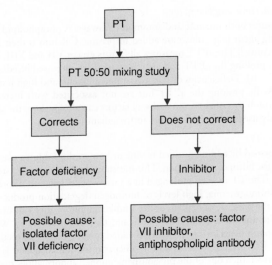

FIGURE 5-2. General workup of an elevated PT in the setting of a normal aPTT.

Lupus Anticoagulants

LAs or antiphospholipid antibodies may occur in the presence or absence of systemic lupus erythematosus or other autoimmune diseases and have been associated with various complications including recurrent fetal loss and venous or arterial thromboembolic disease. Routine aPTT and PT reagents are not sensitive enough to be used to screen for LA, so modifications have been made to develop LA-sensitive clotting tests,

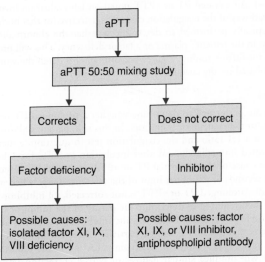

FIGURE 5-3. General workup of an elevated aPTT in the setting of a normal PT.

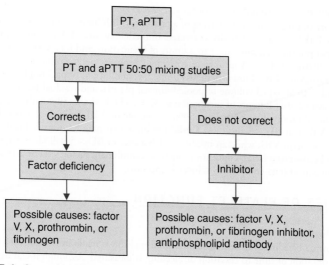

FIGURE 5-4. General workup of an elevation of both the PT and the aPTT.

and the following steps are used to demonstrate (a) a prolonged phospholipid-dependent clotting time (such as modified aPTT, PT, or common pathway clotting test), (b) persistent prolongation of the clotting time after mixing with normal pooled plasma, (c) neutralization of the inhibitor by addition of excess phospholipid, and (d) ruling-out of a specific factor inhibitor (such as anti-factor VIII autoantibody). Since no LA test will detect 100% of LAs, current guidelines require using at least two different sensitive clotting tests to screen for and confirm the presence of LA. If one or both tests are positive, testing should be repeated at least 12 weeks later to determine if the inhibitor activity was temporary (and not clinically significant) or persistent and associated with an increased risk of future thrombotic complications. Please see Chapter 6 for further details on LAs.

Coagulation Factor Assays

These are clot-based assays to determine the functional levels of the factors in the coagulation cascade. They are appropriate when there is a prolongation of the appropriate screening test (PT or aPTT) that is corrected, or nearly corrected, with a 1:1 mix of the patient's sample with normal pooled plasma.

Factor VIII Assay

The determination of factor VIII is necessary for diagnosing hemophilia A and von Willebrand disease (vWD) and for monitoring response to therapy in hemophilia. The ability of dilutions of the patient's plasma to correct the prolonged aPTT of factor VIII-deficient plasma is compared to that of similar dilutions of normal pooled plasma in factor VIII-deficient plasma. The same procedure is used to determine the activity of other intrinsic pathway coagulation factors, using the corresponding deficient plasma for dilutions. The extrinsic and common pathway factor activities are determined by comparing PT results for patient and normal pooled plasma diluted in plasma depleted of factor VII, X, or V or prothrombin.

Factor VIII Inhibitor Quantitation (Bethesda Units)

Laboratory findings seen in the setting of a factor VIII inhibitor are (a) a normal PT, (b) a prolonged aPTT that is partially corrected immediately after 1:1 mixing with normal plasma but prolonged again after 1 to 2 hours of incubation, and (c) a very low factor VIII activity (usually <1%). Appropriate treatment requires determining the titer of the inhibitor (measured as arbitrary Bethesda units). Serial dilutions of patient plasma in saline are mixed with an equal volume of pooled normal plasma, and residual factor VIII activity is measured after 2 hours of incubation at 37°C. The Bethesda titer is the reciprocal of the plasma dilution that neutralizes 50% of the factor VIII activity of normal pooled plasma. A titer of BU <5 indicates a mild inhibitor that may be overwhelmed by larger infusions of factor VIII, while an inhibitor with a titer of BU >5 will likely require infusion of a bypass coagulation concentrate such as recombinant factor VIIa or activated prothrombin concentrate complex to achieve hemostasis.

STUDIES OF PLATELET FUNCTION

Bleeding Time

To perform a bleeding time test, a standardized incision is made in the patient's forearm, and the duration of time to cessation of bleeding is measured. Although it can be a useful test for identifying problems with primary hemostasis, many variables may artificially prolong the bleeding time, such as medications that interfere with platelet function, differences in operator procedure and interpretation, and subcutaneous edema or thinning of the skin. The bleeding time is of some utility for detecting primary hemostasis defects (vWD and qualitative platelet disorders) in patients with histories of recurrent mucosal bleeding. On the other hand, it is not an accurate predictor of surgical bleeding risk in asymptomatic subjects, and its use is declining.

Platelet Function Analyzer-100

The PFA-100 (Dade-Behring, Deerfield, IL) is an in vitro screening test of primary hemostasis. The test principle is as follows: citrated whole blood is aspirated through a microscopic hole in a piece of nitrocellulose paper coated with collagen and epinephrine (COL/EPI) or collagen and ADP (COL/ADP). The flow conditions mimic the shear stress in a capillary bed. vWF adheres to the collagen, and platelets adhere to the vWF, followed by agonist-mediated activation, aggregation, and eventual closure of the hole. The time to occlusion is reported as the **closure time**. The COL/EPI cartridge is sensitive to qualitative platelet disorders, especially aspirin effect, and vWD. The COL/ADP cartridge is less sensitive to aspirin but remains sensitive to vWD. Neither cartridge is sensitive to ADP receptor inhibitors such as clopidogrel (Plavix). Normal PFA-100 closure times do not rule out mild qualitative platelet disorders, and if clinical suspicion is high, platelet aggregation studies should be performed. Like the bleeding time, the PFA-100 has not been validated for preoperative assessment of bleeding risk in asymptomatic patients. A hematocrit of <30% or a platelet count of <100,000/μL can produce false-positive results.

Platelet Aggregation Studies

This battery of tests is indicated when an inherited qualitative defect in platelet function is suggested by the clinical and/or family history. The principle is that, when an aggregating agent is added to the initially turbid platelet-rich plasma specimen, the platelets clump, permitting more light to pass through the plasma. Aggregation agents usually include arachidonic acid, collagen, ADP, epinephrine, and ristocetin. The results with each agent are displayed graphically and interpreted as normal or abnormal. This qualitative test is very labor intensive and should only be performed in selected cases. As many prescription or over-the-counter medications can affect in vitro measurements of platelet function, almost all inpatients should be excluded. Outpatients must discontinue aspirin-containing medications and clopidogrel (Plavix) for at least 7 days and NSAIDs for at least 72 hours prior to testing to avoid false-positive results.

LABORATORY EVALUATION OF SUSPECTED VON WILLEBRAND DISEASE

In addition to a CBC, PT, and aPTT (the aPTT may be mildly prolonged as a result of decreased factor VIII activity), patients suspected of a primary hemostasis disorder such as vWD should have the following testing: (1) vWF antigen (vWF:Ag), (2) factor VIII activity, and (3) ristocetin cofactor activity or collagen binding assay (Table 5-1). No single test is adequate to diagnose vWD. When abnormal tests are found suggesting vWD, these tests should be repeated to confirm the diagnosis. If two sets of tests do not agree, testing symptomatic first-degree relatives for vWD may be appropriate.

von Willebrand Factor Antigen Concentration

Several immunoassay methods are available to measure the concentration of vWF in the patient's plasma, but they will not measure the function of vWF and therefore will not detect qualitative defects. vWF:Ag levels are measured against a normal reference sample and typically levels >50% of reference are considered normal. However, vWF:Ag reference intervals are blood type dependent. Healthy type O subjects may have vWF concentrations as low as 40% compared to pooled normal plasma, while the lower limit of the reference range for non-O controls will be ≥50%. Most laboratories do not provide blood type-specific reference intervals and are likely to have a lower limit ~50%. As a result, some healthy individuals with blood type O and unimpressive personal and family histories of abnormal bleeding may have vWF:Ag, vWF activity, or factor VIII activity <50% due to their blood type but are incorrectly diagnosed with type 1 vWD. The vWF:Ag concentration will be abnormally low in all type 3, most type 1, and some type 2 vWD.

Ristocetin Cofactor Assay

The ability of the patient's plasma specimen to aggregate normal platelets in the presence of ristocetin (an antibiotic that causes severe thrombocytopenia due to in vivo agglutination of platelets to vWF) is compared with that of a normal pooled plasma specimen (>50% is considered normal but healthy blood type O patients may have lower activity; see discussion above). Patients with type 2A, 2B, 2M, and 3 vWD will usually have abnormal values. Type 1 may also be abnormal. This test is useful when used with the vWF:Ag test in the vWF ristocetin cofactor/vWF:Ag ratio. A ratio ≤0.7 suggests a diagnosis of vWD type 2A, 2B, or 2M and requires further specialized testing for discrimination.

Collagen Binding Assay

This ELISA is especially useful for identifying the presence of high molecular weight forms of vWF. Collagen is immobilized in the test well, and following incubation with plasma and washing, bound vWF is measured. Because patients with types 2A and 2B vWD are deficient in high molecular weight vWF, this test is useful in their diagnosis. As described earlier, reference comparison with >50% levels are considered normal. This test is used in comparison with the vWF:Ag test in the vWF collagen binding/vWF:Ag ratio (normal, >0.7).

von Willebrand Factor Multimer Assay

The multimer assay involves labor-intensive gel electrophoresis techniques to separate vWF into bands that normally range in size from 0.5 million to 20 million daltons. Multimer patterns provide qualitative information and are primarily used to confirm the loss of large and intermediate multimers in types 2A and 2B vWD. This test is not routinely performed at most institutions.

TABLE 5-1	LABORATORY EVALUATION OF VON WILLEBRAND DISEASE

	Factor VIII Activity	vWF Antigen	Ristocetin Cofactor Assay	RIPA	Multimer Pattern
Type 1: decrease in antigen and activity	Decreased /normal	Decreased	Decreased	Decreased or normal response	Normal
Type 3: absence of vWF	Markedly decreased	Very low or absent	Very low or absent	Absent	Absent
Type 2A: failure to make full length or increased cleavage	Decreased or normal	Usually low	Decreased	Decreased	Absent large + intermediate multimers
Type 2B: increased binding to platelets, enhanced clearance	Decreased or normal	Usually low	Decreased	Increased response	Absent large multimers
Type 2M: mutant vWF fails to bind platelets in the presence of shear stress or ristocetin	Decreased or normal	Usually low	Decreased	Decreased	Normal
Type 2N: mutant vWF fails to bind factor VIII	Decreased	Normal	Normal	Normal	Normal
Platelet type: GP1b defect on platelets, spontaneous vWF binding	Decreased or normal	Decreased or normal	Decreased	Increased response	Absent large multimers

vWF, von Willebrand factor; RIPA, ristocetin-induced platelet aggregation.

Ristocetin-Induced Platelet Aggregation (RIPA) Analysis

This is really one component of the more comprehensive platelet aggregation study panel. It tests the aggregation of the patient's platelets in the presence of different concentrations of ristocetin. It is used to assist in the diagnosis of types 2B (increased sensitivity to ristocetin) and 2A or 2M (decreased ristocetin sensitivity) vWD. RIPA is used only after the diagnosis of vWD is made and further clarification of subtype is necessary.

Other Tests

- The factor VIII binding ELISA is used to help diagnose type 2N vWD, which is characterized by impaired binding of vWF to factor VIII.
- PFA-100 closure time can be used to screen for vWD in patients with an appropriate bleeding history, and to monitor response to 1-desamino-8-D-arginine vasopressin (DDAVP; which stimulates release of vWF stored in endothelial cells) or infusion of vWF concentrate (Humate-P), since other vWF tests may not be available on a STAT basis.

KEY POINTS TO REMEMBER

- The initial step in evaluation of asymptomatic laboratory abnormalities in coagulation is to repeat the abnormal tests and evaluate for causes of falsely abnormal results (e.g., heparin in IV lines or incomplete filling of collection tubes).
- Evaluation of the PT, aPTT, and CBC is the first step in the determination of the abnormality in the hemostatic process.
- Mixing studies help distinguish between acquired factor inhibitor states and factor deficiencies when evaluating an elevated PT or aPTT.
- At least two different tests should be used to screen for and confirm the presence of LA. If one or both tests are positive, testing should be repeated at least 12 weeks later to determine whether the inhibitor activity was temporary or persistent.
- PFA-100 is replacing bleeding time as the primary screening test for platelet function. Like the bleeding time, the PFA-100 has not been validated for preoperative assessment of bleeding risk in asymptomatic patients.
- No single test is adequate to diagnose vWD. Patients suspected of vWD should have the following testing: (a) vWF:Ag, (b) factor VIII Activity, and (c) ristocetin cofactor activity or collagen binding assay.

REFERENCES AND SUGGESTED READINGS

Hayward CP, Harrison P, Cattaneo M, et al. Platelet function analyzer (PFA)-100 closure time in the evaluation of platelet disorders and platelet function. *J Thromb Haemost.* 2006;4(2):312–319.

Hoffman R, Benz EJ, Shattil SJ, et al. *Hematology. Basic Principles and Practice.* 4th ed. Philadelphia, PA: Elsevier; 2005.

Kamal AH, Tefferi A, Pruthi RK. How to interpret and pursue an abnormal prothrombin time, activated partial thromboplastin time, and bleeding time in adults. *Mayo Clin Proc.* 2007;82(7):864–873.

Kjeldsberg CR. *Practical Diagnosis of Hematologic Disorders.* 4th ed. Chicago, IL: ASCP Press; 2006.

Miyakis S, Lockshin MD, Atsumi T, et al. International consensus statement on an update of the classification criteria for definite antiphospholipid syndrome (APS). *J Thromb Haemost.* 2006;4(2):295–306.

Sadler JE, Budde U, Eikenboom JC, et al. Update on the pathophysiology and classification of von Willebrand disease: a report of the Subcommittee on von Willebrand Factor. *J Thromb Haemost.* 2006;4(10):2103–2114.

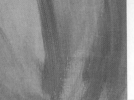

Thrombotic Disease

6

Meagan A. Jacoby and Nathan Martin

INTRODUCTION

Thrombotic disease involves the inappropriate formation of a clot in the venous or arterial circulation. Arterial and venous thrombi form in the presence of Virchow triad: hypercoagulability, stasis, and endothelial damage. Embolism of these clots can occur, causing a pulmonary embolus (PE) when arising from the venous circulation or a systemic embolus when arising in the arterial circulation. Risk factors for venous thrombosis include immobility, surgery, increasing age, obesity, pregnancy, and an inherited or acquired hypercoagulable state (Table 6-1).

Often thrombotic disease results from an interaction of genetic predisposition and environmental factors. Hypercoagulable states can predispose a patient to primarily venous thrombosis or both venous and arterial thrombosis. Evaluation of patients presenting with thrombosis may include workup for a thrombophilia or hypercoagulable state, as well as recommendations on appropriate anticoagulant management and duration of therapy.

DEEP VENOUS THROMBOSIS AND PULMONARY EMBOLUS

Definition
The term venous thromboembolic (VTE) disease encompasses both deep venous thrombosis (DVT) and PE.

Epidemiology
The annual incidence of DVT is approximately 100 per 100,000 persons per year. The most feared complication of DVT is PE. About 40% to 50% of people with a symptomatic DVT will have a silent PE, and 1% to 8% of persons with a PE will die of its complications. The major morbidity associated with DVT other than PE is the postthrombotic syndrome. Treatment of DVT is largely aimed at preventing fatal PE and the postthrombotic syndrome.

Clinical Presentation
Clinical diagnosis of both DVT and PE is highly unreliable and inaccurate, and therefore, objective tests should guide the diagnosis. Clinical findings suggestive of DVT include unilateral calf tenderness and swelling. Symptoms of acute PE include dyspnea, pleuritic chest pain, cough, anxiety, and hemoptysis. Physical exam may reveal tachypnea, tachycardia, and inspiratory crackles, but these findings are nonspecific.

Management
Diagnosis of DVT
Doppler ultrasonography is the test of choice for diagnosing DVT. In most studies, the sensitivity and specificity for DVT are >97%, with venography considered the gold

TABLE 6-1	CAUSES OF HYPERCOAGULABILITY LEADING TO VENOUS THROMBOEMBOLISM

Acquired Cause	Inherited Cause
Surgery/trauma	Factor V Leiden mutation
Malignancy	Prothrombin G20210A mutation
Myeloproliferative disorders	Hyperhomocysteinemi[a]
Pregnancy	Protein C deficiency
Oral contraceptives	Protein S deficiency
Immobilization	Antithrombin deficiency
Congestive heart failure	Increased factor VIII activity
Nephrotic syndrome	
Obesity	
Antiphospholipid antibodies[a]	
Lupus anticoagulant	
Anticardiolipin antibodies	

[a]Hyperhomocysteinemia and antiphospholipid antibodies are considered risk factors for both venous and arterial thrombosis.

standard. A positive Doppler study should lead one to treat the patient. A negative study largely rules out the diagnosis, and alternative diagnoses should be considered. In cases of very high suspicion and negative Doppler study, venography, or CT (or MR) venogram can be considered.

The D-dimer test can be used to aid in the diagnosis of VTE. The sensitivity of the D-dimer test in clinical trials ranges from 93% to 100%; however, the specificity ranges from 35% to 75%. The D-dimer is the result of fibrin breakdown and is generated in many other circumstances including infections, tumors, surgery, trauma, extensive burning, bruises, ischemic heart disease, stroke, peripheral artery disease, aneurysms, inflammatory disease, and pregnancy. Therefore, the D-dimer test can be effective for ruling out the diagnosis if negative, but a positive D-dimer assay requires additional workup. In cases of very high clinical suspicion, however, testing should be pursued despite a negative D-dimer.

Diagnosis of PE
The most useful algorithms and radiographic tests used to diagnose acute PE are still debatable and the subject of ongoing trials. Determining a clinical pretest probability of PE is necessary before performing any diagnostic tests. Objective criteria such as the Wells Criteria can be used to determine a pretest probability, but experienced clinicians can place patients into low, intermediate, or high pretest probabilities just as accurately.

The initial PIOPED trial in 1990 utilized **ventilation/perfusion scans** (V/Q scans) in the diagnosis of acute PE. In that trial, a high probability scan in a patient with a high clinical pretest probability was diagnostic in 96% of cases, and a low probability scan in a patient with a low pretest probability showed PE in only 4% of cases. However, all the other combinations were less diagnostic and required further testing. In addition, in the setting of an abnormal chest x-ray, V/Q scanning is diagnostic in only about 50% of patients.

More recently, the PIOPED II trial has led to recommendations regarding diagnostic algorithms. This trial focused on the use of **CT angiography (CTA) of the lungs** and **CT venography of the lower extremities** to diagnose PE. The gold standard for PE in this trial was either a positive V/Q scan, a positive angiogram (not performed in every patient due to risks), or a positive finding on venous ultrasound of lower extremity in the setting of a nondiagnostic V/Q. The authors suggest that for patients with low and moderate pretest probability, a D-dimer assay should be performed. A negative value gives a posttest probability for PE of <2%. For the majority of patients with positive D-dimers, CTA with protocols searching for PE with or without CT venography of lower extremities should be performed. For patients with a low pretest probability and negative CTA, PE was present only 4% of the time. On the other hand, for patients with a low pretest probability and a positive CTA, PE was determined to be present in only 58% of patients. The reason for the low positive predictive value in these patients was questionable diagnoses of segmental and subsegmental PE. The algorithm for patients with a moderate pretest probability is similar. In these patients, a positive CTA was diagnostic of a PE in 92% of cases.

Patients with a high pretest probability who undergo CTA with negative results should then undergo venous compression ultrasonography of the lower extremities or CT venogram of lower extremities. In patients with a negative CTA and a high pretest probability, PE was actually present in 40% of patients.

In special cases such as patients in renal failure, patients with allergy to contrast dye, women of childbearing age, and pregnant women, the recommendations are guided by expert opinion. In these patients, the algorithm should begin with D-dimer testing followed by venous ultrasonography in the majority of cases. Patients with a positive D-dimer and a negative ultrasound will then need additional testing. Ventilation/perfusion scanning can then be used, with the realization that the testing may be largely nondiagnostic.

While PIOPED and PIOPED II have given clinicians data to rely on when attempting to diagnose acute PE, there are still unanswered questions and limitations to these trials. For example, the majority of the CT scanners used in PIOPED II were only four-slice multidetector CT scanners. At many centers now, 16-slice, 64-slice, and higher scanners are now used to diagnose PE, with precise sensitivities and specificities still undetermined. While pulmonary angiography is still considered the gold standard for diagnosing PE, some radiologists claim that the newest CT scanners are more accurate. Further trials should help clarify these and other issues. Other important considerations include the relative amounts of radiation from each of the various diagnostic modalities and the cost of the different tests. The reader is referred to the recent review by Stein et al. for further details.

DVT Prophylaxis

Primary prevention of VTE in the hospitalized patient with risk factors is essential. These risk factors include an acute infectious disease, congestive heart failure, malignancy, stroke, acute pulmonary disease, acute rheumatic disease, inflammatory bowel disease, and critical illness. Expert opinion suggests that all medical patients older than 40, who are expected to have at least 3 days of inpatient stay and have one risk factor, should be provided with DVT prophylaxis. In addition, patients older than 75, with increased immobility, obesity, and a history of VTE or a thrombophilia, should also receive prophylaxis. Prophylaxis can be nonpharmacologic, with compression stockings or pneumatic compression devices. However, there are no large, blinded trials proving that these interventions prevent VTE in medical patients. Therefore, in patients without a contraindication to low-dose anticoagulation who need prophylaxis, pharmacologic agents are recommended. Subcutaneous heparin three times a day, low molecular weight heparin (LMWH) daily, and fondaparinux daily have been shown to have equal efficacy in preventing VTE with minimal increased bleeding risk.

Complications

In addition to mortality from acute PE, significant morbidity can result from chronic PE. Chronic PEs can result in pulmonary hypertension leading to right-sided heart failure.

Postthrombotic syndrome occurs in at least one third of patients with previous DVT. The symptoms vary from venous stasis pigment changes and/or slight pain and swelling to more severe manifestations such as chronic pain, intractable edema, and leg ulcers. Treatment of the syndrome is largely supportive and often inadequate. Therefore prevention by appropriately treating initial DVT is important.

Treatment

Initial Therapy. Treatment of VTE with unfractionated heparin or LMWH should begin promptly after the diagnosis is established or, in situations of high clinical suspicion, while awaiting confirmatory studies. Thrombolytics may be considered in selected patients with hemodynamically significant PE as mentioned below. Individuals who are actively bleeding or at high risk for bleeding should be considered for inferior vena cava (IVC) filter placement.

- **Unfractionated heparin** involves an initial bolus followed by a continuous intravenous infusion. The dose is usually adjusted according to the aPTT, as heparin has a narrow therapeutic range and a large variability in patient response. The target aPTT should be 1.5 to 2.5 times the control value. Achieving therapeutic aPTT levels quickly is desirable, as persistently subtherapeutic levels increase the risk of recurrence and propagation. Heparin nomograms assist in more rapid attainment and maintenance of therapeutic heparin levels.

- **LMWHs** have longer half-lives and a more predictable dose response than standard unfractionated heparin. Routine lab monitoring in patients with adequate renal function is not necessary. A recent meta-analysis concluded that LMWH is superior to unfractionated heparin for the treatment of DVT, with a lower overall mortality over the first 3 to 6 months and a reduced incidence of major bleeding during initial therapy. In addition, LMWHs are generally more cost-effective than unfractionated heparin whether used in the outpatient or inpatient setting. As LMWHs are partially renally excreted, patients with severe renal failure (estimated GFR <30 mL/h) should receive unfractioned heparin. Anti-factor Xa levels can be followed in patients with minor renal impairment and in patients with extremes in weight (either morbidly obese or very thin) to assist with proper dosing.

Long-Term Treatment

- Long-term anticoagulation is achieved with oral vitamin K antagonists. **Warfarin** is the most widely used of the oral coumarins. The INR, an adjustment of the PT to control for variations in testing reagents, is monitored and the warfarin dose adjusted accordingly. Treatment should be started within 24 hours of the initiation of heparin, with a goal INR of 2 to 3. In rare cases of treatment failure, a higher target INR may be used.

- In patients with cancer, LMWH for the duration of therapy is superior to oral coumarins in reducing the risk of recurrent thromboembolism without increasing the bleeding risk.

- The duration of warfarin therapy is variable and depends on a number of factors including underlying thrombotic risk and risk of bleeding. Current recommendations suggest that 3 months of treatment is adequate for provoked venous thromboembolism (i.e., an identifiable and reversible risk factor, such as trauma). On the other hand, unprovoked VTE or a recurrent episode should be treated for an extended duration. The precise length of treatment is still debatable. Many trials have treated patients for 3 months to 1 year after an initial unprovoked VTE. However, recurrent events occurred in similar numbers after treatment was stopped, regardless of the initial length of treatment. Therefore, most experts recommend treatment for 3 to 6 months for unprovoked VTE, with the realization that after completion of therapy

there may be a recurrence. For patients with recurrent VTE, the recommendation is lifelong anticoagulation.
- The incidence of postthrombotic syndrome can be reduced with prompt anticoagulation and the use of compression stockings. Two trials have suggested that the use of compression stockings for 2 years after the diagnosis of DVT can cut the incidence of postthrombotic syndrome in half.

Inferior Vena Caval Filters. The use of IVC filters has increased significantly in the past 10 to 20 years even as evidence supporting their use remains largely insufficient. Only one randomized controlled trial has compared the use of IVC filters with anticoagulation to the use of anticoagulation alone. At 2 years of follow-up, there was a mild increase in PEs (largely asymptomatic) in those without the filters and an increase in DVT and postthrombotic syndrome in those with the filters. There was no difference in mortality. Unfortunately, neither this study nor any other study has addressed the usual indication for filter placement: patients with a contraindication to anticoagulation. An observational study actually showed that patients receiving IVC filters had a higher mortality rate than those not receiving filters and, in fact, had similar numbers of recurrent PEs. There were likely unidentified comorbid factors contributing to the increase in mortality, but any physician contemplating the use of IVC filters needs to be aware of this data.

Retrievable IVC filters have recently been studied with some encouraging results for patients with temporary contraindications to anticoagulation. These filters can be retrieved up to 2 months after initial placement with minimal adverse effects. The ability to remove the filters would be expected to decrease the incidence of recurrent DVT. However, larger studies are needed before retrievable filters can be recommended on a large scale.

The only currently recommended indication for IVC filter placement is in patients with an absolute contraindication to anticoagulation. Potential indications that require additional study include the following: patients who have failed adequate anticoagulation (for example, patients who have a PE while on therapeutic warfarin), patients undergoing pulmonary thromboembolectomy, prophylaxis in high-risk trauma patients, patients with extensive free-floating iliofemoral thrombus, and patients undergoing thrombolysis of an iliocaval thrombus.

Thrombolytics. The role of thrombolytics in the management of VTE disease has not been fully elucidated. Thrombolytics dissolve clot faster than conventional anticoagulation does; however, the risk of bleeding is significantly increased. A recent meta-analysis suggested that thrombolytics should be reserved for patients with PE and circulatory shock, as there is data demonstrating a survival advantage in these patients. At this point, no studies have shown a survival benefit of using thrombolytics in hemodynamically stable patients, regardless of the extent of PE or findings of right ventricular dysfunction on echocardiogram. Some experts also recommend thrombolytics for patients with refractory hypoxemia secondary to a large PE, though this has never been formally investigated. Prior to use, the clinician must evaluate the patient for any relative contraindication to thrombolytic therapy including recent surgery, bleeding diathesis, recent stroke, active intracranial disease (including neoplasm, aneurysm), pregnancy, uncontrolled hypertension, etc. A careful risk/benefit analysis is warranted in every patient.

Special Cases
Acute Recurrent Thrombosis. The diagnosis of recurrent venous thrombosis in the same vein can be difficult to make. Diagnostic tests currently available have difficulty differentiating between a venous occlusion caused by the initial venous thrombosis and a recurrence. The risk of new thrombosis in adequately anticoagulated patients is very low. However, recurrence can occur, particularly in patients with cancer, heparin-induced thrombocytopenia, and the antiphospholid antibody syndrome. The diagnosis of recurrent

DVT can be made with certainty only if there is a lack of compressibility on ultrasound or a filling defect on venography in an area that was documented to be free of thrombus on prior studies. D-dimer testing may be beneficial; however, this test has not been validated in diagnosing DVT recurrence.

Calf Vein Thrombosis. The treatment of isolated calf vein thrombosis remains controversial due to the fact that these thromboses rarely cause significant PE or postthrombotic complications. However, the risk of clot propagation into proximal veins is ~20%. Current recommendations for patients with calf vein thrombosis and transient risk factors suggest anticoagulation for 6 to 12 weeks. An alternative approach is to repeat the ultrasound in 3 to 7 days and anticoagulate only if the thrombosis has propagated into a proximal deep vein.

Venous Thrombosis during Pregnancy. The risk of VTE is five times higher in pregnant women than nonpregnant women. However, there are few published data to support the choice of anticoagulant or role of IVC filters. As warfarin is teratogenic and can cause fetal hemorrhage, heparins have been the mainstay of therapy. According to a recent review, only ~200 pregnant women have been followed in observational studies using LMWH as treatment. Even fewer women have been studied using either intravenous or subcutaneous heparin. Currently, the general recommendation is to use LMWH for the duration of pregnancy and then continue therapy with warfarin after delivery.

Thrombosis of Cerebral Veins and Sinuses. Although rare, thrombosis of cerebral veins and sinuses is important to identify because, with appropriate treatment, patients often have a good neurological outcome. Occlusion of cerebral veins leads to localized brain edema and venous infarction, whereas occlusion of the venous sinuses leads to intracranial hypertension. About 85% of patients have an identifiable risk factor including a thrombophilia, oral contraceptive use, recent trauma (including lumbar puncture), and infection. The most common presenting symptom is unrelenting headache. The diagnosis can be difficult to make, with an average delay of 7 days from initial presentation to diagnosis. Venography is the current recommended diagnostic modality. Even with the theoretical risk of causing cerebral hemorrhage, the limited evidence suggests a benefit of rapid initiation of anticoagulation, with therapy continuing for at least 6 months. Endovascular thrombolysis has been attempted in some patients. In patients who develop intracranial hypertension, therapy including repeated lumbar punctures, acetazolamide, and possibly surgical creation of a lumboperitoneal shunt may be warranted. More than 80% of patients have a good neurologic outcome if appropriately treated. A search for a thrombophilia should be pursued in these patients.

Budd-Chiari Syndrome. Budd-Chiari syndrome encompasses a variety of disease states that result in hepatic vein occlusion. Typically, thrombosis of the hepatic veins leads to hepatomegaly, right-upper quadrant pain, and other sequelae of acute or chronic liver disease. The most common causes of Budd-Chiari syndrome in the Western world are the myeloproliferative disorders. All patients should undergo screening for thrombophilia and age-appropriate malignancy including myeloproliferative disorders. The decision to use anticoagulation should be based on the extent of liver disease and subsequent risk of bleeding. In certain cases, liver transplantation is the treatment of choice.

Mesenteric and Portal Venous Thrombosis. Portal vein thrombosis often presents after the disease has caused splenomegaly and both esophageal and gastric varices. The main risk factors include local causes (pancreatitis, tumor, infection) as well as thrombophilic states such as myeloproliferative disorders. Treatment involves anticoagulation, assuming that the degree of thrombocytopenia related to splenomegaly and the extent of varices is minimal.

Mesenteric venous thrombosis presents acutely, with a mortality rate ranging from 20% to 50%. The usual presentation is severe abdominal pain and bloody diarrhea. Risk factors include intra-abdominal inflammation and thrombophilias. It is interesting, however, that myeloproliferative disorders are rarely associated with thrombosis of the mesenteric veins. Treatment involves anticoagulation and surgery if the bowel becomes necrotic.

Renal Vein Thrombosis. While frequently asymptomatic and incidentally discovered, patients diagnosed with renal vein thrombosis should be evaluated for nephrotic syndrome as well as the other more common thrombophilias. Treatment involves anticoagulation, with thrombolysis reserved for patients with acute and marked deterioration in renal function due to the thrombosis.

Upper Extremity Deep Venous Thrombosis. DVT of upper extremity veins accounts for 10% of all DVTs. Risk factors specific to upper extremity DVT include indwelling central venous catheters and local trauma. Patients typically present with unilateral upper extremity edema, and diagnosis can be made with Doppler ultrasonography or venography. Approximately one third of upper extremity DVTs will cause PE, so treatment is essential. While there are limited studies guiding treatment, it is generally recommended to fully anticoagulate patients for at least 3 months. The use of thrombolytics is controversial.

Anticoagulation in Patients with Brain Metastases or Primary Brain Tumors. The use of anticoagulation for patients with either primary brain malignancies or metastases to the brain has been controversial. In the past, it was thought that due to the risk of hemorrhage, anticoagulation should be absolutely contraindicated in these patients. However, the limited evidence currently available suggests that anticoagulation is preferable to IVC filters in the majority of cases. Highly vascular tumors such as melanoma, thyroid, and renal cell metastases are still felt to be contraindications to anticoagulation. Further study would be of benefit in strengthening recommendations.

Cancer. Patients with cancer have an increased risk of thrombotic events. In a recent cohort study, the incidence of VTE within the first 6 months of diagnosis was ~12%; the risk increased with chemotherapy and metastatic disease. Cancer of the ovary, pancreas, lung, and hematological cancers are associated with a high rate of VTE in the year prior to diagnosis. Thus, occult malignancy as a cause of VTE should always be a consideration in the appropriate clinical scenario. Trousseau syndrome is a hypercoagulable state associated with malignancy and is characterized by DIC and recurrent arterial or venous thrombotic events. As discussed above, LMWH may be superior to oral coumarins in the treatment of VTE in patients with cancer.

THROMBOPHILIA

Introduction

The presence of inherited thrombotic disorders (thrombophilia) has been appreciated for only a few decades. Inherited causes of thrombophilia can be either gain of function disorders, in which mutations lead to prothrombotic activity (activated protein C resistance/factor V Leiden, prothrombin G20210A), or loss of function disorders, which result in deficiencies of endogenous anticoagulants (antithrombin, protein C, and protein S). Factor V Leiden and prothrombin G20210A mutations are common, while antithrombin, protein C, and protein S deficiencies are rare. Thrombophilias predispose patients to primarily venous thrombosis and likely interact with environmental factors to cause VTE.

Causes

Activated Protein C Resistance/Factor V Leiden

Activated protein C resistance/factor V Leiden is the most common hereditary thrombophilia. The allele frequency among persons of European heritage is 4%, but it is much less common in other populations. More than 90% of patients with activated protein C resistance have the G1691A mutation in the factor V gene (factor V Leiden), which decreases its rate of proteolytic cleavage by activated protein C. Screening is performed by a clotting assay in which patient plasma diluted in factor V-deficient plasma results in the failure of activated protein C to prolong the PTT in vitro. Diagnosis is often confirmed by detection of the factor V Leiden mutation by a DNA-based assay. The relative risk of thrombosis for carriers of the factor V Leiden mutation is thought to be four- to fivefold for heterozygotes and is between 24- and 80-fold for homozygotes. Factor V Leiden is detected in 20% of consecutive, unselected patients with a venous thrombosis, and 40% of patients selected to be at high risk for hereditary thrombophilia. The risk for VTE in heterozygous patients who use oral contraceptives is increased 35-fold.

Prothrombin G20210A

The prothrombin G20210A mutation is a substitution mutation that results in increased levels of plasma prothrombin, leading to increased generation of thrombin. However, assays of prothrombin time or prothrombin antigen are neither specific nor sensitive enough for diagnosis, which is made by DNA analysis. The relative risk of thrombosis in heterozygotes is 2.8. Patients who are homozygous may be at increased risk. The allele frequency among persons of European heritage is 2%, and like factor V Leiden, it is extremely uncommon among the nonwhite population. It is detected in 7% of unselected and 16% of selected patients with venous thrombosis. Since neither the prothrombin G20210A nor the factor V Leiden mutation is uncommon, patients may co-inherit these genes with other thrombophilic genes, with resultant increased risk of thrombosis.

Antithrombin Deficiency

Antithrombin is a plasma protease inhibitor that irreversibly binds and neutralizes thrombin and factors Xa, IXa, and XIa. This reaction is accelerated by heparin. Type I antithrombin deficiency is characterized by both decreased levels and decreased activity, while type II is characterized by decreased protease activity, with defects in either the active center or the heparin binding site. Thus, resistance to the anticoagulant effects of heparin is seen in some patients. There is no difference in clinical severity between type I and type II. Antithrombin activity assays and antigen levels are used to make the diagnosis. Of note, acute thrombosis, heparin, liver disease, DIC, nephrotic syndrome, and pre-eclampsia can all decrease antithrombin levels. Overall, antithrombin deficiency is relatively rare but is considered one of the more severe thrombophilias. Deficiencies in antithrombin (type I) have been identified in 0.02% of healthy subjects and in ~2% of unselected patients with venous thrombosis. The relative risk of thrombosis in these patients is 5.0. Prospective studies indicate that the incidence of VTE in these patients is 4% per year. Nearly 70% of patients present with the first thrombotic event before age 35.

Protein C and S Deficiency

Proteins C and S are vitamin K-dependent endogenous anticoagulants. Protein C deficiency is found in 0.2% to 0.4% of healthy subjects and 3.7% of unselected patients with VTE, and the relative risk of thrombosis in protein C deficiency is 3.1. Protein S deficiency is found in 0.16% to 0.21% of healthy subjects and in 2.3% of unselected patients with VTE. Homozygous protein C deficiency can cause neonatal purpura fulminans. Patients with heterozygous protein C deficiency can present with warfarin skin necrosis at the initiation of anticoagulation due to a transient hypercoagulable state. Warfarin skin necrosis has also been reported in protein S deficiency. Protein C deficiency is diagnosed by an assay to detect activity followed by immunoassays to differentiate type I (reduced antigen and activity) and type II (reduced activity) defects. DNA-based assays are not practical given that more than 150 mutations in the protein C gene have been described. Protein S binds to a plasma protein so that free protein S antigen and activity are used to screen for protein S deficiency and differentiate among type I (decreased antigen and activity), type II (decreased activity), and type III (low free protein S). Similarly to protein C, DNA-based assays are not practical given the number of mutations that have been described in the protein S gene. Protein S levels are affected by oral contraceptives, pregnancy, and hormone replacement therapy. Protein C and S levels are affected by liver disease, anticoagulation with warfarin, nephrotic syndrome, DIC, and vitamin K deficiency.

Elevated Factor VIII Levels

Increased factor VIII levels have been associated with an increased risk of thrombosis (relative risk = 4.8). An increased factor VIII level was found in 25% of patients with a first VTE event, versus 10% of controls, and has been associated with recurrent VTE episodes. Elevated levels are found with increased age, obesity, pregnancy, surgery, inflammation, liver disease, hyperthyroidism, and diabetes. No gene alteration has yet been described, although familial clustering of increased factor VIII levels has been noted. It is unclear how increased factor VIII levels lead to increased thrombotic risk and how elevated factor VIII levels may affect treatment of thromboembolism.

Hereditary Thrombotic Dysfibrinogenemia

The dysfibrinogenemias are qualitative defects in the fibrin molecule that may lead to VTE in 20% of patients, to bleeding tendency in 25% of patients, and are asymptomatic in 55%. Normal or low levels of fibrinogen and a prolonged thrombin time may be observed. Multiple genetic defects have been described. This disorder is rare, and testing for it in patients with suspected thrombophilia is considered low priority.

Management

Workup of the Hypercoagulable State

The presence of thrombophilia increases the risk of a first-time thrombotic event. In addition, the risk of recurrence after a thromboembolic event is more common in patients with antithrombin deficiency, in patients with protein C or protein S deficiency, in those with more than one inherited abnormality, and in those homozygous for factor V Leiden or the prothrombin G20210A mutation. The risk of a recurrent thromboembolic event among heterozygotes for factor V Leiden and the prothrombin G20210A mutation has been equivocal in many studies. However, a recent meta-analysis demonstrated an increased risk of recurrence among heterozygotes for factor V Leiden (odds ratio [OR] = 1.41) and the prothrombin G20210A mutation (OR = 1.72).

Furthermore, in studies of patients with first symptomatic VTE, the risk of recurrence at 5 years was lower when the initial event corresponded with a reversible risk factor. It is estimated that the overall risk of recurrence is about 5% per year after standard therapy. In patients without identifiable risk factors, studies found that patients had a much higher rate of recurrence. Thus, screening for thrombophilia could potentially be helpful in predicting which patients without readily identifiable risk factors are at increased risk of recurrence.

However, there are few clinical trial data available to guide the management of symptomatic or asymptomatic thrombophilic patients in different clinical scenarios. Consequently, there is debate about which patients should be screened. Screening symptomatic and asymptomatic individuals and their family members for the presence of thrombophilia has both benefits and drawbacks. In addition to prevention of recurrence, benefits include a focus on prophylaxis with anticoagulant therapy during high-risk situations, such as surgery, immobilization, and pregnancy to prevent a first-time event, and an awareness of increased risk associated with oral contraceptive use, pregnancy, and hormone replacement therapy. Drawbacks may include difficulties in obtaining life insurance coverage and overanticoagulation, with exposure to unnecessary bleeding risk. In general, consideration of a hypercoagulable workup is usually recommended in patients with recurrent

VTE, unprovoked thrombosis, thrombosis at a young age (<50), thrombosis at unusual sites (cerebral sinus, mesenteric vein, portal vein, hepatic vein), recurrent fetal loss, placental abruption, or severe pre-eclampsia. Of note, some experts do not recommend screening for protein C, protein S, or antithrombin in patients older than 50 with an unremarkable family history presenting with their first VTE, as this is likely to be low yield. Universal screening, even for women considering hormonal therapy, oral contraceptives, or pregnancy, is not currently recommended, as it is not cost-effective and may deny women birth control options.

The optimal time for testing patients for hereditary defects is not well defined but performing the thrombophilic evaluation at the time of thrombosis can result in misleading test results. For example, acute thrombosis can cause low levels of antithrombin, protein C, and protein S. Therapy with heparin reduces antithrombin levels, and warfarin reduces protein C and S levels.

Treatment
There are few clinical trial data to provide evidence-based recommendations for the duration of anticoagulation in patients with hereditary thrombophilia. These patients are often excluded from clinical trials, or the effects of thrombophilia are limited to subgroup analysis. However, many experts would recommend a longer duration of anticoagulation in patients with active cancer, multiple allelic abnormalities, antithrombin deficiency, protein C or S deficiency, more than one thrombotic event, or antiphospholipid antibody syndrome (see below). Some experts recommend lifelong anticoagulation for two or more unprovoked VTEs, unprovoked VTE with antithrombin deficiency or multiple genetic abnormalities, or one life-threatening VTE. Of note, one clinical trial noted a significant risk reduction in patients with idiopathic VTE continued on long-term low-intensity warfarin (INR, 1.5 to 2.0) after standard initial therapy. Specific drug information regarding anticoagulation may be found in Chapter 12. In all patients with a history of a thromboembolic event, regardless of the presence or absence of hereditary thrombophilia, prophylaxis should be pursued with unfractionated heparin or LMWH during high-risk situations, including surgery, trauma, and immobilization. Women should also be advised of the increased risk of recurrent thrombotic events with oral contraceptives, hormone replacement therapy, and pregnancy.

ARTERIAL THROMBOEMBOLISM

Introduction
Arterial thromboses are those that eventually lodge in the arterial side of the circulatory system. They may either occur in situ due to a damaged artery (e.g., by trauma, vasculitis, or foreign body) or be the result of embolization from a proximal source (e.g., from the atria in atrial fibrillation, a ventricular or arterial aneurysm, a proximal clot formed in an area of damaged artery, or a venous clot that passes into the arterial circulation through a heart defect).

Presentation
Symptoms
The symptoms are typically related to the acute ischemia of the organ in which the clot forms or lodges.

Risk Factors
Risk factors for arterial thrombosis are smoking, hypertension, atherosclerosis, turbulent blood flow, diabetes, chronic inflammation, and hyperlipidemia.

Causes

The initial management of an arterial thrombus includes a search for either its source as an embolus from a distant site or its origin as a clot that formed in situ. The reader is referred to the *Washington Manual Cardiology Subspecialty Consult* for more information about atrial fibrillation and to the *Washington Manual Rheumatology Subspecialty Consult* regarding vasculitis.

The presence of a hypercoagulable state as the etiology of the arterial thrombus may be considered if there are no readily identifiable risk factors. Arterial thromboses may be associated with hyperhomocysteinemia and antiphospholipid syndrome, discussed below, as well as heparin-induced thrombocytopenia, myeloproliferative disorders, and paroxysmal nocturnal hemoglobinuria, discussed elsewhere. Of note, these disorders may present with either venous or arterial thrombosis.

Hyperhomocysteinemia

Homocysteine is an intermediate formed in the metabolism of methionine. Elevated levels of homocysteine are associated with arterial and venous thrombosis. Hyperhomocysteinemia can be due to inheritance of enzyme defects involved in the homocysteine metabolic pathways or can be acquired. Severe hyperhomocysteinemia (plasma levels >100 μmol/L) is most commonly due to defects in cystathionine B-synthase (CBS) and results in homocystinuria, mental retardation, and thromboses at a young age. The most common genetic defect in mild homocystinemia (plasma levels, 15 to 40 μmol/L) results in reduced activity of the enzyme methylenetetrahydrofolate reductase. Acquired causes include vitamin B_{12}, vitamin B_6, and folate deficiencies; chronic renal failure; hypothyroidism; cancer; increasing age; smoking; inflammatory bowel disease; psoriasis; rheumatoid arthritis; and the use of methotrexate, phenytoin, and theophylline. The diagnosis is made by measuring fasting homocysteine plasma levels. Prospective studies show that the relative risk for VTE in patients with hyperhomocysteinemia is 3.4. Patients deficient in folate, vitamin B_6, or vitamin B_{12} can be supplemented with these vitamins at sufficient doses to achieve normal levels. In the absence of specific deficiencies, plasma homocysteine levels can be reduced by up to 50% by administration of folate at doses of 1 to 2 mg/day, although it is uncertain whether this ultimately leads to a decreased frequency of adverse events. In patients with severe hyperhomocysteinemia due to CBS deficiency, treatment with vitamin B supplements improves homocysteine levels and delays thrombotic events. However, this may not extend to other patient populations. In several recent studies, patients with first-time events, either arterial (stroke, MI) or VTE, treated with vitamin supplementation had reductions in homocysteine levels but no protection from recurrent MI, recurrent venous thrombosis, or progression of peripheral vascular disease.

Antiphospholipid Syndrome

Antiphospholipid syndrome is characterized by recurrent venous or arterial thrombosis, pregnancy morbidity/fetal loss, and the presence of antiphospholipid antibodies (anticardiolipin antibodies, lupus anticoagulants, anti-B_2glycoprotein 1), which are autoantibodies that recognize phospholipids and/or phospholipid binding proteins. Diagnosis relies on meeting at least one of the clinical and one of the laboratory criteria that follow.

Clinical:
- One or more episodes of venous, arterial, or small vessel thrombosis
- Pregnancy morbidity:
  - At least one unexplained death of a morphologically normal fetus beyond the 10th week of gestation
  - At least three unexplained spontaneous abortions before the 10th week of gestation
  - One or more premature births secondary to eclampsia, pre-eclampsia, or placental insufficiency before the 34th week of gestation

Laboratory:

- The presence of lupus anticoagulant on two or more occasions at least 12 weeks apart
- The presence of anticardiolipin antibody of IgG or IgM isotype at medium or high titer on two or more occasions at least 12 weeks apart
- The presence of anti-B_2 glycoprotein 1 of IgG or IgM isotype on two or more occasions at least 12 weeks apart

Lupus anticoagulants are IgG or IgM antibodies that react with negatively charged phospholipids. Thus, in vitro they act as anticoagulants and interfere with membrane surfaces in clotting assays, resulting in false prolongation of the aPTT and, occasionally, the PT. The presence of the lupus anticoagulant may be confirmed with the dilute Russell's viper venom assay or phospholipid neutralization assay. **Anticardiolipin** and **anti-B_2 glycoprotein 1** are detected by immunologic assays. The pathogenesis of antiphospholipid antibodies is thought to involve the binding and subsequent activation of endothelial cells, platelets, and complement to promote thrombosis and the inhibition of the fibrinolytic pathway. The syndrome is considered primary if there is no accompanying autoimmune disease and secondary if the patient has SLE. Approximately 30% to 50% of patients develop DVT of the legs within 6 years of follow-up. Although venous thrombosis is more common, patients may present with arterial occlusions, the most frequent involving the brain, followed by coronary occlusions. Importantly, any vessel or vascular bed may be involved and diverse presentations, such as intestinal, pancreatic, or splenic infarction, ARDS, retinitis, and acute renal failure, may occur. Other features occasionally seen include thrombocytopenia, hemolytic anemia, and livedo reticularis. The treatment of antiphospholipid syndrome is lifelong anticoagulation, typically with warfarin, with the goal INR 2.0 to 3.0. Some clinicians use a higher target INR but this is associated with a higher risk of bleeding. Hydroxychloroquine and ASA may be used as adjunct therapy. Catastrophic antiphospholipid syndrome, characterized by multiple simultaneous thromboses, occurs in <1% of patients and is associated with multiorgan failure and death. Plasma exchange and rituximab have been used to treat these patients, although these approaches are based on case studies and not on clinical trials.

KEY POINTS TO REMEMBER

- Keep in mind all components of Virchow triad (endothelial damage, stasis, hypercoagulability) as possible sources of thrombi.
- The clinical diagnosis of DVT is highly unreliable. Use Doppler ultrasonography to exclude it when the diagnosis is entertained.
- PE and DVT may be treated acutely with unfractionated heparins or LMWH. They should be continued for at least 5 days and until therapeutic oral anticoagulation is achieved.
- IVC filters are an important alternative to anticoagulation for treatment of DVT/PE but are clinically inferior and should be used only when absolutely necessary.

REFERENCES AND SUGGESTED READINGS

Ageno W, Squizzato A, Garcia D, et al. Epidemiology and risk factors of venous thromboembolism. *Semin Thromb Hemost.* 2006;32(7):651–658.
Arcasoy SM, Vachani A. Local and systemic thrombolytic therapy for acute venous thromboembolism. *Clin Chest Med.* 2003;24:73–91.

Bauer K. The thrombophilias: well-defined risk factors with uncertain therapeutic implications. *Ann Intern Med.* 2001;135:367–373.

Bounameaux H, Perrier A. Diagnosis of pulmonary embolism: in transition. *Curr Opin Hematol.* 2006;13(5):344–350.

Cushman M. Epidemiology and risk factors for venous thrombosis. *Semin Hematol.* 2007;44:62–69.

Decousus H, Leizorovicz A, Parent F, et al. A clinical trial of vena caval filters in the prevention of pulmonary embolism in patients with proximal deep-vein thrombosis. *N Engl J Med.* 1998;338: 409–415.

Francis CW. Clinical practice. Prophylaxis for thromboembolism in hospitalized medical patients. *N Engl J Med.* 2007;356(14):1438–1444.

Gatt A, Makris M. Hyperhomocystinemia and venous thrombosis. *Semin Hematol.* 2007;44;70–76.

Hann CL, Streiff MB. The role of vena caval filters in the management of venous thromboembolism. *Blood Rev.* 2005;19(4):179–202.

Lee AY, Levine MN, Baker RI, et al. Low-molecular-weight heparin versus a coumarin for the prevention of recurrent venous thromboembolism in patients with cancer. *N Engl J Med.* 2003;349: 146–153.

Levine S. The antiphospholipid syndrome. *N Engl J Med.* 2002;346:752–763.

Palareti G, Cosmi B. Diagnosis of deep vein thrombosis. *Semin Thromb Hemost.* 2006;32(7): 659–672.

Pesavento R, Bernardi E, Concolato A, et al. Postthrombotic syndrome. *Semin Thromb Hemost.* 2006;32(7): 744–751.

Segal JB, Streiff MB, Hofmann LV, et al. Management of venous thromboembolism: a systematic review for a practice guideline. *Ann Intern Med.* 2007;146(3):211–222.

Seligsohn U, Griffin J. Hereditary thrombophilia. In: Lichtman MA, Beutler E, Kipps TJ, et al., eds. *Williams hematology.* 7th ed. New York: McGraw-Hill; 2006:667–700.

Seligsohn U, Lubetsky A. Genetic susceptibility to venous thrombosis. *N Engl J Med.* 2001;334:1222–1229.

Stam J. Current concepts: thrombosis of the cerebral veins and sinuses. *N Engl J Med.* 2005;352:1791–1798.

Stein PD, Woodard PK, Weg JG, et al. Diagnostic pathways in acute pulmonary embolism: recommendations of the PIOPED II investigators. *Am J Med.* 2006;119(12):1048–1055.

Stein PD, Fowler SE, Goodman LA, et al. Multidetector computed tomography for acute pulmonary embolism. *N Engl J Med.* 2006;354:2317–2327.

Streiff MB, Segal JB, Tamariz LJ, et al. Duration of vitamin K antagonist therapy for venous thromboembolism: a systematic review of the literature. *Am J Hematol.* 2006;81(9):684–691.

Coagulopathy

7

Lee Demertzis

HEMOPHILIA A

Introduction

Hemophilia A is an inherited coagulation disorder caused by alterations of the gene encoding factor VIII (FVIII), leading to impaired intrinsic pathway function. The incidence is approximately 1 in 5000 live male births. The inheritance pattern is X-linked recessive; the gene that encodes FVIII is located on the long arm of the X chromosome (Xq28). Thirty percent of cases are the result of spontaneous mutations.

Presentation

Hemophilia A is a clinically heterogeneous disorder classically characterized by joint and muscle hemorrhages, easy bruising, and prolonged bleeding after trauma or surgery. Patients do not bleed excessively after minor cuts or abrasions. Chronic disability can result from hemarthrosis-induced arthropathy and intramuscular bleeding. The severity of the disease depends on the patient's FVIII level, with mild disease classified as a level 6% to 30% of normal, moderate as 2% to 5% of normal, and severe as ≤1% of normal.

Management

Diagnosis

Hemophilia A should be suspected whenever unusual bleeding is encountered in a male patient. Supportive laboratory data include a normal platelet count, a normal PT, and a prolonged aPTT. The diagnosis is confirmed by obtaining a FVIII level. Genetic analysis is used for carrier detection and prenatal diagnosis; fetal samples are acquired by amniocentesis or chorionic villus sampling.

Treatment

Both the severity of the disease and the type of hemorrhage determine the treatment of bleeding episodes.

DDAVP (Desmopressin)

An analogue of antidiuretic hormone (vasopressin) that lacks vasoactive properties, DDAVP acts by releasing endothelial stores of von Willebrand factor (vWF), thereby transiently increasing plasma levels of FVIII and vWF by a factor of 3 to 5 within 30 to 60 minutes of administration. Patients with mild or moderate disease and minor bleeding episodes may be treated with DDAVP alone. Dosing is 0.3 μg/kg IV or SC or 300 μg/kg intranasally. Dosing frequency is guided by the half-life of FVIII after DDAVP administration, which is 8 to 10 hours. Benefits of DDAVP use include ease of administration (suitable even for home use) and avoidance of blood products and costly synthetic factors. DDAVP should not be used in patients with unstable coronary artery disease, due to concern for ultralarge vWF multimer-mediated platelet aggregation in regions of high shear stress near atherosclerotic plaques.

Factor VIII Replacement

Patients with severe hemophilia require FVIII replacement for both minor and major bleeding. Options consist of either purified FVIII concentrate from pooled plasma or recombinant FVIII. The choice of therapy is determined by availability, the patient's history of exposure to pooled plasma products, and patient preference. In general, each unit per kilogram of FVIII replacement will raise the plasma FVIII level by 2%. The goal of therapy is determined by the clinical situation. The target FVIII level is ≥30% for minor bleeding, ≥50% for more severe bleeding (e.g., muscle and joint hemorrhages), and ≥80% for surgical procedures or life-threatening bleeding. The half-life of FVIII replacement is 8 to 12 hours; therefore, following a loading dose, repeat doses are usually administered every 12 hours. Alternatively, FVIII replacement can be provided by continuous infusion. Therapy should continue until hemostasis is achieved; postoperative therapy is usually continued for 10 to 14 days. Measuring peak and trough FVIII levels after the first dose and selected subsequent doses permits dose adjustments to ensure cost-effective therapy.

Recombinant Factor VIIa

Recombinant factor VIIa promotes hemostasis by activating the extrinsic pathway. It is currently approved for use in hemophilia A and B patients who have developed inhibitors to FVIII or factor IX (FIX). This costly agent is dosed at 90 μg/kg every 2 to 3 hours until hemostasis is achieved.

Gene Therapy

Current studies in gene therapy involve using either adenoviral or retroviral vectors to introduce the gene for FVIII or FIX into somatic cells or, alternatively, culturing a patient's dermal fibroblasts ex vivo, transfecting the cells with FVIII or FIX cDNA, and then reimplanting the cells in the patient. To date, these efforts have met with limited success. The most promising approach appears to be viral vector-mediated gene therapy. Aside from the difficulty in achieving significant factor levels in the host using this technique, concerns have arisen regarding inhibitor formation and the risk of cancer from insertional mutagenesis.

HEMOPHILIA B

Hemophilia B (Christmas disease) results from abnormalities of the gene encoding FIX, which is located on the long arm of the X chromosome (Xq27). Inheritance is X-linked recessive, and the incidence is ~1 in 30,000 live male births. The clinical syndrome and laboratory studies are indistinguishable from hemophilia A, except that specific factor assays reveal decreased FIX levels. Principles of FIX replacement therapy are similar to those for treatment of hemophilia A. Two differences are that each unit per kilogram of FIX replacement will raise the plasma FIX level by 1% and that the half-life of FIX replacement is 16 to 17 hours.

VON WILLEBRAND DISEASE (vWD)

Introduction

vWD is caused by quantitative or qualitative abnormalities of vWF, resulting in disorders of primary and secondary hemostasis. The usual inheritance pattern of vWD is autosomal dominant; incomplete penetrance may lead to phenotypic variability. The incidence is ~1 in 100 to 400.

vWF is a glycoprotein synthesized by endothelial cells and platelets. It is stored in the Weibel-Palade bodies of endothelial cells as well as platelet alpha granules. vWF plays a role in both primary and secondary hemostasis. It mediates the adhesion of platelets at sites of vascular injury and stabilizes and transports FVIII in the circulation. vWF is synthesized as a 300-kD monomer, which then assembles into multimers of various sizes. The largest multimers mediate platelet adhesion.

Classification

vWD is a group of disorders that are classified into types 1, 2, and 3 on the basis of the associated vWF abnormality (see Table 5-1).

- **Type 1 vWD** is the most common form of vWD, accounting for ~70% of cases. The disease occurs as a result of *quantitative* deficiencies of vWF and FVIII, with levels of both factors reduced to 5% to 30% of normal. The inheritance pattern is autosomal dominant.
- **Type 2 vWD** represents a group of vWF *qualitative* abnormalities. In these disorders, the plasma levels of vWF protein are typically mildly reduced, but platelet adhesion is disproportionately low. *Type 2A vWD* is the most common qualitative abnormality of vWF, characterized by loss of high molecular weight vWF multimers and ensuing platelet dysfunction. In *Type 2B vWD*, the abnormal vWF has an increased affinity for the platelet glycoprotein Ib surface receptor, leading to more avid binding of vWF to platelets. The vWF:platelet complexes are cleared from plasma, resulting in both mild thrombocytopenia and diminished plasma levels of large vWF multimers. During pregnancy, elevated estrogen levels result in increased vWF levels, which may worsen thrombocytopenia in this disorder. *Pseudo-vWD* is a similar disorder in which platelet GPIb possesses an increased affinity for vWF. *Type 2M vWD* is characterized by a mutation that impairs binding of vWF to GPIb, leading to ineffective platelet binding. In contrast to type 2A, normal multimer patterns are preserved. *Type 2N* (Normandy) *vWD* is caused by mutations of the vWF FVIII binding region, leading to FVIII deficiency. vWF-dependent platelet function is normal. The resulting clinical picture is similar to that of mild or moderate hemophilia A.
- **Type 3 vWD** is an autosomal recessive disorder characterized by very low vWF levels (<1% of normal), low FVIII levels (1% to 10% of normal), and a phenotype resembling moderate or severe hemophilia A.

Presentation

Clinically, a diagnosis of vWD is suspected in patients with recurrent mucocutaneous bleeding or prolonged bleeding after trauma or surgery. A family history of a bleeding disorder is common. In contrast to hemophilia, musculoskeletal bleeding is rare. Although the majority of affected patients have mild vWD and minor bleeding, patients with the most severe form may suffer life-threatening hemorrhage.

Management

Workup
- Initial tests include a CBC, PT, and aPTT, which may be mildly prolonged as a result of decreased FVIII levels. These tests are most useful in suggesting alternate diagnoses. Confirmation of the diagnosis of vWD is often difficult; see Chapter 5 for a full discussion of the different laboratory tests available to evaluate for vWD.
- In brief, in suspected vWD, a recommended initial laboratory panel would include CBC, PT, aPTT, the quantitative vWF antigen (vWF:Ag) and FVIII level assays, and at least one qualitative vWF assay: Ristocetin cofactor assay (vWF:RCof) and/or vWF collagen binding assay (vWF:CBA). When abnormal tests are found suggesting

vWD, these tests should be repeated after 2 weeks to confirm the diagnosis. Similarly, if there is a moderate or strong clinical index of suspicion of vWD, all normal or borderline tests should be repeated to confirm the original findings.

Treatment

Treatment of bleeding episodes and **prophylaxis for surgery** are the main indications for treatment of vWD.

DDAVP. Details regarding mechanism of action, dosing, and precautions are given above (see Treatment, under Hemophilia A). At the time of vWD diagnosis or before elective treatment, a test dose of DDAVP should be administered to establish the individual pattern of response. FVIII levels and vWF:RCof or vWF:CBA should be measured at 1 and 4 hours after drug administration to determine peak factor levels and clearance rate, respectively. DDAVP is effective in treating most patients with type 1 vWD. Type 2 vWD does not respond as well as type 1, but a trial of DDAVP in these patients is reasonable. The exception is type 2B vWD, in which DDAVP is contraindicated due to transient thrombocytopenia after drug administration. In general, DDAVP is entirely ineffective in type 3 vWD.

FVIII and vWF Concentrates. These are the primary treatment for all vWD subtypes when significant bleeding or major surgery is involved. Virus-inactivated FVIII + vWF concentrates, such as **Humate-P** and **Alphanate**, are the products of choice, when available. Cryoprecipitate, which contains significantly higher concentrations of FVIII and vWF than fresh-frozen plasma, can also be used, although techniques of virus inactivation are not routinely applied to this product. Concentrate dosing ranges from 25 to 50 IU/kg. FVIII levels should be obtained every 12 hours on the day concentrates are administered and every 24 hours thereafter. Target FVIII levels are similar to those detailed for hemophilia A (see Treatment, under Hemophilia A, above). Monitoring vWF:RCof as a measure of vWF activity is also reasonable; target levels are similar to those for FVIII. Therapy is continued until bleeding stops or healing is complete postoperatively. When hemorrhage is not controlled despite adequate FVIII levels, platelet transfusion often achieves hemostasis. DDAVP can be used as adjunctive therapy in patients in which it is effective. **Antifibrinolytic amino acids (aminocaproic acid, tranexamic acid)** are also potential therapeutic adjuncts. They are contraindicated in patients with gross hematuria, because clots that do not lyse may cause ureteral obstruction.

ACQUIRED DISORDERS OF COAGULATION

Vitamin K Deficiency

Vitamin K is a fat-soluble vitamin that is involved in the posttranslational modification of procoagulant factors II, VII, IX, and X, and anticoagulant proteins C, S, and Z (a cofactor for the inhibition of activated factor X). These reactions take place in the liver, where vitamin K serves as a cofactor for the conversion of glutamic acid residues to gamma-carboxyglutamic acid, which facilitates binding of coagulation factors to phospholipid, an essential step in coagulation. Vitamin K must then be recycled by vitamin K epoxide reductase (VKOR) for further gamma-carboxylation to occur. It follows that vitamin K deficiency would render these so-called vitamin K-dependent coagulation factors ineffective. Disorders of vitamin K most commonly result from use of warfarin, a VKOR inhibitor. Vitamin K deficiency may occur secondary to inadequate dietary intake, which may deplete vitamin K stores in as little as 7 days, malabsorption syndromes, or use of antibiotics, which may eliminate vitamin K-producing bowel flora. On laboratory investigation, vitamin K antagonism/deficiency results in a prolonged PT that corrects during mixing studies. Vitamin K repletion may be provided PO, SC, or IV, with the preferred route being PO. IV vitamin K is effective but carries the risk of anaphylaxis. To minimize this risk, vitamin K may be diluted in a dextrose or saline solution and slowly administered via an infusion pump. SC administration is rarely necessary. With adequate replacement therapy, the PT should begin to normalize within 12 hours and should normalize completely in 24 to 48 hours. If bleeding is significant or does not respond to vitamin K therapy, factor replacement in the form of fresh-frozen plasma should be administered.

Liver Disease

All coagulation factors, with the exception of vWF and, possibly, FVIII, are produced in the liver. Liver dysfunction leads to a number of coagulation abnormalities secondary to decreased factor synthesis, decreased clearance of activated factors, dysregulation of fibrinolytic pathways, and production of abnormal fibrinogen. The coagulopathy of liver disease is usually stable unless the liver synthetic function is rapidly worsening, such as in fulminant hepatic failure. Patients with liver synthetic dysfunction frequently also have thrombocytopenia secondary to portal hypertension and splenic sequestration.

Disseminated Intravascular Coagulation

Disseminated intravascular coagulation is a hemostatic derangement of multiple etiologies characterized by small- and medium-vessel thrombosis with consumption of platelets and coagulation factors. It leads to microangiopathic hemolytic anemia, thrombocytopenia, and coagulation abnormalities. See Chapter 4 for a complete discussion.

Acquired Inhibitors of Coagulation

Acquired inhibitors of coagulation are immunoglobulins, usually IgG, which exert their effects by inhibiting the activity or increasing the clearance of coagulation factors. They can be directed against any of the coagulation factors, with inhibitors of FVIII being most common. A significant proportion of patients with inherited disorders of coagulation, especially hemophilia, develops inhibitors due to extensive blood product exposure. De novo inhibitor formation has also been well described; there is a variety of associated conditions, including malignancy, rheumatoid arthritis, lupus, drug reactions, and the postpartum state. The chief clinical manifestation of inhibitor formation is a bleeding diathesis, which can be severe. Laboratory evaluation will reveal prolongation of the PT, the aPTT, or both. To assess for the presence of an inhibitor, a mixing study is performed. If the abnormal coagulation studies do not correct with mixing, an inhibitor is likely, and the Bethesda assay can be run to quantify the inhibitor. If antiphospholipid antibodies are suspected, a source of phospholipid (such as dilute Russell's viper venom) can be added to mixed plasma. Correction of the abnormal coagulation tests suggests the presence of antiphospholipid antibodies (see Chap. 6 for more information on antiphospholipid syndrome). Treatment varies depending on the type of inhibitor and severity of bleeding. Therapeutic options consist of factor concentrates, recombinant factor VIIa, immunosuppression with corticosteroids and/or cyclophosphamide, and plasma exchange.

Disorders of Fibrinogen

Fibrinogen is a precursor to fibrin that is produced in the liver and is an acute phase reactant. Disorders of fibrinogen may be either qualitative (dysfibrinogenemia) or quantitative (afibrinogenemia, hypofibrinogenemia) and may be inherited or acquired, with acquired abnormalities far outnumbering congenital cases. The chief cause of acquired disorders is liver disease, namely, cirrhosis, acute and chronic hepatitis, and hepatocellular carcinoma. Clinically, bleeding episodes of varying severity are the most common manifestations, although paradoxical thrombotic events have also been described. Pregnancy may be complicated by excessive bleeding at delivery and an increased miscarriage rate. The thrombin time (TT) is the most sensitive screening test for fibrinogen disorders. The PT and aPTT may be prolonged but are less sensitive than the TT. However, the TT suffers from poor specificity, and care should be taken to exclude heparin as the etiology of a prolonged TT before continuing the workup (see Chap. 5). Diagnostic confirmation involves quantitative and qualitative fibrinogen assays and, in the case of congenital disorders, demonstration of a molecular defect. The therapeutic armamentarium consists of fibrinogen concentrates, cryoprecipitate, topical fibrin glue, and antifibrinolytic amino acids.

Unsuspected, Surreptitious, or Accidental Use of Anticoagulants

When abnormal coagulation test results are present and an organic cause cannot be established, unsuspected exposure to an anticoagulant drug may be the culprit. For example, hospitalized patients frequently receive heparin during routine venous catheter flushes. Similarly, patients may have had blood drawn from lines through which heparin is being infused. Patients with coagulation studies consistent with warfarin effect and an otherwise negative evaluation may be surreptitiously ingesting warfarin. Ingestion of anticoagulant rodenticides containing "superwarfarins" (e.g., brodifacoum) causes a prolonged elevation of the PT, lasting up to 1 year. Blood products are indicated for patients with associated bleeding, along with high-dose vitamin K replacement (e.g., 50 to 800 mg PO daily), as standard doses of vitamin K do not usually correct the coagulopathy. Vitamin K should be continued until the PT normalizes. Serum assays for warfarin and superwarfarins are available and may provide diagnostic assistance in challenging cases.

KEY POINTS TO REMEMBER

- In an asymptomatic patient, the initial steps in evaluation of coagulation laboratory abnormalities are to repeat the tests and evaluate for falsely abnormal studies (e.g., related to heparin exposure).
- Hemophilia A is a rare inherited disorder characterized by decreased FVIII levels. Use of DDAVP and transfusion of plasma products are the mainstays of management.
- vWD is a family of disorders characterized by quantitative or qualitative abnormalities of vWF, with ensuing defects in primary and secondary hemostasis. Laboratory workup is complex; an initial panel should include CBC, PT, aPTT, vWF:Ag, FVIII:C, and either vWF:RCof or vWF:CBA.
- Liver disease, vitamin K antagonism, and vitamin K deficiency are important acquired causes of coagulopathy.

REFERENCES AND SUGGESTED READINGS

Blanchard RA, Furie BC, Jorgensen M, et al. Acquired vitamin K-dependent carboxylation deficiency in liver disease. *N Engl J Med.* 1981;305:242–248.

Bolton-Maggs PHB, et al. The rare coagulation disorders—review with guidelines for management from the United Kingdom Haemophilia Centre Doctors' Organization. *Haemophilia.* 2004;10:593–628.

Budde U. Laboratory diagnosis of congenital von Willebrand disease. *Semin Thromb Hemost.* 2002;28:173–189.

Butenas S, Brummel KE, Branda RF, et al. Mechanism of factor VIIa-dependent coagulation in hemophilia blood. *Blood.* 2002;99:923–930.

Chua JD, Friedenberg WR. Superwarfarin poisoning. *Arch Intern Med.* 1998;158: 1929–1932.

Dawson NA, Barr CF, Alving BM. Acquired dysfibrinogenemia. *Am J Med.* 1985;78: 682–686.

Favaloro EJ. Laboratory assessment as a critical component of the appropriate diagnosis and sub-classification of von Willebrand's disease. *Blood Rev.* 1999;13:185–204.

Hoyer L. Hemophilia A. *N Engl J Med.* 1994;330:38–47.

Lackner H. Hemostasis abnormalities associated with dysproteinemias. *Semin Hematol.* 1973;10:125–133.

Lechner K, Niessner H, Thaler E. Coagulation abnormalities in liver disease. *Semin Thromb Hemost.* 1977;4:40–56.

Levi M, Ten Cate H. Disseminated intravascular coagulation. *N Engl J Med.* 1999;341: 586–592.

Mannucci PM. Desmopressin (DDAVP) in the treatment of bleeding disorders: the first 20 years. *Blood.* 1997;90:2515–2521.

Mannucci PM. How I treat patients with von Willebrand disease. *Blood.* 2001;97: 1915–1919.

Mannucci PM. The hemophiliac—from royal genes to gene therapy. *N Engl J Med.* 2001;344:1773–1779.

Mannucci PM. Treatment of von Willebrand's disease. *N Engl J Med.* 2004;351:683–694.

Ponder KP. Gene therapy for hemophilia. *Curr Opin Hematol.* 2006;13:301–307.

Sadler JE, et al. Update on the pathophysiology and classification of von Willebrand disease: a report of the subcommittee on von Willebrand factor. *J Thromb Haemost.* 2006;4:2103–2114.

Sahud MA. Laboratory diagnosis of inhibitors. *Semin Thromb Hemost.* 2000;26:195–203.

Schwaab R, Oldenburg J. Gene therapy of hemophilia. *Semin Thromb Hemost.* 2001;27:417–424.

Zehnder JL. Clinical use of coagulation tests. Available at: www.utdol.com.

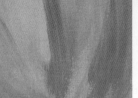

Myelodysplasia, Bone Marrow Failure Syndromes, and Other Causes of Pancytopenia

8

Giridharan Ramsingh and Robert Schwartz

PANCYTOPENIA

Pancytopenia is characterized by a reduction in all blood cell lines: RBCs, WBCs, and platelets. Patients with pancytopenia usually present with symptoms of anemia, bleeding secondary to thrombocytopenia, or recurrent infections as a result of leukopenia.

Etiology and Classification

Pancytopenia may be the result of processes that either directly affect the bone marrow (BM) or result from processes outside of it. Those that occur as a result of an insult to the marrow itself may be characterized by a decrease in hematopoietic elements (aplasia) or by ineffective hematopoiesis or infiltration of the BM.

Causes

The causes of pancytopenia are outlined below. Aplastic anemia (AA) is associated with decreased BM cellularity. The other causes are usually associated with increased BM cellularity, although hypoplastic BM can be seen in myelodysplastic syndrome, leukemia, lymphoma, paroxysmal nocturnal hemoglobinuria (PNH), vitamin B_{12} and folate deficiency, autoimmune diseases, and sepsis.

- Decreased production of blood cells
  - AA
  - Vitamin B_{12} and folate deficiency
  - BM infiltration due to aleukemic leukemia, lymphoma, metastatic carcinoma, myelofibrosis, sarcoidosis, tuberculosis, myeloma, hairy cell leukemia, or storage disorder (Gaucher, Niemann-Pick)
- Ineffective erythropoiesis
  - Myelodysplastic syndrome
- Increased destruction of blood cells
  - Hypersplenism
  - Autoimmune disorders: systemic lupus erythematosus, Sjögren syndrome
  - Paroxysmal nocturnal hemoglobinuria
  - Overwhelming sepsis

Presentation

Evaluation

The evaluation of pancytopenia is presented in Figure 8-1. Initial lab evaluation should involve a peripheral smear and reticulocyte count. HIV status, folate and B_{12} levels, and viral, bacterial, and fungal studies should also be obtained. If no etiology is clear, a BM aspirate should be obtained. Viral studies (CMV, EBV, hepatitis panel, HIV, parvovirus)

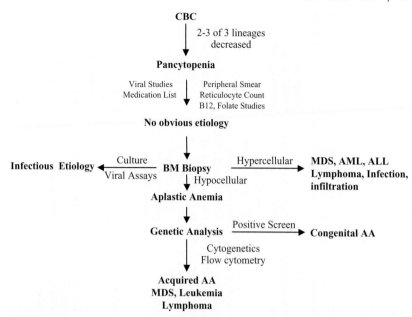

FIGURE 8-1. Workup of pancytopenia. AA, aplastic anemia; ALL, acute lymphocytic leukemia; AML, acute myeloid leukemia; BM, bone marrow; CBC, complete blood count; MDS, myelodysplastic syndrome.

may be appropriate in the setting of a patient with a hypocellular marrow. Cytogenetics and flow cytometry of the BM aspirate are useful when a hematologic malignancy is suspected. The medication list of the patient should be studied, as medications may often be the culprit and removal of the offending medication may be curative. After other more common diagnoses have been excluded, the diagnoses of acquired and inherited AA should be considered.

Clinical Presentation

Patients can present in innumerable ways depending on the severity and type of cell lineages affected. Anemia can cause fatigue, shortness of breath, or lightheadedness. Patients with significant thrombocytopenia can present with bleeding, hemorrhage, and bruising. Neutropenia is associated with infections including pneumonia, sepsis, and urinary tract infections.

BONE MARROW FAILURE

BM failure is defined as the inability of the BM to produce an adequate number of circulating blood cells. The causes can be inherited and acquired. Inherited BM failure syndromes are detailed in Table 8-1. Acquired BM failure states include myelodysplasia, acquired AA, and PNH.

Myelodysplasia

Introduction

Myelodysplastic syndromes (MDSs) are neoplastic clonal stem cell disorders manifest clinically by BM failure and pathologically by the presence of dysplastic morphology in one or

TABLE 8-1   INHERITED BONE MARROW FAILURE SYNDROME

	Fanconi Anemia	Dyskeratosis Congenita	Shwachman-Diamond Syndrome	Diamond-Blackman Anemia	Congenital Amegakaryocytic Thrombocytopenia
Inheritance	AR, rarely X-linked recessive	X-Linked recessive, AD, AR	AR	80% sporadic AD, AR, X-linked	AR
Genetics	Polygenic etiology leading to spontaneous chromosomal breakage and increased sensitivity to DNA cross-linking agents	X-Linked recessive Dyskerin gene (DKC1) mutation; AD TERC gene; AR, not identified: all lead to defective telomerase activity	Shwachman-Diamond syndrome gene mutation predicted to cause changes in RNA metabolism and/or ribosome biogenesis	Ribosomal protein S19 and S24 gene mutation leading to ribosomal dysfunction in a subset of patients; other mutations unidentified	c-mpl (thrombopoietin receptor) gene mutation leading to impaired stem cell survival
Bone marrow failure	Aplastic anemia	Aplastic anemia	Aplastic anemia	Pure red cell aplasia	Thrombocytopenia followed by aplastic anemia
Other abnormalities	Microcephaly, thumb abnormalities, hypogonadism, skin changes	Triad of skin pigmentation, nail dystrophy, and mucosal leukoplakia	Exocrine pancreatic deficiency, skeletal abnormalities, skin changes	Craniofacial, thumb, and growth abnormalities	Cardiac and neurological abnormalities

Diagnostic tests	DNA cross-linking agent induced chromosomal breakage	Mainly clinical; genetic testing for DKC1 and TERC genes available	Mainly clinical; SBDS gene testing available	Mainly clinical; RPS19 and RPS24 gene mutation studies in a subset of patients	c-mpl gene testing confirmatory
Complications	Infection and hematological and solid organ malignancies	Hematological malignancies, pulmonary complications, infections	Infection, myelodysplasia, hematological malignancies	Myelodysplasia and hematological and solid organ malignancies; iron overload from transfusion	Infections
Treatment	Supportive, AHSCT	AHSCT	Supportive, pancreatic enzyme supplementation, AHSCT in bone marrow failure	Supportive, steroids, AHSCT in some	AHSCT

AD, autosomal dominant; AR, autosomal recessive; AHSCT, allogenic hematopoietic stem cell transplantation.

more cell lines in BM or peripheral blood. There is increased apoptosis despite increased cell proliferation causing discrepancy between the cellular BM and peripheral cytopenias.

Epidemiology
MDS is considered a disease of the elderly. The annual incidence of MDS ranges from 2 to 12 cases per 100,000 people but increases to 50 cases per 100,000 among people aged ≥70 years. The mean age at diagnosis of MDS is 70 years. In Asia the disease is evident at a younger age, with a mean of 53 years. Other known risk factors include exposure to chemotherapy (alkylating agents and topoisomerase II inhibitors), chloramphenicol, radiation, benzene and other solvents, petroleum products, smoking, and immunosuppression. Inherited BM failure syndromes are a significant risk factor for MDS in the pediatric age group.

Pathogenesis
MDS exhibits cytopenia or cytopenias despite a cellular BM. The malignant stem cell possesses increased proliferative potential but accelerated apoptosis, resulting in ineffective maturation. Apoptosis is more marked in the earlier stages of the disease. As the disease progresses there is less cell apoptosis, which may be one of the mechanisms leading to disease progression. The exact inciting event is unknown but it is considered to be a multiple hit process at both the genetic and the epigenetic level. Overproduction of inflammatory cytokines contributes to increased apoptosis at the earlier stages. There is also evidence to suggest involvement of the BM microenvironment through the release of vascular endothelial growth factor (VEGF), which increases apoptosis through the release of various other cytokines. VEGF has also been shown to increase leukemic stem cell multiplication. Cellular immunological response mediated by T cells has been implicated in a subset of MDS patients who present at a younger age and have hypocellular BM. These patients may respond to immunosuppressive therapy with antithymocyte globulin.

Classification
The classification of MDSs has evolved with progress in the understanding of its pathogenesis. The World Health Organization (WHO) classification established in 1997 has replaced the previous French-American-British (FAB) classification (Table 8-2). There are several distinct clinical entities worth discussing in more detail.

5q⁻ Syndrome. 5q⁻ syndrome includes the presence of a severe hypoplastic anemia, a normal or elevated platelet count, atypical marrow megakaryocytes, and a comparatively indolent clinical course, accompanying an isolated chromosome 5q deletion. The WHO category of MDS with deletion 5q incorporates the above criteria and requires a blast count of <5% in the peripheral blood or BM.

Hypoplastic MDS. A minority of MDS patients has a hypocellular marrow. There is evidence to suggest a T cell immune-mediated mechanism of BM failure in these patients. They may respond to treatment with antithymocyte globulin and cyclosporine.

Therapy-Related MDS (tMDS). tMDS occurs most frequently in patients diagnosed with tumors that are associated with a good prognosis such as breast cancer, non-Hodgkin lymphoma, Hodgkin lymphoma, and testicular cancer. For instance, 1.7% of patients with breast cancer develop secondary BM disease, with a mean time of 18 months. tMDS and acute myelogenous leukemia occur in about 5% to 20% of patients with Hodgkin lymphoma and non-Hodgkin lymphoma. tMDS differs from sporadic MDS in that it tends to be associated with distinct chromosomal abnormalities. tMDS after exposure to alkylating agents is associated with deletions of chromosome 5 or 7 and occurs 3 to 5 years after therapy. Topoisomerase II inhibitors such as daunorubicin, etoposide, and tenoposide cause tMDS/acute myelogenous leukemia with translocations involving the MLL gene at 11q23, usually manifesting 1 to 3 years after treatment.

TABLE 8-2 WHO CLASSIFICATION OF MYELODYSPLASTIC SYNDROMES

Category	Peripheral Blood	Bone Marrow
Refractory anemia (RA)[a]	Anemia No blasts	<5% blasts <15% ringed sideroblasts
RA with ringed sideroblasts (RARS)[a]	Anemia No blasts	<5% blasts ≥15% erythroid ringed sideroblasts
RA with excess blasts-1 (RAEB-1)	Cytopenias <5% blasts Absence of Auer rods	5%–9% blasts Absence of Auer rods
RA with excess blasts-2 (RAEB-2)	Cytopenias <5% blasts Auer rods may be present <1000/μL monocytes	10%–19% blasts Auer rods may be present
MDS, unclassified (MDS-U)	Cytopenias No blasts Absence of Auer rods	Dysplasia in granulocytes or mega-karyocytes <5% blasts Absence of Auer rods
MDS with isolated del(5q)	Anemia <5% blasts Absence of Auer rods	Normal or increased mega-karyocyte number Absence of Auer rods del(5q) the only cytogenetic abnormality

[a]This is the classification of RA and RARS *only* if there are anemia and erythroid dysplasia on bone marrow exam (i.e., *only* the RBC line is affected). If RA and RARS are associated with more than one cell line affected, the phrase "with multilineage dysplasia" is added to the classification.

Adapted from Vardiman J, Harris N, Brunning R. The World Health Organization classification of the myeloid neoplasms. *Blood*. 2002;100:2292–2302.

Presentation
MDS is clinically a heterogeneous disorder. Its clinical manifestations result from BM failure: anemia causing pallor, fatigue, and shortness of breath; thrombocytopenia causing abnormal bleeding and purpura; and leukopenia causing infections, usually bacterial. Sometimes the diagnosis is made retrospectively after transformation to acute leukemia. Lymph node involvement and hepatosplenomegaly are rare.

Management
   Diagnosis. In the absence of other causes, BM failure (cytopenia) with BM findings of normal or increased cellularity with dysplastic myeloid cells is a cornerstone in establishing the diagnosis of MDS. In a subgroup of patients the diagnosis may remain unresolved, as with cytopenia without evidence of dysplasia. The **CBC** often reveals decreased reticulocyte count and elevated mean corpuscular volume. **Peripheral blood smear** may show oval macrophytic red cells, hypogranular neutrophils, and giant platelets.

BM biopsy is essential in the diagnostic evaluation. The cellularity is normal or increased except in rare cases where it can be hypocellular. Dysplastic morphological changes may not be present in all patients with MDS and the subjectivity of the findings may pose a significant diagnostic challenge. Morphological abnormalities include megaloblastic red cell precursors with multiple nuclei and asynchronous maturation of the nucleus or cytoplasm. Ringed sideroblasts (erythroid precursors with iron-laden mitochondria) are occasionally identified. There is often a predominance of immature myeloid cells, and granulocytic precursors may show asynchronous maturation of the nucleus and cytoplasm. Mature granulocytes are often hypogranular and hypolobulated. Megakaryocytes may be smaller and have fewer nuclear lobes.

The incidence of a recurrent cytogenetic abnormality is about 40% to 70% in de novo MDS and 95% in secondary MDS. In cases where morphological features are ambiguous, **cytogenetics** becomes very useful in diagnosis of MDS. Chromosomal deletions are the most common defects found. The most frequent deletions involve the long arms of chromosomes 5, 7, 20, 11, and 13 and the short arms of chromosomes 12 and 13. Loss of a whole chromosome is the second most frequent abnormality. The most common monosomies involve chromosomes 5, 7, and Y. Trisomies are the third most common cytogenetic abnormality and most frequently involve chromosomes 8, 11, and 21. Balanced translocations that are common in acute myelogenous leukemia are very rare in MDS; however, unbalanced translocations are common.

Fluorescent in situ hybridization (FISH) is becoming an important diagnostic tool in the evaluation of MDS. Unlike cytogenetics, which can be performed only in mitotic cells, FISH can be performed in mitotic cells as well as cells in interphase. It also has the advantage of quick results and a high sensitivity and specificity. It can detect clonal cryptic defects in about 3% to 15% of MDS patients with normal cytogenetics and may detect chromosomal abnormalities earlier in the course of the disease. However FISH will only detect what is being looked for and hence cannot replace cytogenetics.

Prognosis. Evolution to acute myelogenous leukemia occurs in 10% to 50% of all cases of MDS, and it varies with the MDS subtypes and correlates with the survival duration. Prognosis can also be roughly gauged by the International Prognostic Scoring System for MDS (Tables 8-3 and 8-4). This system assigns points to certain lab features. The patient's total point score can then be used as a rough gauge of risk level.

Treatment
- **Supportive treatment.** Blood transfusion is given when a patient has symptomatic anemia, and platelet transfusions when the platelet count falls below 10,000.

TABLE 8-3	INTERNATIONAL PROGNOSTIC SCORING SYSTEM FOR MDS RISK FACTOR CATEGORIES[a]		
Points	Bone Marrow Blasts (%)	Karyotype	Cytopenias
0	<5	Good	0 or 1
0.5	5–10	Intermediate	2 or 3
1.0		Poor	
1.5	11–20		
2.0	21–30		

[a]Percentage marrow blasts, karyotype, and cytopenias are each assigned point values. These are then added together to come up with the patient's risk score. Good prognosis = normal, −Y only, del(5q) only, del(20q) only; intermediate = trisomy 8; poor = complex defects, monosomy 7. Hemoglobin, <10 g/dL; absolute neutrophil count, <1.5 × 10^9; platelet count, <100 × 10^9/L.

Modified from Greenberg P, Cox C, LeBeau MM, et al. International Scoring System for evaluating prognosis in myelodysplastic syndromes. *Blood.* 1997;89:2079–2088.

TABLE 8-4	INTERNATIONAL PROGNOSTIC SCORING SYSTEM BY MDS RISK LEVEL	
Risk Level (total points)	**Median Survival (years)**	
Low (0)	5.7	
Intermediate-1 (0.5–1.0)	3.5	
Intermediate-2 (1.5–2.0)	1.2	
High (≥2.5)	0.4	

Adapted from Greenberg P, Cox C, LeBeau MM, et al. International Scoring System for evaluating prognosis in myelodysplastic syndromes. *Blood.* 1997;89:2079–2088.

Erythropoietin (EPO) at 40,000 U once or twice weekly is shown to produce a response in about 15% to 20% of patients, with patients with lower EPO levels responding better. Myeloid growth factors such as granulocyte colony-stimulating factor (G-CSF) and granulocyte/macrophage colony-stimulating factor (GM-CSF), either alone or in combination with EPO, tend to produce a response rate of 25% to 70% in neutrophil counts. In patients with refractory anemia with ringed sideroblasts (RARS) resistant to EPO alone, adding myeloid factors may improve the response. Patients with blood transfusion requirements of <2 U per month and EPO levels of <500 U/L show the best response to growth factors.

- **Immunomodulators**
  - **Thalidomide** inhibits angiogenesis, alters cellular immune responses, modulates various cytokines, and has direct antileukemic antiproliferative effects. It has been shown to cause independence from blood transfusion or significantly reduce transfusion requirements in about 18% of MDS patients; however, it was poorly tolerated due to sedation, constipation, neuropathy, and thrombosis. It has no effect on cell lines other than red cells.
  - **Lenalidomide** is a derivative of thalidomide and has a similar mechanism of action, with the additional property of enhancing EPO receptor signaling. It is more potent and has a favorable side-effect profile compared to thalidomide. Its dose-limiting side effects include neutropenia and thrombocytopenia. It induces substantial hematopoietic and cytogenetic responses in patients with MDS. Patients with MDS of low to intermediate-1 risk level and patients with normal cytogenetics have a better response rate. The results are best in patients with deletion 5q⁻ abnormalities, of whom 70% experience transfusion independence or a decline in transfusion needs.
- **Demethylating agents**
  - **Azacytidine** has shown an overall response rate of 60% with a complete remission rate of 7% in patients with MDS, irrespective of the subtype of MDS. Major side effects include nausea and vomiting, neutropenia, and thrombocytopenia.
  - There is no study comparing **decitabine** with azacytidine, but it appears that the responses in phase III trials are roughly equivalent.
- **Hematopoietic Stem Cell Transplantation (HSCT)**
  - **Allogeneic HSCT** is the primary curative treatment for patients with MDS. Disease-free survival ranges from 29% to 40%, with a nonrelapse mortality of 37% to 50% and a rate of relapse ranging from 23% to 48% with an HLA-identical sibling donor. It is the treatment of choice for young patients with a suitable donor. The prognostic factors include age, disease duration, disease state, and percentage of blasts in BM, cytogenetic abnormalities, type of donor, and intensity of the pretransplant conditioning. In patients with advanced stages, chemotherapy to suppress blast count prior to transplant is a reasonable strategy. The role of

reduced-intensity regimens in patients of advanced age or with other comorbidities remains to be determined.

APLASTIC ANEMIA

Introduction
AA is characterized by pancytopenia and a hypocellular BM in the absence of BM infiltration and increased reticulin deposition.

Epidemiology
The incidence of AA is 2 cases per 1 million population in Western countries, and it is three times more common in Asia. The incidence of AA peaks at 2 to 3 years due to inherited causes, with a second peak at 20 to 25 years. The majority of patients present after age 50.

Etiology
The etiology of AA is stem cell failure, although three distinct mechanisms play a role: DNA instability, toxic injury, and immune-mediated destruction. Inherited forms of AA are presented in Table 8-1. The inciting factor for acquired AA has not been elucidated. Several associations have been described, listed below. These risk factors are observed in only about 20% of patients.

- Chemicals
  - Benzene
  - Pesticides
  - Lubricating agents
  - Recreational drugs
- Drugs
  - Antibiotics: chloramphenicol, sulfonamides
  - Anti-inflammatory agents: diclofenac, indomethacin, naproxen, phenylbutazone
  - Antidepressants: dothiepin
  - Anticonvulsants: carbamazepine, phenytoin
  - Antithyroids: thiouracil
  - Antipsychotics: phenothiazines, clozapine
  - Antirheumatics: gold, penicillamine
  - Others: allopurinol
- Idiopathic
- Immune disorders: eosinophilic fascitis, SLE
- PNH
- Viruses: viral hepatitis, EBV, parvovirus
- Others: anorexia nervosa, thymoma, pregnancy

Pathogenesis
The pathophysiology of acquired AA is immune-mediated attack on the hematopoietic stem cells in most cases, caused by activated cytotoxic T cells expressing Th_1-type cytokines such as interferon-gamma and tumor necrosis factor-alpha. The reason for T cell activation remains unclear. It is possible that an inciting event like a virus, toxin, or medical drug provokes an aberrant immune response, causing activation of cytotoxic T cells that destroy hematopoietic stem cells. HLA-DR2 is overexpressed in patients with AA. There is also evidence to suggest a genetic basis for aberrant T cell activation. Telomere shortening is observed in one third to one half of patients with AA, but mutations involving the genes controlling telomere repair or protection are seen in only 10% of patients. It is unclear whether this is the cause of or result of AA.

Classification

Acquired AA is classified as moderate, severe, and very severe based on degree of BM cellularity and pancytopenia.

- **Very severe:** BM cellularity <25% and two of the following: absolute neutrophil count (ANC) of <200, platelet count of <20,000, reticulocyte count of <60,000
- **Severe:** BM cellularity <25% and two of the following: ANC of <500, platelet count of <20,000, reticulocyte count of <60,000
- **Moderate:** Hypocellular marrow with pancytopenia not meeting criteria for severe AA

Presentation

Symptoms are related to pancytopenia. Weight loss, pain, loss of appetite, or fever suggests another diagnosis. Physical examination usually reveals pallor, mucosal bleeding, petechiae, and ecchymoses. The presence of lymphadenopathy, hepatomegaly, or splenomegaly strongly suggests another diagnosis such as lymphoma, leukemia, or BM infiltration.

Management

Diagnosis

The diagnosis is established by BM aspiration and biopsy. The findings include a profoundly hypocellular marrow with a decrease in all cellular elements, with marrow space being replaced by fat cells and stromal elements. The residual hematopoietic elements are morphologically normal. There is no increased reticulin formation or infiltrative elements. In addition, some degree of dyserythropoiesis is sometimes present, requiring chromosomal analysis (normal in AA, abnormal in MDS).

- Etiological causes need to be worked up, which will include viral serologies for hepatitis, CMV, EBV, parvovirus, HIV, and herpes; serum B_{12} and folate levels; screening for Fanconi anemia and PNH; BM cytogenetics; and drug screening.

Treatment

Supportive Care. Patients with symptomatic anemia will need transfusion. Patients with symptomatic thrombocytopenia or a platelet count of <10,000 should be given platelets. Blood products should be irradiated to prevent transfusion-associated graft-versus-host disease. In patients who are considered for stem cell transplantation, only CMV-negative products should be administered to CMV IgG-negative patients, and blood products from family members should be avoided to prevent alloimmunization.

EPO and myeloid factors are not used as a mainstay of treatment. They are usually used following immunosuppressive therapy until counts recover, but they have not been shown to improve survival.

Immunosuppression. Antithymocyte globulin with cyclosporine is used in patients not eligible for stem cell transplantation because of age or lack of matched sibling donor. The 5-year survival in patients treated with immunosuppression is similar to that after stem cell transplantation. However, most patients do not recover to normal blood counts and many relapse (40%). Also, there is risk of evolution to PNH (13%) and MDS (15%) in patients treated with immunosuppression.

Hematopoietic Stem Cell Transplantation. Allogeneic transplantation is the treatment of choice in a young patient who has a matched donor. HSCT has been shown to have a 77% 5-year survival, with a higher survival in children. Patients older than 40 years have a much higher transplant-related mortality, primarily from a higher incidence of graft-versus-host disease. Unrelated transplants are offered to children who have failed a single course of immunosuppression and adults who have failed multiple courses of antithymocyte globulin and alternative therapies.

PAROXYSMAL NOCTURNAL HEMOGLOBINURIA

Introduction
PNH is an acquired disease characterized by nonmalignant clonal expansion of one or more hematopoietic stem cells that have undergone somatic mutation of the PIG-A gene.

Pathogenesis
Protein encoded by the PIG-A gene is essential for the synthesis of glycosyl phosphatidylinositol (GPI), and therefore GPI-linked proteins are lacking in the PIG-A mutant clone. Two of the GPI-linked proteins, CD55 (decay accelerating factor; DAF) and CD 59 (membrane inhibitor of reactive lysis; MIRL), that inhibit the activity of complement are absent in the PNH clone, resulting in complement-mediated lysis of RBCs. The PNH clone is present in a considerable proportion of the general population without symptoms. In patients with PNH, the clone is expanded significantly. It is postulated that PNH patients have some degree of BM failure and the PNH clone is selectively protected from BM injury as result of the lack of GPI-linked proteins. The pathogenesis of thrombosis in PNH is poorly understood.

Presentation
The clinical manifestations of PNH are intravascular hemolytic anemia, BM failure, and thrombosis. BM failure can be transient, mild, or severe. Thrombosis usually involves the venous system. Thrombosis can occur in unusual sites such as intra-abdominal veins. The clinical course is unpredictable and patients can have spontaneous remissions. PNH can present with or without (classic PNH) evidence of another specified BM disorder such as AA or MDS. Subclinical PNH (without clinical or laboratory evidence of hemolysis) can occur in association with other BM failure syndromes.

Management
Diagnosis
Flow cytometry using antibodies against GPI-linked proteins is the most sensitive and specific test to identify the PNH clone. The hemolysis is intravascular (high reticulocyte count, increased lactate dehydrogenase and unconjugated bilirubin, and decreased haptoglobulin) and is Coombs negative. Iron studies need to be completed to evaluate for iron-deficiency anemia, which can result from renal loss of hemoglobin. BM biopsy is essential in assessing BM failure.

Treatment
Treatment of Anemia. Anemia can result from hemolysis and BM failure. Transfusions are given for symptomatic anemia. If hemolysis is considered to be the contributing factor for anemia, then options include steroids, androgens, and complement inhibitors. **Corticosteroids** are used for treating acute as well as chronic hemolysis, but long-term use is limited because of toxicity. Steroids work by inhibiting complement. **Danazol** can be used alone or in conjunction with steroids for hemolytic anemia in PNH. Danazol can also be used for hypoproliferative anemia associated with PNH. **Eculizumab**, a monoclonal antibody against complement C5, has been approved for use in PNH. It controls hemolysis and improves quality of life. Its serious adverse effects include infection by encapsulated organisms. Iron-deficiency anemia can result from chronic hemoglobinuria, and iron replacement may be necessary. However, most patients are iron overloaded from chronic blood transfusion. Folic acid deficiency can result from chronic hemolysis, and replacement is required in all patients with hemolysis.

Thrombosis. Prophylactic anticoagulation is controversial. Patients who experience thrombosis should be anticoagulated indefinitely. Eculizumab has been shown to decrease the incidence of thrombosis.

Hematopoietic Stem Cell Transplantation. Indications for HSCT remain unresolved because of the unpredictable course of the disease. Currently there is no definite indication for transplantation. Patients with life-threatening thrombosis and underlying severe BM failure should be considered for transplantation.

KEY POINTS TO REMEMBER

- Pancytopenia is caused by aplasia of BM, ineffective hematopoiesis, or BM infiltration.
- Myelodysplasia is a clonal stem cell disorder resulting in ineffective hematopoiesis, causing cytopenias with a cellular BM.
- Cytogenetics, blast percentage, and level of cytopenia are important prognostic markers for MDS.
- Immunomodulators and demethylating agents can be used to treat MDS.
- AA can be acquired or congenital.
- Acquired AA may respond to immunosuppressive agents.
- PNH is an acquired disease with nonmalignant clonal expansion of a hematopoietic stem cell with PIG-A gene mutation.
- Clinical manifestations of PNH include nonimmune hemolysis, cytopenia, and thrombosis.

REFERENCES AND SUGGESTED READINGS

Brodsky RA, Jones R. Aplastic anemia. *Lancet.* 2005;365:1647–1656.

Cherian S, Bagg A. The genetics of myelodysplastic syndrome: classical cytogenetics and recent molecular insights. *Hematology.* 2006;11:1–13.

Dokal I. Fanconi's anemia and related bone marrow failure syndrome. *Br Med Bull.* 2006;77:37–53.

Komrokji RS, Bennett JM. Evolving classifications of myelodysplastic syndromes. *Curr Opin Hematol.* 2007;14:98–105.

Melchert M, et al. The role of lenalidomide in the treatment of patients with chromosome 5q and other myelodysplastic syndromes. *Curr Opin Hematol.* 2007;14:123–129.

Parker C, et al. Diagnosis and management of paroxysmal nocturnal hemoglobinuria. *Blood.* 2005;106:3699–3709.

Parker CJ. Pathophysiology of paroxysmal nocturnal hemoglobinuria. *Exp Hematol.* 2007;35:523–533.

Shadduck RK, et al. Recent advances in myelodysplastic syndromes. *Exp Hematol.* 2007;35:137–143.

Young NS, et al. Current concepts in the pathophysiology and treatment of aplastic anemia. *Blood.* 2006;108:2509–2519.

Myeloproliferative Disorders

John S. Welch and Mike G. Martin

INTRODUCTION

The myeloproliferative disorders (MPDs) are a group of clonal diseases characterized by overproduction of mature, largely functional cells arising from the transformation of a clonal hematopoietic stem cell. The World Health Organization (WHO) has designated seven conditions as MPDs (Table 9-1). Philadelphia chromosome-positive chronic myeloid leukemia (CML) is discussed in the chapter on the leukemias (Chap. 29), while the Philadelphia chromosome-negative chronic MPDs, polycythemia vera (PV), essential thrombocythemia (ET), chronic idiopathic myelofibrosis (CIMF), and chronic eosinophilic leukemia/hypereosinophilic syndrome (CEL/HES), are discussed here. Collectively, these disorders are uncommon. They share the signs and symptoms of hepatosplenomegaly, hypercatabolism, clonal marrow hyperplasia without dysplasia, and increased numbers of one or more cell lines. They are typically indolent and chronic in nature but may evolve into acute leukemia. Recent description of the activating Janus kinase2 (JAK2) mutation V617F in many of these disorders links them with a common pathophysiologic thread. While of clear clinical importance, this mutation is still being incorporated into current diagnostic, prognostic, and treatment algorithms, and international consensus has not yet been reached.

POLYCYTHEMIA VERA

Background

PV is a monoclonal stem cell disease characterized by proliferation of a multipotent stem cell with trilineage hyperplasia resulting primarily in expansion of the RBC line. Recently, the activating JAK2 V617F mutation has been noted in nearly all patients. JAK2 is an essential kinase in the erythropoietin (EPO) receptor signal transduction pathway. Constitutive JAK2 kinase activity results in EPO-independent proliferation of erythrocyte precursors. JAK2 is also involved in the JAK2-STAT5 pathways of the thrombopoietin receptor (MPL) and the granulocyte colony-stimulating factor receptor (GCSF-R). The V617F mutation can thus lead to proliferation of multiple cell lines, and patients with PV often have elevated platelets and leukocytes as well.

Epidemiology

PV is the most common of the MPDs, with an incidence of ~2 in 100,000 people. The average age of PV patients is 60 years, but it occurs across all age groups, with a slight male predominance. While familial clustering does exist, it is uncommon, and the JAK2 mutation is acquired somatically, suggesting a separate predisposition pathway.

TABLE 9-1	MUTATIONAL AND WHO CLASSIFICATION OF MYELOPROLIFERATIVE DISORDERS	
BCR-ABL Positive	**BCR-ABL Negative**	*JAK2V617F*
Chronic myeloid leukemia	Polycythemia vera	~95%
	Essential thrombocythemia	50%–60%
	Chronic idiopathic myelofibrosis	35%–55%
	Chronic neutrophilic leukemia	1%–5%
	Chronic eosinophilic leukemia/hypereosinophilic syndrome	
	Myeloproliferative disease, unclassifiable	

Clinical Presentation

Patients are commonly asymptomatic at presentation; however, they may present with symptoms related to increased RBC mass and hyperviscosity. Symptoms may include headache, weakness, peptic ulcer disease, hyperhydrosis, vision changes, tinnitus, and vertigo. In addition, many patients experience pruritus, especially with exposure to hot water. Erythromelalgia, due to microarteriolar occlusion, is characterized by a burning sensation in the digits and may be severe. Patients are also predisposed to thrombosis and, less often, hemorrhage. Many of these symptoms have been attributed to hyperviscosity, but dysfunction of leukocytes and platelets may also play an important role. Physical exam findings include splenomegaly, hepatomegaly, hypertension, and plethora.

Management

Diagnosis

The diagnosis is suspected when blood counts reveal an elevated hematocrit (Hct). The **EPO level is low** (<20 mU/mL) and often undetectable. The **JAK2 V617F mutation** is seen in nearly all patients. Leukocyte alkaline phosphatase scores, vitamin B_{12}, and uric acid levels may be elevated but are nonspecific findings. These patients also have an elevated RBC mass as demonstrated by ^{51}Cr labeling of RBCs and isotope dilution, although this is rarely tested now. In addition, ~60% of patients have elevated granulocyte counts, and 50% have thrombocytosis.

The **peripheral smear** may show microcytic, hypochromic RBCs with anisocytosis and poikilocytosis, reflecting exhaustion of iron stores due to increased hemoglobin (Hgb) synthesis. WBCs generally have normal morphology, but there are often increased basophils, eosinophils, and immature forms. Platelets occasionally have an abnormal morphology, with megathrombocytes seen on the smear.

Bone marrow biopsy findings are not diagnostic of PV, but biopsy is frequently performed to evaluate fibrosis and cytogenetics even when the diagnosis is not in question. Findings include hypercellular marrow with trilineage hyperplasia and clustered megakaryocytes with hypolobulated nuclei. Approximately 10% to 20% of PV patients will have an abnormal karyotype. Common karyotype changes include trisomy 9 (amplification of JAK2), trisomy 8 (also found in other MPDs, myelodysplastic syndrome, acute myeloid leukemia [AML]), trisomy 1q (unclear significance), del 5q and del 7q (more often seen after cytotoxic therapy), and del 13q (also associated with idiopathic myelofibrosis and chronic lymphocytic leukemia).

TABLE 9-2	DIAGNOSTIC CRITERIA FOR POLYCYTHEMIA VERA AND ESSENTIAL THROMBOCYTHEMIA

Polycythemia Vera	Essential Thrombocytosis
JAK2 positive	
Hct >52%, males Hct >48%, females	Platelets >450 × 10⁶/mL No other malignancy
JAK2 negative	
4 major or 3 major + 2 minor: *Major:* • Hct >60% (males) or >56% (females) • No secondary erythrocytosis • Palpable splenomegaly • Acquired genetic abnormalities (excluding JAK2 and BCR-ABL) *Minor:* • Platelets >450 × 10⁶/mL • Neutrophils >10 × 10⁶/mL • Radiographic splenomegaly • Low serum erythropoietin	All of the following: • Platelets >600 × 10⁶/ml on 2 occasions 1 month apart • No cause for reactive thrombocytosis • Ferritin >20 μg/L • No other myeloproliferative disease or myelodysplasia

Adapted from Campbell PJ, Green AR. The myeloproliferative disorders. *N Engl J Med.* 2006; 355:2452–2466.

Diagnostic Criteria. The Polycythemia Vera Study Group established diagnostic criteria >30 years ago. These are currently in flux, as they include neither EPO levels nor the JAK2 mutation. At Washington University we have adopted the Campbell proposed criteria based on JAK2 status with modifications of the Polycythemia Vera Study Group criteria (Table 9-2). Patients with JAK2-positive PV have a hematocrit >52% in men or >48% in women or an increased red cell mass (>25% above predicted) and a documented mutation. JAK2-negative PV, being much less common, must be carefully examined for secondary causes of polycythemia.

Differential Diagnosis. Patients with secondary polycythemia typically have elevated EPO levels caused by chronic hypoxemia, heavy smoking, renal disease, or malignancies such as renal cell cancer, hepatocellular cancer, and hemangioblastoma. Relative polycythemia, or pseudopolycythemia, is associated with a normal red cell mass and decreased plasma volume secondary to causes such as dehydration, diuretics, and burns. In cases of JAK2-negative polycythemia with low-normal EPO levels, *BCR-ABL* rearrangements should be evaluated, as CML may present with many of the same features.

Clinical Course

PV is a chronic disorder and may be characterized as having phases during its course. The **pre-erythrocytic phase** is generally asymptomatic, with an isolated increase in platelets or in RBCs. Patients may experience trivial pruritus and may have mild splenomegaly. This progresses to the **erythrocytic phase**, characterized by erythrocytosis requiring regular phlebotomy as well as increased granulocytes and platelet counts. Splenomegaly, pruritus, thrombosis, and hemorrhage may be present. This may last for a number of years. The **spent phase** is characterized by a reduced need for phlebotomy. Thrombocytosis and leukocytosis persist, and splenomegaly is progressive.

Up to 50% of patients may progress to a clinical picture difficult to differentiate from that of idiopathic myelofibrosis. Anemia develops, and the peripheral smear shows a leuko-erythroblastic picture with teardrop poikilocytes, nucleated red cells, and anisocytosis. Immature granulocytes are seen, with a slight increase in basophils, and platelets are often abnormal in morphology. Splenomegaly worsens, and there are increased systemic symptoms. AML may occur in up to 20% of patients, and the risk is increased in patients treated with alkylating agents. The incidence of progression to AML is higher in patients with myelofibrosis.

Thrombotic risk is present throughout the course of PV and may be linked to elevated, dysfunctional leukocytes or platelets. Reduction of thrombotic risk is a mainstay of therapy and recurrent thrombosis can be common.

Treatment

The goals of treatment are to reduce the blood volume to normal and to prevent thrombotic and hemorrhagic complications. Thrombotic risk has been associated with an age >60 years, prior thrombosis, and a platelet count >1000 × 10^9/L. Thrombocytosis clearly increases thrombotic risk, and this risk appears to be a continuum, with increased risk starting at 400 × 10^9/L and peaking at 900 × 10^9/L. Hemorrhagic risk increases with platelet counts >1500 × 10^9/L. Emerging risk factors include leukocyte counts >15 × 10^9/L and cardiovascular factors including smoking, obesity, hypertension, hypercholesterolemia, diabetes, and coronary artery disease (Table 9-3).

- *Low-risk patients* are <60 years old and have no history of thrombosis, no cardiovascular risk factors, and platelet counts <1500 × 10^9/L. These patients are managed with phlebotomy to a Hct of <45% and low-dose aspirin. Iron deficiency via phlebotomy is a goal of treatment.
- *High-risk patients* are ≥60 years old or have a history of a thrombotic event, or cardiovascular risk factors, or platelet counts >1500 × 10^9/L. These patients typically require cytoreductive agents in addition to phlebotomy, and aspirin is usually held off until platelet counts are <1500 × 10^9/L.
- Treatment for *intermediate-risk patients* must be individualized, as data are insufficient to clearly support either a conservative (low-risk) or an aggressive (high-risk) treatment plan. Typically, these patients are treated with phlebotomy, aspirin, and management of cardiovascular risk factors to limit thrombotic risk. Patients with

TABLE 9-3	THROMBOTIC RISK FACTORS IN POLYCYTHEMIA VERA AND ESSENTIAL THROMBOCYTHEMIA

Thrombotic risk factors typically requiring cytoreduction
   Age >60
   Prior thrombosis
   Platelets >400 × 10^9 to 600 × 10^9/L

Emerging thrombotic risk factors: treatment is individualized
   Cardiovascular risk factors: smoking, obesity, hypertension, hypercholesterolemia, diabetes, coronary artery disease
   Leukocytes >15 × 10^9/L: polycythemia vera
   Leukocytes >8.7 × 10^9/L: essential thrombocythemia

elevated platelets ($>400 \times 10^9$ to 600×10^9/L) or elevated leukocytes ($>15 \times 10^9$/L) may need to be treated more like high-risk patients, but data and consensus are still developing here.

Pharmacologic Agents

- Hydroxyurea, interferon-alpha, and anagrelide are the most commonly used cytoreductive agents. Hydroxyurea acts to decrease all three blood lines. It has been particularly useful in patients with extensive pruritus. Long-term use of hydroxyurea has been suggested to increase the risk of leukemogenesis (mean time to transformation, ~15 years). This has been difficult to assess in MPD patients, who already have an underlying propensity toward leukemic evolution. However, in other diseases, such as sickle cell anemia, leukemogenic risk has not been seen. Long follow-up of prospective trials will be required to definitively answer this question, and some authors currently prefer its use in the elderly more than in those younger than 60. Hydroxyurea is generally well tolerated but may also cause erythema, hyperpigmentation, and distal leg ulcers. Gastrointestinal symptoms of nausea, vomiting, constipation, and diarrhea are very common with doses >60 mg/kg.
- **Interferon-alpha** decreases both the red cell number and the frequency of thrombohemorrhagic events. As in CML, it effects the stem cell compartment, and reversal of JAK2 mutational status can be seen. It must be administered subcutaneously and can cause fever, arthralgias, myalgias, alopecia, anorexia, peripheral neuropathies, and depression. ACE inhibitors should be avoided with interferon-alpha, as this may lead to granulocytopenia and thrombocytopenia.
- **Anagrelide** primarily effects platelet production and is more commonly used in PV for thrombocytosis. Side effects include palpitations, tachycardia, nausea, diarrhea, and fluid retention.
- Agents such as **radioactive phosphorus** and **alkylating agents** also are cytoreductive agents but are associated with increased transformation to AML and are rarely used today.
- Additional agents can be useful in symptom management. Hyperuricemia may be treated with allopurinol. Erythromelalgia may be treated with ASA or other NSAIDs. Hemorrhage should be managed with platelet transfusion, since platelets have abnormal function in PV. Pruritus is often poorly responsive to antihistamines but may respond to cimetidine or cyproheptadine. If these agents fail, cytoreductive agents may be needed.

Prognosis
Patients with PV who are treated have a mortality rate similar to that of age-matched controls. Death is secondary to thrombosis in 30% to 40% of patients. Myelofibrosis is the cause of death in ~5% of patients, and hemorrhage is the cause in 2% to 10% of patients.

Special Topics
   Surgery. Elective surgery should be avoided in patients with poorly controlled polycythemia, as 75% will have hemorrhagic or thrombotic complications, and mortality is high. Platelet counts and Hct should be controlled for at least 2 months before surgery, if possible. Thromboembolic prophylaxis should be used as well. Splenectomy is rarely recommended in PV patients because of the high risk of surgical complications.
   Polycythemia Vera and Pregnancy. There is an increased incidence of premature births, pre-eclampsia, and hemorrhage in PV patients. Management should include phlebotomy and low-dose ASA. ASA should be discontinued ~5 days prior to delivery to limit hemorrhagic risk. If cytotoxic treatment is needed, interferon-alpha is the agent of choice, as it has not been shown to be teratogenic or leukemogenic.

ESSENTIAL THROMBOCYTHEMIA OR
ESSENTIAL THROMBOCYTOSIS

Background

ET is a stem cell disorder whose distinguishing characteristic is a markedly elevated platelet count caused by excessive megakaryocyte proliferation. The activating JAK2 V617F mutation is seen in nearly half of patients with ET, and patients also may have other clinical features of PV. Studies of X chromosome inactivation suggest that ET is a heterogeneous disease and both monoclonal and polyclonal evolution has been noted.

Epidemiology

ET occurs at an incidence of between 1.5 and 2.5 per 100,000 with most patients >50 years old and an equal male:female distribution. There is a bimodal distribution with a second population of younger and predominantly female patients.

Clinical Presentation

Symptoms generally are related to hemorrhage and vasoocclusion, although most patients are asymptomatic at diagnosis. Bleeding is commonly from mucous membranes, skin, and GI tract and is rarely life-threatening. Vaso-occlusion may cause erythromelalgia (burning pain, increased skin warmth, and erythema of the feet and hands), transient ischemic attacks, visual disturbances, headache, seizures, and dizziness. Large vessel involvement has also been reported with MI and cerebrovascular accidents. A small percentage of patients may experience pruritus. Physical exam findings are generally limited to splenomegaly and easy bruising.

Management

Diagnosis

Patients have an elevated platelet count, with large platelets visible on peripheral smear. Granulocytes may be increased, with mild basophilia and rare early forms. Serum B_{12} and leukocyte alkaline phosphatase scores are generally normal. Iron deficiency must be ruled out. Bone marrow findings are commonly nondiagnostic and include hypercellularity with granulocyte hyperplasia and increased megakaryocytes. The megakaryocytes are large, are often clustered, and may exhibit mild atypia. JAK2 V619F is seen in nearly half of ET patients.

Diagnostic Criteria. At Washington University we have begun incorporating JAK2 status into the diagnostic criteria (Table 9-2). Other causes of reactive (secondary) thrombocytosis should be carefully sought and include splenectomy, trauma, cancer, acute and chronic inflammation, infection, and iron deficiency. C-reactive protein and sedimentation rate can be useful in this evaluation. If iron stores are absent, iron replacement is initiated, which may uncover PV in some patients. Philadelphia chromosome also should be evaluated to rule out CML. Ultimately, bone marrow biopsy may be required to differentiate ET from other myelodysplastic syndromes.

Clinical Course

The natural history of untreated patients with ET is frequently benign but may include recurrent thrombotic and hemorrhagic events for some high-risk patients.

Treatment

- The goals of treatment focus on maintaining platelet counts of $<600 \times 10^9/L$ ($<400 \times 10^9/L$ if possible) and limiting thrombohemorrhagic risk. Thrombotic risk has been linked to age (>60 years old), prior thrombosis, and platelet count $>400 \times 10^9$ to $600 \times 10^9/L$. Other risk factors that are still emerging and being validated include elevated leukocytes ($>8.7 \times 10^9$/L), positive JAK2 V617F mutation, and cardiovascular risk factors including diabetes, obesity, smoking, hypertension, hyperlipidemia, and hypercholesterolemia (Table 9-3). Thus treatment can be risk stratified into:

- *Low-risk patients* are <60 years old, with no prior thrombotic event and a platelet count <400 $\times$ 10^9 to 600 $\times$ 10^9/L. These patients are managed with low-dose aspirin and observation.
- *High-risk patients* are ≥60 years old or have a history of thrombosis. These patients require cytoreductive agents such as hydroxyurea, interferon-alpha, and anagrelide, with aggressive treatment of reversible risk factors.
- *Intermediate-risk patients* require individualized therapy.
- Aspirin is commonly used to prevent thrombosis but should be withheld once platelet counts are >1500 $\times$ 10^9/L due to bleeding risk. As discussed in the PV section above, hydroxyurea has been suggested to increase the risk of leukemic transformation in MPD patients (mean time to transformation, ~15 years). However, patients with MPDs are already at risk of transformation. Accurately assessing a small, increased risk by hydroxyurea treatment is difficult and the data remain murky. In young patients, it is not unreasonable to start with anagrelide, which has not been linked to leukemogenesis. However, the combination of anagrelide and aspirin has been shown to increase the risk of bleeding compared to hydroxyurea and aspirin. In patients who require aspirin, especially those >60 years, hydroxyurea is still typically the first-line agent. In younger patients, alternatives include anagrelide monotherapy and interferon-alpha.
- Management of thrombosis typically requires either lifelong aspirin, for arterial thrombosis, or Coumadin, for venous thrombosis. In addition, other risk factors should be aggressively managed including platelet count, leukocyte count, and cardiovascular risk factors.
- Rarely, symptomatic, extreme thrombocytosis may be managed with thrombopheresis, although the results are short-lived and must be combined with other modalities of therapy.
- Symptoms of gout may be managed with allopurinol. Vaso-occlusive symptoms may respond to ASA alone. Like PV, pruritus may respond to cimetidine or cyproheptadine.

Prognosis

Patients generally have an excellent prognosis and appear to have median survivals similar to those of age-matched controls. Morbidity and mortality are related to thrombotic and hemorrhagic events. Transformation to AML is relatively rare, but risk is increased in patients treated with multiple cytotoxic drugs.

Special Topics

Surgery. Splenectomy poses a high risk for patients with ET and an increased platelet count and is contraindicated.

Essential Thrombocythemia and Pregnancy. Pregnant patients are at higher risk of early miscarriage complications and are often treated with ASA. As the pregnancy progresses, the platelet count usually decreases toward the normal range but may rebound quickly after delivery. Aspirin should be discontinued ~5 days prior to delivery to limit hemorrhagic risk.

CHRONIC IDIOPATHIC MYELOFIBROSIS (AGNOGENIC MYELOID METAPLASIA)

Background

CIMF is a clonal disorder thought to arise from a primitive lymphohematopoietic precursor. Patients have clonal circulating red cells, granulocytes, and platelets and their marrow is fibrotic due to a reactive, polyclonal proliferation of fibroblasts and other mesenchymal cells induced by the neoplastic cells. The neoplastic cells also emigrate from the marrow and establish sites of extramedullary hematopoiesis (myeloid metaplasia) in various sites throughout the body. One third of cases of CIMF harbor cytogenetic abnormalities at diagnosis and often transform to AML. Common genetic abnormalities found in CIMF are mutations in JAK2 (35% to 55%), the retinoblastoma susceptibility gene, and the p53 gene as well as abnormalities of the RAS family of proto-oncogenes. Neoangiogenesis is particularly active in CIMF compared with the other myeloproliferative syndromes.

Epidemiology

CIMF is the least common of the MPDs, with an annual incidence of 0.2 to 1.5 cases per 100,000. The typical case is a male older than age 50. The median age at diagnosis ranges from 54 to 65, and 70% of cases are diagnosed after age 60. No common etiologic factor has been identified, though there are sporadic reports of an association with radiation and benzene exposure.

Presentation

Symptoms and Physical Exam

Two thirds of patients are symptomatic at diagnosis from the effects of hypercatabolism, cytopenias or extramedullary hematopoiesis (Table 9-4). Bone pain may also be a prominent feature. Splenomegaly is very common, with 85% to 100% of patients having it at diagnosis, and it is frequently progressive, with up to 35% of patients developing massive splenomegaly (extending into the pelvis). Two thirds of patients will have hepatomegaly and 10% will have peripheral lymphadenopathy. A minority of patients will develop portal hypertension, with the associated signs and symptoms.

Lab Analysis

The CBC is usually abnormal in CIMF. Fifty to seventy percent of persons will be anemic at presentation, some severely, with 25% of persons having a Hgb of <8 g/dL. Other abnormalities are variably present: leukocytosis (50%), leucopenia (7%), thrombocytosis (28%), and thrombocytopenia (37%). The peripheral smear shows a leukoerythroblastic picture with teardrop poikilocytes, nucleated red cells, and anisocytosis. Abnormalities in immunologic studies are found in 50% of patients and include autoantibodies, polyclonal hyperglobulinemia, a positive Coombs test, and monoclonal antibodies.

Management

Diagnosis

In contrast to the other myeloproliferative syndromes, there are no universally accepted diagnostic criteria for CIMF. During bone marrow biopsy, marrow may not be attainable by aspiration secondary to fibrosis, resulting in a "dry tap." Findings on marrow exam include increased cellularity, granulocyte hyperplasia, and megakaryocyte dysplasia.

TABLE 9-4	CLINICAL MANIFESTATION OF CIMF	
Hypercatabolic State	**Extramedullary Hematopoiesis**	**Cytopenias**
Fatigue	Splenomegaly	Anemia
Weight loss	Portal hypertension	Thrombocytopenia
Nocturnal sweating	Tumor mass effects	
Pruritus	Pulmonary hypertension	
Hyperuricemia		

Reticulin staining is increased, and variable degrees of fibrosis are present. The diagnosis is usually made by the constellation of increased marrow reticulin or collagen fibrosis, typical leukoerythroblastic peripheral blood findings, and splenomegaly in the absence of other known disorders such as ET, PV, CML, and AML-M7.

Diagnostic Criteria

- Diagnostic criteria consist of splenomegaly, a leukoerythroblastic smear, a normal red cell mass, bone marrow with fibrosis that is not secondary to an identifiable cause, and absence of the Philadelphia chromosome.
- Other causes of bone marrow fibrosis, including cancers metastatic to the marrow, CML, myelodysplasia with fibrosis, other MPDs, infection, and lymphoma, must be ruled out. In addition, the marrow may not be fibrotic early in the course of the disease, further complicating the diagnosis. Careful morphologic exam of the bone marrow, as well as cytogenetic studies, may help to differentiate among disorders.
  - The diagnosis of *osteosclerosis* is made when sclerotic lesions by x-ray are present along with the criteria for CIMF. These lesions occur in up to 50% of patients and may cause severe pain.

Clinical Course

The course of CIMF is highly variable and most of the morbidity and mortality is due to progressive marrow failure, thrombosis, hypersplenism, advanced age, and evolution into AML. Approximately 7% of patients will develop portal hypertension related to increased portal flow from massive splenomegaly as well as intrahepatic obstruction related to thrombosis in small portal veins. Associated ascites and variceal bleeding may occur. Progressive splenomegaly may lead to **splenic infarction**, which presents acutely with fever, nausea, and left upper quadrant pain. Patients may develop neutrophilic dermatoses, which appear as tender plaques. Extramedullary hematopoiesis may develop in many sites, including the spleen, liver, lymph nodes, serosal surfaces, paraspinal or epidural spaces, and urogenital system.

Treatment

- Conventional therapy, including **supportive care,** does not alter the natural history of CIMF. Low-risk patients with only mild splenomegaly should initially be observed. Those with progressive organomegaly and/or leukocytosis or thrombocytosis should be initially managed with hydroxyurea. Those with painful or massive splenomegaly and those with portal hypertension should be considered for either splenic irradiation or splenectomy. Those who develop anemia in the setting of cytopenias should be treated with androgens, transfusion, and exogenous erythropoietin. Those who develop anemia and increased WBC and/or platelet counts should be managed with corticosteroids and transfusions.
- **Splenectomy** may alleviate mass-related symptoms, portal hypertension, refractory anemia, and thrombocytopenia. Prolonged benefit has been seen; however, serious perioperative complications, including bleeding, thrombosis, and infection, occur in nearly 30% of persons. Therefore, it should be reserved for patients who have not responded to more conservative management for these symptoms. The median survival for patients undergoing splenectomy is 2 years. There is an increased risk for leukemic transformation in those individuals who undergo splenectomy.
- **Splenic irradiation** usually controls pain and other symptoms related to splenomegaly (94% of the time for a median of 6 months). But the associated toxicity is not trivial. Severe cytopenias may develop in up to 43% of irradiated patients, of which 13% may be fatal due to infections and hemorrhage. Toxicity is not related to radiation dose, so blood counts must be monitored closely with

treatment. In addition, radiation therapy does not improve the anemia and, therefore, is generally used for patients who are not surgical candidates.

- **Thalidomide**, with or without a tapering course of steroids, has shown some promise in ameliorating both splenomegaly and cytopenias. Unfortunately it is poorly tolerated, with up to two thirds of persons stopping the medication within 6 months. **Lenalidomide** may have similar benefits, with better tolerability. These and other targeted therapies have been associated with a hyperproliferative syndrome requiring rescue hydroxyurea for leukocytosis and/or thrombocytosis.
- **Allogeneic stem cell transplantation** is the only therapy that offers the chance to eliminate marrow fibrosis and potentially cure patients. With standard myeloablative conditioning regimens there is significant morbidity and mortality. Reduced-intensity conditioning regimens may abrogate some of these complications. Transplantation should be considered in young patients with a poor prognosis and a histocompatible donor.

Prognosis
CIMF carries the worst prognosis of all the MPDs, with a median survival of ~3.5 to 5.5 years. However, the prognosis is variable and ranges from <3 to >10 years. Poor prognostic features include advanced age and anemia (Hgb < 10 g/dL). Additional findings that indicate a poor prognosis include thrombocytopenia, leukocytosis, systemic symptoms, immature granulocytes, certain karyotype abnormalities, and circulating blasts. The degree of fibrosis does not appear to be related to prognosis. The median survival of patients <56 years old with none or one of these factors is 176 months, as opposed to 33 months for those with two or three factors. Patients with CIMF die of infection, hemorrhage, heart failure, and leukemic transformation. The rate of progression to acute leukemia is ~20% over 10 years.

HYPEREOSINOPHILIC SYNDROMES

Background

Two syndromes compose this category: chronic eosinophilic leukemia (CEL) and idiopathic hypereosinophilic syndrome (HES). They should be suspected when the peripheral eosinophil count is persistently >1500/μL. The diagnosis of these disorders requires ruling out other causes of eosinophilia, such as underlying infection, allergy, autoimmune disease, pulmonary disease, clonal lymphoid disorder, and other MPDs. Also, the peripheral eosinophilia should be accompanied by an elevated eosinophil count in bone marrow and characteristic end-organ damage.

Epidemiology

The incidence of these disorders is unknown. There is a striking male predilection, with a male:female ratio of 9:1. The peak incidence is in the fourth decade.

Clinical Presentation

Ninety percent of patients will have symptoms at diagnosis. Characteristically, patients will complain of various nonspecific constitutional symptoms such as fever, fatigue, cough, pruritus, diarrhea, angioedema, and muscle pains. Infiltrating eosinophils will produce end-organ damage in the majority of patients within 3 years of diagnosis. Cardiac disease is the major cause of death but virtually every organ system maybe involved, leading to protean clinical manifestations (Table 9-5).

TABLE 9-5	CLINICAL MANIFESTATION OF CHRONIC EOSINOPHILIC LEUKEMIA/HYPEREOSINOPHILIC SYNDROME (CEL/HES)

Cardiac
  Constrictive pericarditis
  Fibroplastic endocarditis
  Myocarditis
  Intramural thrombosis

Central nervous system
  Mononeuritis multiplex
  Peripheral neuropathy
  Paraparesis
  Cerebellar dysfunction
  Epilepsy
  Dementia
  Cerebral vascular accident
  Eosinophilic meningitis

Pulmonary
  Infiltrates
  Fibrosis
  Pleural effusions
  Pulmonary emboli

Skin
  Angioedema
  Urticaria
  Papulonodular lesions
  Erythematous plaques

Gastrointestinal
  Ascites
  Diarrhea
  Gastritis
  Colitis
  Pancreatitis
  Cholangitis
  Hepatitis

Musculoskeletal
  Arthritis
  Arthralgias
  Myalgias
  Raynaud phenomenon

Management

Diagnosis

The diagnosis is usually suspected based on peripheral eosinophilia and some constellation of the symptoms reviewed in Table 9-4. CEL is due to an autonomous proliferation of clonal cells. HES is diagnosed when the diagnostic criteria for CEL are satisfied, but without evidence of clonality or myeloid cell proliferation. Recently, a molecular defect has been identified in about half of CEL/HES cases. It is a specific interstitial deletion on chromosome

4 that results in the expression of a FIP1L1-PDGFRA fusion tyrosine kinase. This fusion kinase is sensitive to inhibition by imatinib.

Diagnostic Criteria. Diagnosis relies on the exclusion of all possible causes of reactive eosinophilia. Also, patients must be evaluated and ruled out for T cell lymphomas, Hodgkin lymphoma, mastocytosis, ALL, AML, CML, PV, ET, CIMF, and the myelodysplastic syndromes. If all of these exclusions are met, a diagnosis of HES can be made. If there is a clonal chromosomal abnormality or if there are >2% blasts in the peripheral blood or >5% but <19% blasts on bone marrow aspirate, then the diagnosis is CEL. If there are ≥20% blasts on bone marrow aspirate, then the diagnosis is AML.

Treatment
- Treatment is aimed at those with end-organ damage. Corticosteroids reduce peripheral eosinophil numbers and the toxicity of the eosinophilic granules. Steroid-resistant patients are treated with various single-agent or combination therapies, including hydroxyurea, interferon, vincristine, and etoposide.
- Several recent studies have shown the efficacy of imatinib in the treatment of both CEL and HES. Notably, responses are seen both in patients with recognized mutations of the FIP1L1-PDGFRA kinase, the assumed target of imatinib in this disease, and in those without it. These dramatic responses argue that imatinib should be the first-line therapy for symptomatic CEL and HES.

Prognosis
The clinical course of both HES and CEL is markedly variable. Blast transformation may come early or very late in the clinical course. Features that predict a poor prognosis are marked splenomegaly, cytogenetic abnormalities, dysplastic myeloid features, and increased peripheral or marrow blast counts. Long-term survival is possible. In one case series up to 42% of persons were still alive 15 years after diagnosis.

KEY POINTS TO REMEMBER

- The myeloproliferative syndromes are a heterogeneous group of clonal stem cell disorders that can have significant clinical overlap.
- JAK2V617F is seen in nearly all patients with PV and many patients with other MPDs.
- The diagnosis of CIMF, CEL/HES, PV, or ET requires the exclusion of secondary causes.
- MPDs may evolve into acute leukemia.
- Myelofibrosis carries the poorest overall prognosis of the myeloproliferative syndromes.
- Thrombotic risk factors should be carefully sought and reversed.
- Addition of cytoreduction therapy for PV and ET is based on both elevated cell lines and thrombotic risk.
- Treatment for CEL and HES should be reserved for those with end-organ damage.
- Imatinib has shown dramatic activity in CEL/HES and should probably be considered the treatment of choice.

The diagnostic criteria for the myeloproliferative syndromes are not absolute rules, and the patient's entire clinical picture should be taken into consideration.

REFERENCES AND SUGGESTED READINGS

Arana-Yi C, Quintas-Cardama A, Giles F, et al. Advances in the therapy of chronic idiopathic myelofibrosis. *Oncologist.* 2006;11:929–943.

Brito-Babapulle F. The eosinophilias, including the idiopathic hypereosinophilic syndrome. *Br J Haematol.* 2003;121:203–223.

Campbell PJ, Green AR. The myeloproliferative disorders. *N Engl J Med.* 2006;355:2452–2466.

Penninga EI, Bjerrum OW. Polycythaemia vera and essential thrombocythaemia: current treatment strategies. *Drugs.* 2006;66:2173–2187.

Richard R. *Myeloproliferative Disorders. American Society of Hematology Self-Assessment Program.* 2nd ed. Malden, MA: Blackwell; 2006:152–189.

Schwarz J, Pytlik R, Doubek M, et al. Analysis of risk factors: the rationale of the guidelines of the Czech Hematological Society for diagnosis and treatment of chronic myeloproliferative disorders with thrombocythemia. *Semin Thromb Hemost.* 2006;32:231–245.

Transfusion Medicine

10

James C. Mosley, III

INTRODUCTION

Blood product transfusion can be lifesaving in the appropriate situation. However, these products are a limited resource that should be given only in specific indicated situations. The physician ordering a blood product should have a thorough understanding of what is being transfused to ensure the appropriate use of resources.

PRETRANSFUSION TESTING

All donors and recipients of blood products are required to undergo testing to help protect against adverse transfusion reactions. **Donors** must meet minimum requirements for weight, blood pressure, and hematocrit (Hct). Before donation, individuals are screened for high-risk behavior that may put them at risk for transfusion-associated diseases such as Creutzfeldt-Jakob disease, HIV, and hepatitis. Donor units are screened for hepatitis B surface antigen, hepatitis B core antibody, hepatitis C virus antibody, HIV-1 and HIV-2 antibody (anti–HIV-1 and anti–HIV-2), HIV p24 antigen, human T cell leukemia virus (HTLV)-I and HTLV-II antibody (anti–HTLV-I and anti–HTLV-II), and syphilis. Table 10-1 lists the approximate risks of infection from blood transfusion. **Compatibility testing** of blood products is comprised of blood typing, an antibody screen, and crossmatch. Donor and recipient blood are classified by ABO group and Rh blood types. Naturally occurring IgM antibodies against red cell antigens of the ABO system are capable of fixing complement and lead to immediate hemolytic reactions when ABO-incompatible blood is transfused. Before red cell transfusions, an *antibody screen* is performed in which the patient's serum is screened against a panel of red cells containing antigens responsible for most hemolytic reactions via an indirect antiglobulin test. Most alloantibodies are IgG antibodies resulting from previous exposure via transfusion or pregnancy and include antibodies to Duffy, Kell, Kidd, and Rh red cell antigens. A *major crossmatch* is an indirect antiglobulin test in which the patient's serum is incubated with donor blood cells to establish compatibility. Historically, a major crossmatch was performed on all donors but now this is reserved only for individuals with an alloantibody detected on the antibody screen or a history of transfusion reaction suggestive of RBC incompatibility. For individuals without clinically significant alloantibodies, an *immediate spin crossmatch* is performed instead, in which the patient's serum is mixed with donor red cells. The tube is spun and read immediately. The lack of agglutination demonstrates ABO compatibility. As an alternative to the immediate spin crossmatch, a computer crossmatch may be used if the recipient's ABO blood type has been determined on two separate occasions.

TABLE 10-1	APPROXIMATE RISKS OF INFECTION FROM BLOOD TRANSFUSION		
	Risk Factor (per million)	Estimated Frequency (per unit)	No. of Deaths/Million Units
Hepatitis A	1	1/1 million	0
Hepatitis B	7–32	1/30,000 to 1/250,000	0–0.14
Hepatitis C	4–36	1/30,000 to 1/150,000	0.5–17.0
HIV	0.4–5.0	1/200,000 to 1/2 million	0.5–5.0
HTLV-I and -II	0.5–4.0	1/250,000 to 1/2 million	0
Parvovirus B19	100	1/10,000	0

HTLV, human T cell leukemia virus.

Adapted from Goodnough LT, Brecher ME, Kanter MH, et al. Transfusion medicine. First of two parts—blood transfusion. *N Engl J Med.* 1999;340:438–447.

RED CELL TRANSFUSIONS

Indications

The indication for RBC transfusion is the augmentation of O_2 delivery to tissues when O_2 delivery is impaired by anemia. Guidelines for blood transfusion have been issued by several organizations. These guidelines recommend that, among patients without known cardiac risk factors, the threshold for transfusion should be a hemoglobin (Hgb) level of 6 to 8 g/dL. They also indicate that patients with Hgb levels >10 g/dL are unlikely to benefit from, and may be harmed by, blood transfusion. Guidelines advocating a uniform "transfusion trigger" are unrealistic, as measurements of the Hgb and Hct are imprecise measures of the O_2-carrying capacity of blood. The decision for transfusion is dependent on variables such as the patient's cardiopulmonary reserve and O_2 consumption, in addition to the rate and magnitude of blood loss.

Red Cell Products

- **Whole blood** contains physiologic amounts of RBCs, platelets, and plasma proteins. Whole blood is rarely used, because whole blood units are usually divided into their individual components to maximize the use of available blood resources.
- **Packed RBCs** are composed of ~200 mL of red cells suspended in plasma and additives to a final volume of 225 to 350 mL. Each unit is predicted to raise the Hgb of a 70-kg adult by ~1 g/dL.
- **Gamma-irradiated products** are used to prevent graft-versus-host disease by depletion of donor T cells, and are used for immunocompromised patients receiving blood transfusions.

- **Cytomegalovirus (CMV)-negative** products are indicated in individuals who are CMV negative and in whom infection with CMV may produce adverse consequences (e.g., transplant recipients, pregnant women, and other immunocompromised individuals).
- **Leukoreduction** (i.e., leukocyte depletion or leuko-poor) is also considered effective at reduction of transmission of CMV because CMV is highly associated with white cells. Leukocyte depletion may prevent alloimmunization to platelets and should be used in patients who are expected to need platelet transfusions during multiple courses of chemotherapy and do not have pre-existing HLA antibodies.
- **Washed RBCs** that are processed with normal saline have a reduced content of plasma proteins. Washed blood is indicated (a) if the plasma contains antibodies known to be harmful for the intended recipient or (b) to remove constituents to which the intended recipient is known to have severe side effects. Washed RBCs are indicated when the removal of antibodies such as anti-IgA and anti-HPA-1 is needed. *The most common indication for washed RBCs is IgA deficiency in the recipient.* Washed blood is also indicated in rare recipients experiencing anaphylactic reactions to plasma components.

Dosing and Administration

Packed RBCs are stored at 1° to 6°C for up to 42 days. Red cell transfusions are given over a maximum of 4 hours through a standard 170- to 260-μm filter. Premedication with acetaminophen, 650 mg PO or PR, and diphenhydramine, 25 to 50 mg PO or IV, is used for many patients to reduce the frequency and severity of urticaria and febrile nonhemolytic reactions. Hydrocortisone, 50 to 100 mg IV, may benefit patients with recurrent febrile nonhemolytic reactions. Each unit of blood will typically **raise the Hgb by 1 g/dL** or the **Hct by 3%**. Whenever possible, transfusion should be withheld until blood typing and antibody screens are performed. In **emergency situations**, type O, Rh-negative red cells may be used when a type and screen are not available.

Complications

- **Viral infection** via blood transfusion was a great concern even before the identification of HIV in 1982. The development of highly sensitive screening assays has greatly reduced the frequency of viral transmission via transfusion over the past 20 years. All blood products are now screened for the *hepatitis B virus, hepatitis C virus, HIV-1, HIV-2, HTLV-I* and *HTLV-II*, and *syphilis*. Current rates of transmission for viral infections are too low to be measured directly and are estimated using mathematic models based on the window period in which the donor is infectious, but screening tests are negative (Table 10-1). A number of other agents, which are not routinely screened for, may be transmitted via blood transfusion, including CMV, parvovirus B19, and Creutzfeldt-Jacob disease.
- **Bacterial contamination** can result in fever, chills, and hypotension during or immediately after transfusion. The most commonly implicated organism is *Yersinia enterocolitica*, but other gram-negative organisms have been reported. The risk of infection is related directly to the length of storage.
- **Simple allergic reactions** occur from transfused allergens in the plasma, leading to local or generalized urticaria. These reactions are common and usually respond to treatment with diphenhydramine (25 to 50 mg IV q4–6h).
- **Acute hemolytic reactions** occur as a result of IgM antibodies against ABO-incompatible donor red cells. Approximately one half of acute transfusion reactions are due to clerical error and occur at frequencies estimated at 1 in 250,000 to 1 million. Patients complain of chills, dyspnea, back pain, and chest pain, which may begin immediately after commencement of transfusion. Initial signs include fever and

tachycardia, with severe reactions resulting in hypotension, disseminated intravascular coagulation (DIC), and renal failure from acute tubular necrosis. Nonimmunologic hemolysis can rarely occur from hypotonic fluids, coadministered drugs, bacterial toxins, or thermal injury. When an acute hemolytic transfusion is suspected, the **transfusion must be stopped immediately.** The blood product and patient ID should be rechecked and the blood bank notified. Blood should be sent for direct antibody testing and urine sent for free Hgb. Lab tests for DIC and hemolysis should be ordered including PT, PTT, fibrinogen, and fibrinogen degradation products, as well as bilirubin, lactate dehydrogenase, and haptoglobin. Therapy consists of aggressive hydration to maintain a urine flow >1 mL/kg/h and may require the use of loop diuretics and/or mannitol.

- **Delayed hemolytic reactions** result from reactions to minor red cell antigens in alloimmunized individuals when circulating antibodies from an amnestic response react with circulating donor red cells. Hemolysis occurs at a much slower rate than in acute reactions, with a delay of 2 to 14 days posttransfusion. Signs include an unexpected decrease in the Hgb concentration with evidence of hemolysis and development of a positive direct antibody test. Treatment is supportive, with minimal adverse effects in most patients.

- **Febrile nonhemolytic reaction** manifests as a temperature elevation occurring during or shortly after a transfusion and in the absence of any other pyrexic stimulus. It may reflect the action of antibodies against WBCs or the action of cytokines present in the transfused component or those generated by the recipient in response to transfused elements. Febrile reactions occur in ~1% of transfusions. They are more frequent in patients previously alloimmunized by transfusion or pregnancy. No routinely available pre- or posttransfusion tests are helpful in predicting or preventing these reactions. Antipyretics usually provide effective symptomatic relief. Patients who experience repeated, severe, febrile reactions benefit from receiving leukocyte-reduced components.

- **Transfusion-related acute lung injury (TRALI)** is a poorly understood and infrequently recognized form of acute respiratory distress syndrome. Donor anti-HLA, antineutrophil antibodies, or lipid products from donor red cell membranes have been postulated to react with recipient neutrophils to damage pulmonary epithelium. Transfusion-related acute lung injury is characterized by dyspnea, hypotension, and fever with bilateral pulmonary infiltrates within 1 to 8 hours of transfusion, without evidence of cardiac compromise or fluid overload. Therapy is supportive, but patients may require intensive monitoring and support that necessitates transfer to the ICU.

- **Iron overload.** One unit of packed RBCs contains 200 to 250 mg of elemental iron. In patients with thalassemia or bone marrow failure, chronic transfusions can saturate macrophages from the reticuloendothelial system, resulting in iron deposition in the liver, myocardium, and endocrine tissues, leading to organ dysfunction. Concern for iron overload occurs typically after ~100 units.

- **Transfusion-associated graft-versus-host disease** results when donor lymphocytes remain viable in the host and react with host tissue. The reaction occurs in HLA homozygous, haplotype-identical donors or in immunocompromised recipients. Rash, fever, cytopenias, and GI symptoms appear 4 to 10 days after transfusion. This condition is almost universally fatal. Gamma-irradiation of blood products effectively inactivates donor lymphocytes in the blood products.

- **Other adverse effects** associated with red cell transfusions include volume overload, especially in patients with congestive heart failure or renal failure. In these patients, frequent respiratory exams and inquiries to breathing status should be assessed. The clinician should have a low threshold for furosemide administration in patients with any suspicion of fluid overload. Hyperkalemia is a consideration, as RBCs leak potassium during storage. Hypocalcemia may result from massive transfusion due to calcium binding with the citrate preservative in the bag.

PLATELET TRANSFUSIONS

Indications

Platelet transfusions reduce the risk of spontaneous hemorrhage in individuals with thrombocytopenia secondary to impaired bone marrow function or in those with dilutional thrombocytopenia secondary to the massive transfusion of red cells. In general, transfusions are *not indicated* in conditions in which there is increased platelet destruction, such as idiopathic thrombocytopenic purpura (ITP), thrombotic thrombocytopenic purpura (TTP), and DIC, except in the presence of active bleeding. In stable patients, a transfusion threshold of <10,000 cells/μL is similar in outcome to a threshold <20,000 cells/μL with respect to bleeding complications. In contrast, patients with myelodysplasia or aplastic anemia can often be observed without transfusion. Therapeutic transfusions are *indicated* in individuals with bleeding secondary to thrombocytopenia. In surgical patients, a transfusion trigger at 50,000 cells/μL is adequate for most surgical and invasive procedures, and a trigger at 100,000 cells/μL for neurosurgical procedures is generally accepted. The trigger for platelet transfusion must be considered within the clinical context of each individual patient and factors such as fever, infection, qualitative platelet defects (e.g., von Willebrand disease [vWD], uremia, cirrhosis), a precipitous drop in platelet count, and planned procedures all can contribute to the decision for transfusion.

Platelet Products

- **Pooled platelets** or **random donor platelets** are concentrates of platelets separated from single units of whole blood and suspended in 40 to 70 mL of the original plasma. Random donor units are required to contain >5.5 × 10^{10} platelets in 75% of tested units. Usually, 6 donor platelet units (often called a "six-pack") is used at a time.
- **Single-donor platelets** or **apheresis platelets** are produced by cell separator systems that remove platelets and cellular components while returning blood and plasma to the donor. One single donor unit replaces 4 to 8 units of random donor platelets and is suspended in between 100 and 500 mL of plasma. Units are required to contain >3 × 10^{11} platelets in 75% of tested units and have been shown to be equivalent to pooled platelets. The use of apheresis platelets may reduce disease transmission by reducing the number of donor exposures but costs 50% to 100% more than pooled platelets.
- **Leukocyte-reduced platelets** are derived from either a single or a random donor source and contain <5 × 10^{6} leukocytes. As with red cell transfusions, leukocyte-reduced platelets are indicated for the prevention of recurrent febrile, nonhemolytic transfusion reaction, HLA alloimmunization, and transfusion-transmitted CMV infection.

Dosing and Administration

Platelets are stored at room temperature for a maximum of 5 days. Crossmatching is generally not required. Premedication is not necessary, and each unit must be transfused over a maximum of 4 hours. The usual dose in an adult patient is 4 to 8 units of pooled platelets or 1 apheresis platelet unit. In general, 1 unit of random donor platelets is expected to increase the platelet count of a 70-kg adult by 5000 to 10,000 cells/μL for a period of 2 to 3 days. Dosing of platelets is often imprecise, because the number of platelets contained within each unit is not standardized.

Complications

- **Platelet-related sepsis** results from bacterial contamination of platelet products. As a consequence of storage at room temperature, the incidence is much higher than in red cell transfusion and is estimated to be 1 in 12,000, with a mortality rate of 26%. Implicated organisms include *Staphylococcus aureus*, *Klebsiella pneumoniae*, *Serratia marcescens*, and *Staphylococcus epidermidis*. No accepted method exists for identifying contaminated products, but it should be considered in individuals who develop fever within 6 hours of transfusion.
- **Platelet refractoriness** results in a platelet response less than predicted and is thought to be the result of HLA alloantibodies in transfusion recipients. Platelet response is assessed by measuring the platelet count before and 10 to 60 minutes after transfusion. A corrected count increment (CCI) of <5000 is indicative of platelet refractoriness.

$$CCI = [(\text{posttransfusion platelet count} - \text{pretransfusion platelet count})/ \text{number of platelets transfused}] \times \text{body surface area}$$

- Platelet transfusions from HLA-matched donors or platelet crossmatching techniques may reduce refractoriness in selected patients.

PLASMA PRODUCTS

Indications

Plasma products contain various amounts of the coagulation factors necessary for hemostasis. Plasma products are available for use in replacement of some or all plasma proteins. In addition, a number of products created by recombinant DNA technologies are available for the replacement of factors VIII and IX in patients with hemophilia.

Whole-Plasma Products

- **Fresh-frozen plasma** (FFP) consists of the fluid portion of blood that is separated and placed at $-18°C$ or below for ≤1 year and is available in units of ~200 mL. By definition, 1 mL of undiluted plasma contains 1 IU of each coagulation factor.
- **Donor-retested FFP** is produced from single units of plasma, and the donor must come back and test negative for transfusion-associated viral infections on a second donation 112 days later before the first donation is released. This practice reduces the risk of viral transmission, because testing spans the window period in which an individual may be infected but possess negative serologies.
- **Solvent/detergent-treated plasma** is produced from single units of FFP that are pooled in lots of 2500 units and treated with the solvent tri-*N*-butyl phosphate and the detergent Triton X-100 to destroy any lipid-bound viruses, including HIV, hepatitis B virus, hepatitis C virus, and HTLV-I and -II. The process does not destroy nonenveloped viruses such as parvovirus and hepatitis A.
- **Transfusion of FFP** is indicated for patients who are actively bleeding or about to undergo surgery and have clinically significant coagulation abnormalities requiring replacement of multiple plasma coagulation factors. Patients on warfarin (Coumadin) who require immediate reversal, patients with thrombotic thrombocytopenic purpura, and patients with factor deficiencies for which no concentrates are available may all benefit from transfusion of FFP. The initial transfusion is 2 units, followed by repeat measurement of the patient's PT/PTT to gauge the need for further FFP.

Fractionated Products

- **Cryoprecipitate** is prepared by thawing FFP at 1° to 6°C and recovering the cold-insoluble precipitate. Each unit of cryoprecipitate should contain 80 IU of factor

VIII activity units and 150 mg of fibrinogen in ~15 mL of plasma and is a source of factor VIII, fibrinogen, von Willebrand factor, and factor XIII. Cryoprecipitate is indicated for bleeding associated with fibrinogen deficiency and factor XIII deficiency. After administration of cryoprecipitate, periodic measurement of the fibrinogen level should be performed. Prophylactic fibrinogen administration is typically not performed until the fibrinogen level is <100. The cryoprecipitate component may be used as second-line therapy for vWD and hemophilia A if virally inactivated factor concentrates are unavailable.

- **Factor VIII** and **factor IX concentrates** are available from a number of different manufacturers and differ in the method of preparation and activity. Plasma-purified products are virally inactivated in some manner (pasteurization, solvent-detergent treatment, immunoaffinity purification) to reduce the risk of transmission of HIV and hepatitis B and C. Factor concentrate products produced by recombinant technology are also available and seem to pose no risk for viral transmission.
- **Von Willebrand factor–containing factor VIII concentrates** are indicated in type 2B, 2N, and type 3 vWD. In addition, these products may be used in type 1 or 2A vWD, unresponsive to desmopressin (DDAVP). Only humate-P has been licensed by the FDA for use in vWD. Alphanate and Koate DVI are factor VIII concentrates that are not specifically licensed for vWD but also contain von Willebrand factor.
- **Prothrombin complex concentrates** can be used to treat patients with deficiencies of factors II, VII, and X. These products vary considerably in the amounts of these factors that they contain—both between the different preparations and even between individual lots.

GRANULOCYTE TRANSFUSIONS

Granulocytes collected by pheresis are rarely indicated or used because of the availability of granulocyte colony-stimulating factor and granulocyte/macrophage colony-stimulating factor. Because these products contain lymphocytes that can cause graft-versus-host disease, they are typically gamma-irradiated. Granulocytes must be transfused as soon as possible after collection, as their function deteriorates rapidly with storage. Indications for granulocyte transfusions include patients with severe neutropenia and infection who do not respond to antibiotic treatment.

BLOOD CONSERVATION

Autologous Blood Donations

Autologous blood donation may be used in patients having elective surgical procedures for which blood is usually crossmatched. Patients donate a unit of blood 1 or 2 times per week before surgery. Advantages of autologous donation include the prevention of transfusion-transmitted disease and red cell alloimmunization. Disadvantages include substantially higher costs than allogeneic donations and the discarding of blood that is not transfused. In addition, many transfusion-associated risks, such as clerical error, bacterial contamination, and volume overload, are still present with autologous transfusions.

Acute Normovolemic Hemodilution

Acute normovolemic hemodilution is the removal of blood with simultaneous infusion of acellular solutions to maintain intravascular volume before surgical blood loss. Hemodilution results in less overall RBC loss during surgery. The removed blood is held in the OR and is reinfused during or after surgery to maintain the desired Hgb concentration.

Intraoperative Blood Recovery

Intraoperative recovery of blood involves the collection and reinfusion of red cells lost during surgery using cell-washing devices. Contraindications for the use of these devices include bacteria or other contaminants in the operative field, as they are not completely removed by the washing devices. Cancer is a relative contraindication because of the potential for aspiration and dissemination of malignant cells. Although recovery of blood has not been shown to reduce transfusion requirements in several controlled trials, blood salvaged during surgery is readily available and less costly than donor units.

KEY POINTS TO REMEMBER

- Blood products are a limited resource and should be infused only when clinically indicated.
- The most common indication for washed RBCs is IgA deficiency in the recipient.
- Although there are some guidelines regarding red cell transfusions, they are imprecise and consideration must be given to the clinical situation of each individual patient.
- Infectious complications from blood products are exceedingly rare today, but these risks must still be weighed when deciding to transfuse the patient.
- When an acute hemolytic transfusion is suspected, the transfusion must be stopped immediately.
- When a plasma product is indicated, the product most directly targeted to the hematologic defect should be used.

REFERENCES AND SUGGESTED READINGS

American Association of Blood Banks. Circular of information for the use of human blood and blood components. Available at: http://www.aabb.org. Accessed: March 25, 2003.

American College of Physicians. Practice strategies for elective red blood cell transfusion. *Ann Intern Med.* 1992;116:403–406.

American Society of Anesthesiologists. Practice guidelines for blood component therapy. A report by the American Society of Anesthesiologists Task Force on Blood Component Therapy. *Anesthesiology.* 1996;84:732–747.

College of American Pathologists. Practice parameter for the use of red blood cell transfusions. *Arch Pathol Lab Med.* 1998;122(2):130–138.

Consensus Conference. Perioperative red blood cell transfusion. *JAMA.* 1988;260:2700–2703.

Expert Working Group. Guidelines for red blood cell and plasma transfusions for adults and children. *CMAJ.* 1997;156 (Suppl 11):S1–S25.

Goodnough LT, Brecher ME, Kanter MH, et al. Transfusion medicine—blood transfusion—first of two parts. *N Engl J Med.* 1999;340:438–447.

Goodnough LT, Brecher ME, Kanter MH, et al. Transfusion medicine—blood conservation—second of two parts. *N Engl J Med.* 1999;340:525–533.

Hébert PC, Wells G, Blajchman MA, et al. A multicenter, randomized, controlled clinical trial of transfusion requirements in critical care. *N Engl J Med.* 1999;340:409–417.

Rebulla P, Finazzi G, Marangoni F, et al. The threshold for prophylactic platelet transfusions in adults with acute myeloid leukemia. *N Engl J Med.* 1997;337:1870–1875.

Sazaama, K, DeChristopher PJ, Dodd R, et al. Practice parameter for the recognition, management, and prevention of adverse consequences of blood transfusion. *Arch Pathol Lab Med.* 2000;124:61–70.

Schiffer CA, Anderson KC, Bennett CL, et al. Platelet transfusion for patients with cancer: clinical practice guidelines of the American Society of Clinical Oncology. *J Clin Oncol.* 2001;19:1519–1538.

Silliman C. Transfusion-related acute lung injury. *Transfusion.* 1999;13:177–186.

Wu W-C, Rathore SS, Wang Y, et al. Blood transfusion in elderly patients with acute myocardial infarction. *N Engl J Med.* 2001;345:1230–1236.

Sickle Cell Disease

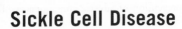

11

Meagan A. Jacoby

INTRODUCTION

Sickle cell disease (SCD) is a term for a group of genetic disorders characterized by the presence of at least one sickle gene and the predominance of hemoglobin (Hgb) S. Examples of SCD include sickle cell anemia (homozygous Hgb SS), sickle beta-thalassemia syndromes (Hgb S-beta$^+$ or S-beta^0), and Hgb SC disease. There is tremendous variability in clinical severity among disease groups and among individual patients with the same Hgb abnormalities. In the United States, these disorders are most commonly observed in African Americans and Hispanics from the Caribbean, Central America, and parts of South America and less commonly in Mediterranean, Indian, and Middle Eastern populations. In African Americans, the incidence of Hgb SS is 1:350 and that of Hgb SC is 1:835. The two hallmark pathophysiologic features of sickle cell disorders are chronic hemolytic anemia and vaso-occlusion, resulting in ischemic tissue injury.

PATHOPHYSIOLOGY

Normal Hgb is a tetramer consisting of two alpha and two beta chains. Hgb S results from the substitution of valine for glutamic acid at the sixth amino acid of the beta-globin gene. The change in the molecular structure of Hgb S results in the polymerization of the Hgb tetramers leading to the sickled shape of the RBC and increased whole-blood viscosity. Factors that contribute to Hgb S polymerization include decreased pH, RBC dehydration, and, most importantly, decreased O_2 tension. The poor deformability of the RBC containing Hgb S results in occlusion of the microvasculature and ischemic tissue injury. It is now appreciated that pro-inflammatory interactions among the sickled cell, the vascular endothelium, and circulating leukocytes and reticulocytes contribute to vaso-occlusion. Sickled RBCs adhere to and activate vascular endothelium, causing further up-regulation of endothelial adhesion molecules and recruitment and activation of WBCs. Adherent WBCs and sickled RBCs form aggregates in the microvasculature, impede blood flow, and lead to continued hypoxia. Abnormal vasomotor tone favoring vasoconstriction also contributes to vaso-occlusion. Organs prone to venous stasis such as spleen and bone marrow are susceptible to frequent vaso-occlusion and infarction.

PRESENTATION

The hallmarks of SCD are anemia due to decreased RBC life span and chronic hemolysis, and vaso-occlusion leading to acute and chronic complications secondary to end-organ dysfunction. The major causes of morbidity are acute vaso-occlusive pain crises, anemia, and infections. The clinical manifestations of SCD vary tremendously both within and among the major genotypes. Even within genotypes regarded as being the most severe for patients with SCD, some patients are entirely asymptomatic, whereas others are disabled by recurrent pain and chronic complications. SCD is associated with a shortened life expectancy due to multisystem failure from acute and chronic vaso-occlusion. One autopsy series reported causes of death in sickle cell patients, in decreasing order of frequency, as infection, stroke, therapy complications, splenic sequestration, pulmonary emboli/thrombi, renal failure, pulmonary hypertension, hepatic failure, red cell aplasia, and left ventricular dysfunction. Of note, death was sudden in 40% of the cases. In 1973, the mean survival was only 14.3 years. Currently, it is reported that the life expectancy is 42 years for men and 48 years for women with sickle cell anemia. Risk factors for mortality in SCD are frequent pain crises, acute chest syndrome (ACS), and renal and pulmonary disease.

Sickle Cell Trait

Sickle cell trait (Hgb AS) has a prevalence of ~8% to 10% in African Americans. Sickle cell trait is a benign carrier condition with no hematologic manifestations. Red cell morphology, red cell indices, and the reticulocyte count are normal. Patients with sickle cell trait have a normal life expectancy. Clinical complications of sickle cell trait have been reported, most typically splenic infarction occurring at high altitudes; hematuria; increased frequency of urinary tract infection, especially in pregnancy; and a mild defect in ability to concentrate urine. Sickle cell trait is also associated with a 30-fold increased incidence of sudden death during basic training of African American military recruits, apparently related to exercise-induced vaso-occlusion and rhabdomyolysis. Risk factors include exertion under extreme conditions, and the risk of sudden death can be reduced with measures to prevent exertional heat illness. Sickle cell trait is not a contraindication to competitive sports and screening prior to participation is not required. In individuals who appear to have sickle cell trait but are symptomatic, the lab diagnosis must be verified. Hemoglobins other than S that polymerize may account for reports of "sickle cell trait" associated with clinical problems, and these patients should be further evaluated.

Hemoglobin SC Disease

Hgb SC disease is approximately one fourth as frequent among African Americans as Hgb SS. Although deoxygenated Hgb C forms crystals, Hgb C does not participate in polymerization with deoxy–Hgb S. This results in a disease that is less severe than homozygous Hgb SS disease, and the degree of anemia and leukocytosis is frequently mild. Splenomegaly may be the only physical finding, and clinical complications may be less frequent than in sickle cell anemia. The lifespan of Hgb SC and Hgb SS red cells is 27 and 17 days, respectively. The predominant red cell abnormality on the peripheral smear is an abundance of target cells and crystal-containing cells. The frequency of acute painful episodes is approximately one half that of sickle cell anemia, and the life expectancy is two decades longer. However, there is a higher incidence of peripheral retinopathy in Hgb SC disease than Hgb SS disease. These patients may present with splenic sequestration and infarct in adulthood.

MANAGEMENT

Diagnosis

Neonatal screening resulting in timely definitive diagnosis and appropriate comprehensive care has been shown to reduce the morbidity and mortality of SCD in early childhood. Forty-four states and the District of Columbia provide universal screening for newborns, and screening upon request is provided in the other six states. When a screening test indicates SCD, a definitive diagnosis is established through further blood testing. SCD is identified through lab testing alone. There are no findings on physical exam that suggest the presence or absence of Hgb S. In adults, there may be findings that correlate with the long-term complications of the disease. The peripheral smear is normal in sickle cell trait (Hgb AS), but sickle cells are seen in each of the major SCD syndromes. Solubility testing is abnormal in all syndromes having at least one sickle cell gene and thus detects all carriers of the Hgb S gene, as well as those with the SS phenotype. Hgb electrophoresis is able to provide the clinician with the exact phenotype of SCD. Typical electrophoretic profiles are listed in Table 11-1.

ACUTE MANAGEMENT

Hematologic Complications

Acute exacerbations of anemia in the patient with SCD are a significant cause of morbidity and mortality. The most common causes of these exacerbations are splenic sequestrations and aplastic crises.

- **Acute splenic sequestration** of blood is characterized by an exacerbation of anemia, increased reticulocytosis, and a tender, enlarging spleen. Acute sequestration can progress to hypovolemic shock and death. It is associated with a 15% mortality rate, accounted for 6.6% of deaths in one autopsy series, and is common in children with SCD-SS. Patients susceptible to splenic sequestration are those whose spleens have not undergone fibrosis (i.e., young patients with sickle cell anemia and adults with Hgb SC disease or S-beta$^+$ thalassemia). The basis of therapy is simple transfusion to restore blood volume and red cell mass. Transfusion can lead to release of sequestered cells and thus overtransfusion and resulting hyperviscosity should be avoided. Because splenic sequestration recurs in 50% of cases, splenectomy is recommended after the event has abated. Acute sequestration can also occur in the liver.

- **Aplastic crises** are transient arrests of erythropoiesis characterized by abrupt falls in Hgb levels and decreased reticulocytosis. Given the decreased life span of RBC in SCD, aplastic crises place patients at risk for severe anemia that is frequently symptomatic. Parvovirus B19 accounts for the majority of aplastic crises in children with SCD, but the high incidence of protective antibodies in adults makes parvovirus a less frequent cause of aplasia. Intravenous immune globulin can be used to treat parvovirus infection. Other infections have been reported to cause transient aplasia. Aplastic crisis can also be the result of bone marrow necrosis, which is characterized by fever, bone pain, reticulocytopenia, and a leukoerythroblastic response. The mainstay of treating aplastic crises is simple transfusion to correct severe anemia. SCD patients in the peri-infection period are at increased risk for complications, including pain crisis, acute chest syndrome (ACS), and stroke. A useful guideline for transfusion is the reticulocyte count. In parvovirus B19 infection, reticulocytopenia lasts 7 to 10 days. A patient having an exacerbation of a chronic anemia with an elevated absolute reticulocyte count is less likely to require urgent transfusion than one with a normal or low absolute reticulocyte count.

- **Hyperhemolytic crisis** is the sudden exacerbation of anemia with increased reticulocytosis and elevated bilirubin level. The usual therapy for a hyperhemolytic crisis is simple transfusion. Most of these patients recover within 14 days. The diagnosis of a delayed hemolytic transfusion reaction should be considered in any patient receiving a recent blood transfusion.

- **Subacute anemia:** The gradual onset of worsening anemia may be due to developing renal insufficiency or folic acid deficiency. Chronic hemolysis results in increased use of folic acid stores and can lead to megaloblastic crises if nutritional supplementation is not undertaken.

TABLE 11-1	CLINICAL AND HEMATOLOGIC FINDINGS IN THE COMMON VARIANTS OF SICKLE CELL DISEASE							
		Hgb Electrophoresis (%)				Hematologic Value[a]		
Morphology	Clinical Severity	S	F	A_2	A	Hgb (g/dL)	MCV (fL)	RBC
SS	Usually marked	>90	<10	<3.5	0	6–11	>80	Sickle cells, target cells
SC	Mild to moderate	50	<5	—[b]	0	10–15	75–95	Sickle cells, target cells
AS	None	40–50	<5	<3.5	50–60	12–15	>80	Normal
S-beta^0	Marked to moderate	>80	<20	>3.5	0	6–10	<80	Sickle cells, target cells
S-beta$^+$	Mild to moderate	>60	<20	>3.5	10–30	9–12	<80	No sickle cells, target cells

Hgb, hemoglobin; MCV, mean corpuscular volume.

[a]Hematologic values are approximate.

[b]Fifty percent Hgb C.

Acute Painful Crisis

Acute pain is the first symptom of disease in >25% of patients. The acute painful episode is the most frequent reason for which patients with SCD seek medical attention. There is tremendous variability of painful episodes within genotypes and within the same patient over time. In one large study of patients with sickle cell anemia, one third rarely had pain, one third were hospitalized for pain approximately two to six times per year, and one third had more than six hospitalizations per year. More frequent pain crises are associated with higher mortality rates. Pain episodes may be precipitated by temperature extremes, dehydration, infection, hypoxia, acidosis, stress, menses, and alcohol consumption. In addition, patients may cite that anxiety, depression, or physical exhaustion may be precipitants. In many instances, no precipitating factors can be identified. The painful episodes can occur in any area of the body, most commonly the back, chest, extremities, and abdomen. In ~50% of painful episodes, patients will present with objective clinical signs such as fever, joint swelling, tenderness, tachypnea, hypertension, nausea, and vomiting. There is no clinical or lab finding that is pathognomonic for painful crisis.

In general, the management of acute painful crises includes the identification and treatment of possible precipitating factors, IV fluid hydration, and analgesics. When a patient presents complaining of pain, the physician is charged with ruling out etiologies other than vaso-occlusion. Acute painful episodes generally last 4 to 6 days but may vary in intensity and duration. The possibility that the pain is precipitated by a concurrent medical condition, such as an infection, should be considered, and the physician should search for a precipitating illness in every instance.

Providing aggressive relief of pain often requires the use of parenteral narcotics. Patients will often be aware of the medications and dosages that have provided adequate relief in the past, and they are often undertreated for pain. Of note, patients with SCD do not respond to conventional doses of analgesia. They typically are on chronic oral narcotics and may have developed a tolerance to conventional doses of narcotics. Patient-controlled anesthesia (PCA) pumps are effective in the treatment of an acute painful crisis. Appropriate conversion between chronic PO medications and IV doses of narcotics must be used to ensure adequate and prompt pain relief. In cases in which there is no nausea or vomiting, patients are continued on the PO regimen prescribed for continuous relief at home, and PCA-demand-only doses can be added. Demerol may be used occasionally but should be avoided if possible. Patients should be monitored frequently and objective pain scores followed closely for titration of effective analgesia.

Painful events are not commonly associated with changes in the patient's Hgb levels, and transfusions are not indicated for simple acute painful crises. Hydroxyurea reduces the frequency of painful crises.

Infections

Infections are a leading cause of morbidity and mortality in SCD patients. Outcomes for children improved with the use of prophylactic penicillin to prevent *Streptococcal pneumoniae* sepsis. Although adults are less susceptible, all patients should receive the pneumonia vaccinations. Adults with Hgb SS disease are functionally asplenic and fever should be worked up aggressively with the appropriate cultures, imaging studies, and consideration of prompt antibiotic coverage. Patients with other genotypes are also at risk for infection, although they are not always functionally asplenic. Sources of fever include sepsis, meningitis, ACS, osteomyelitis, and urinary tract infection. In meningitis, empiric coverage should include *Streptococcus pneumoniae* and *Haemophilus influenzae*. Coverage for acute chest syndrome and osteomyelitis are discussed below.

Neurologic Complications

Neurologic complications are common in patients with SCD, including transient ischemic attacks, cerebral infarction, cerebral hemorrhage, seizures, spinal cord infarction or compression, CNS infections, vestibular dysfunction, and sensory hearing loss. The risk for cerebral infarction, including clinical and silent infarctions, is as high as 30%. The highest stroke rates occur in children, and the risk of stroke by age 20 is 11%. Ischemic strokes are more common in children and those >30 years old, whereas hemorrhagic stroke is more common at between 20 and 30 years of age. **Risk factors** for strokes include severe anemia, low reticulocyte counts, low Hgb F levels, high WBC counts, the Hgb SS genotype, ACS within the previous 2 weeks, and systolic hypertension. Strokes are fatal in ~20% of initial cases, and 70% of patients will have a recurrence within 3 years. Patients with symptoms and signs of an acute stroke should be evaluated immediately. In those with hemorrhage, initial management depends on the site and amount of bleeding. In children with infarcts, prompt partial exchange transfusion is performed to reduce Hgb S to <30%. Chronic exchange transfusion therapy to maintain Hgb S levels below 30% has been shown to prevent recurrent thrombosis. At this time, it is unclear how long chronic transfusion should be maintained. Prophylactic transfusions to reduce Hgb S to <30% in children with abnormal transcranial Doppler velocity measurements in cerebral blood vessels have been shown to reduce the risk of first clinical stroke. Unfortunately, there are few systematic data on primary prevention of stroke in adults with SCD. It is unclear whether acute ischemic stroke in adults should be treated with immediate exchange transfusion as it is in children, or whether it should be approached as it is in adults without SCD (i.e., recombinant tissue plasminogen activator, aspirin, etc.) The role of chronic transfusion for secondary prevention in adults is unclear.

Pulmonary Complications

- One of the most feared acute pulmonary complications in SCD is **acute chest syndrome**. ACS is defined as a new infiltrate on chest x-ray (CXR) and one or more of the following: fever, cough, chest pain, dyspnea, tachypnea, and hypoxemia. Of note, the initial CXR may be negative. The definitive etiology of ACS is not known but infection, vaso-occlusion and infarct, fat embolism from necrotic marrow or a combination of these factors have been implicated. It has been reported to occur in 29% of patients with SCD and can progress to respiratory failure and death. ACS is the second most frequent cause of hospitalization and the most frequent complication of surgery in SCD. It should be noted, however, that nearly 50% of cases occur during hospitalization for other causes. Risk factors include prior episodes of ACS, HgB SS, leukocytosis, hospitalization for acute pain crisis, and high-baseline Hgb concentrations. Atypical and typical bacterial pathogens and viruses, especially respiratory syncytial virus (RSV), have been found in patients with ACS. Antibiotics are indicated as initial therapy, preferably a cephalosporin and a macrolide or fluoroquinolone. Hypoxemia should be corrected by supplemental oxygen. Analgesics and incentive spirometry to correct splinting from chest pain should be initiated. Bronchodilators should be considered. Either simple or exchange transfusion should be considered promptly if there is a change in oxygen status from baseline. Simple transfusion can be used if there is a need for increased O_2-carrying capacity such as mild hypoxemia or worsened anemia. Severe hypoxemia, clinical deterioration, or impending respiratory failure should lead to urgent consideration of exchange transfusion. Care in an intensive care unit and ventilator support may be required. ACS has a mortality rate of ~10%. Chronic therapy with hydroxyurea can reduce the frequency of episodes.
- **Chronic pulmonary disease** is an important cause of morbidity and mortality in patients with SCD. SCD patients may have restrictive and obstructive lung diseases,

pulmonary fibrosis, and pulmonary hypertension. Pulmonary disease is more common in those with a history of ACS. Pulmonary hypertension occurs in up to 32% of SCD patients and carries a poor prognosis, even with mean pulmonary pressure elevations in the mild to moderate range. The etiology of pulmonary hypertension in SCD is unknown, although chronic intravascular hemolysis, which impairs normal vasodilation through its effects on the nitric oxide pathway, may contribute. Diagnosis is made with cardiac catheterization or echocardiogram-Doppler study. Patients presenting with exertional dyspnea and findings of right heart failure should be evaluated promptly. There are few data on the efficacy of different treatment modalities, and maximizing supportive care, treating comorbid conditions, and employing medications used in other patient populations with pulmonary hypertension may be of benefit. These patients may be considered for hydroxyurea, pulmonary vasodilators, anticoagulation, and home O_2 therapy.

Hepatobiliary Complications

- The prevalence of pigmented **gallstones** in SCD is directly related to the rate of hemolysis. In sickle cell anemia, gallstones occur in children as young as 3 to 4 years and are eventually found in ~70% of patients. Patients presenting with fever, nausea, vomiting, and right upper quadrant pain should be evaluated for acute cholecystitis. Cholecystectomy should be considered even for asymptomatic gallstones.
- **Hepatomegaly and liver dysfunction** in SCD can be caused by multiple etiologies, including intrahepatic blood sequestration, transfusion-acquired hepatitis, transfusion-related iron overload, and very rarely autoimmune liver disease. Hepatic sequestration is characterized by a rapidly enlarging liver, decreased hematocrit, and rising reticulocyte count. Diagnosis is difficult, as CT and ultrasound show only a diffusely enlarged liver, liver function tests may be normal to moderately elevated, and the liver is variably tender. Both simple and exchange transfusion have been used to treat hepatic sequestration. As in splenic sequestration, care must be taken not to overtransfuse.
- **Benign cholestasis of SCD** results in severe, asymptomatic hyperbilirubinemia without fever, pain, leukocytosis, or hepatic failure. Progressive cholestasis with right upper quadrant pain, marked elevations in bilirubin and alkaline phosphatase, and progression to liver failure have been reported. These patients are treated with exchange transfusion and supportive care. Another serious complication is the **hepatic crisis**, in which hepatic ischemia results in fever, right upper quadrant pain, leukocytosis, severe hyperbilirubinemia, and abnormal liver function tests. It may progress to fulminant liver failure, which has a dismal prognosis. Because of the nearly uniform mortality of this type of hepatic crisis, exchange transfusion, plasmapheresis, and liver transplantation have been used as therapy, but no controlled data are available to support this approach.

Obstetric and Gynecologic Complications

Delayed menarche, dysmenorrhea, ovarian cysts, pelvic infection, and fibrocystic disease of the breast are more common in women with SCD. However, the major reproductive concern in these patients is pregnancy. The improvement in fetal and maternal outcomes is largely due to improved prenatal and high-risk obstetric care. The incidence of spontaneous abortion, intrauterine growth retardation, pre-eclampsia, placental abruption, low birth weight, and intrauterine fetal death are higher in women with SCD. Maternal complications during pregnancy include increased rates of acute painful episodes, severe anemia, infections, and even death. The course of pregnancy is more benign in Hgb SC disease. Therapeutic interventions for painful crises in pregnant women should be identical to those in nonpregnant women, with IV hydration, attention to complications, and adequate pain control. Opiates can affect fetal movement and heart rate but are not teratogenic. Transfusions are generally reserved for patients with worsening anemia (Hgb <6 g/dL) and in anticipation of surgery. Hydroxyurea has been shown to be teratogenic in animals and should be stopped in pregnancy. There is a very high incidence of acute painful episodes associated with therapeutic abortions. Inpatient IV hydration immediately before the procedure and for the 24 hours after the procedure is recommended. Oral contraceptives containing low-dose estrogen are a safe, recommended method of birth control in women with SCD.

Renal Complications

- The kidney is particularly vulnerable to complications of SCD with manifestations that result from medullary, distal and proximal tubular, and glomerular abnormalities leading to the **inability to concentrate the urine.** Papillary infarction with hematuria, renal tubular acidosis, and abnormal potassium metabolism occur more commonly in patients with SCD or sickle cell trait. Patients with hematuria should be evaluated with ultrasound.
- Patients with SCD cannot excrete acid and potassium normally but usually do not develop systemic acidosis or hyperkalemia without an additional acid load, such as in the setting of renal insufficiency. **Chronic renal insufficiency** may be predicted by albuminuria and should be suspected in the setting of hypertension and worsening anemia. Risk factors for the development of chronic renal failure include hypertension and the use of anti-inflammatory drugs. The average age at onset of chronic renal failure is 23 years in sickle cell anemia and 50 years in Hgb SC disease. The use of ACE inhibitors was found to diminish proteinuria and pathological glomerular changes; it is unclear whether their use slows the progression of sickle nephropathy. Renal transplantation is recommended for patients with end-stage renal failure.

Priapism

Priapism affects 29% to 42% of males with SCD. It peaks in frequency at 1 to 5 and at 13 to 21 years of age. Priapism is most likely to develop in patients with lower Hgb F levels and reticulocyte counts, increased platelet counts, and the Hgb SS genotype. First-line therapy is conservative, including increasing PO fluid intake and analgesia. If the episode persists for 3 hours, the patient should seek medical care. IV fluids, parenteral narcotics, and a Foley catheter to promote bladder emptying are the initial treatments for acute priapism. If the episode lasts 4 to 6 hours, penile aspiration and irrigation as well as intracavernous injection of an alpha-adrenergic agonist by a urologist should be performed. Partial exchange transfusion can be considered, although efficacy has not been proved in randomized controlled trials and it can be associated with complications in this setting. ASPEN syndrome (*a*ssociation of *S*CD, *p*riapism, *e*xchange transfusion, and *n*eurologic events), which involves headache, mental status change, neurologic deficits, and stroke, has been described in SCD patients with priapism undergoing exchange transfusion. It is important that initiation of transfusion does not delay more definitive treatment. If detumescence does not occur with nonsurgical management, a spongiosum-cavernosum or cavernosaphenous vein shunt may be recommended. Despite interventions, impotence remains a frequent complication of priapism. There is a paucity of clinical trials for the secondary prevention of priapism, although chronic transfusion according to stroke protocol, hydroxyurea, and vasoactive agents such as pseudoephedrine are used at some centers.

Ocular Complications

Anterior chamber ischemia, retinal artery occlusion, and proliferative retinopathy with the risk of subsequent hemorrhage and retinal detachment can lead to vision loss in

SCD. Sickle retinopathy is found most frequently between 15 and 30 years of age. Although found in all SCD, it is most frequent in Hgb SC. All patients who sustain eye trauma must be evaluated by an ophthalmologist urgently because they are at increased risk of visual loss. Patients should undergo a yearly retinal exam performed by an ophthalmologist. Sickle cell retinopathy may require vision-improving therapy with laser photocoagulation.

Bone Complications

- Bone and joint problems are a common cause of both acute and chronic pain in SCD. Erythroid hyperplasia secondary to chronic hemolytic anemia leads to widening of the medullary space and thinning of the trabeculae and cortices. This results in bony distortion, especially in the skull, vertebrae, and long bones. Vaso-occlusion and subsequent bone and marrow infarct are common, especially in the spine, ribs, and long bones. **Dactylitis**, painful swelling of the hands and feet, is caused by microinfarcts of the phalanges and metatarsals and usually occurs in early childhood. **Osteonecrosis** occurs in all SCD phenotypes but most frequently in sickle cell anemia with coexistent alpha thalassemia. Osteonecrosis occurs in both the femoral and the humeral heads, as well as in the vertebral bodies. The femoral heads more commonly undergo progressive destruction as a result of chronic weightbearing. MRI is the most accurate imaging study to diagnose avascular necrosis of the femoral head. Core decompression surgery to relieve increased intraosseous pressure can be used in early-stage osteonecrosis. A patient with more advanced disease is a candidate for total hip arthroplasty. This decision must take into account the likelihood that a second hip revision may be required and that there are more complications and a relatively high failure rate in patients with SCD compared to other patient populations. Vertebral infarction also occurs and leads to chronic back pain.

- **Osteomyelitis** must be differentiated from the more common bone infarction, because the two syndromes present with similar clinical and imaging findings but are treated very differently. Staphylococcus and salmonella are common pathogens for osteomyelitis in sickle cell patients. Increasing antibiotic resistance to salmonella is a major problem in SCD. Septic arthritis must also be distinguished from the more common joint effusion associated with acute painful episodes. Bone biopsy and culture are the most reliable tests to establish the diagnosis before starting long-term antibiotics.

Dermatologic Complications

Skin ulcers are major causes of morbidity in SCD. Ulcers occur commonly near the medial or lateral malleolus and are frequently bilateral. About 2.5% of patients age 10 and older develop leg ulcers. Ulcers may begin spontaneously or as a result of trauma. They are commonly infected with *Staphylococcus aureus*, *Pseudomonas*, streptococci, or *Bacterioides* species. Males have a threefold greater risk of developing leg ulcers. Therapy with gentle débridement, wet-to-dry dressings, and compression bandages is typically effective. Compression stockings may be used to prevent recurrence.

Cardiac Complications

An important cardiac consideration in the management of patients with SCD is the high cardiac output related to chronic anemia. Chronic high cardiac output can result in four-chamber enlargement and cardiomegaly. Age-dependent loss of cardiac reserve can lead to a greater risk of heart failure in adult patients during fluid overload, transfusion, or other reduced O_2-carrying capacity states. Acute myocardial infarction in the absence of coronary disease has been reported but is rare.

Chronic Management

Many patients can live for long periods without experiencing acute or severe exacerbations of the disease. Increased awareness of the disease and its long-term complications is contributing to the prolonged survival seen in sickle cell patients today.

Routine Patient Visits

- All patients with SCD should have routine office appointments to establish baseline physical findings, lab data, and a relationship between the patient and the treating physician. Patients with Hgb SS should have regular medical evaluations every 3 to 6 months, depending on the symptoms or manifestations of the disease.
- Preventive care should be initiated and maintained. A vaccination history should also be maintained. Adults should have seasonal influenza vaccines. If the patient has never received the pneumococcal vaccination, it should be offered and given at intervals based on the recommendations of the American Association of Family Physicians. Daily folic acid (1 mg PO daily) is given for the prevention of folate deficiency in the chronic hemolytic state. Retinal evaluation by an ophthalmologist is begun at school age and should be continued to monitor for evidence of retinopathy. Patients with relative hypertension are at increased risk for stroke and should be monitored and treated. Patients should be counseled during routine clinic visits about red flags for which they should seek further medical attention (Table 11-2).

Surgery and Anesthesia

- Surgery and anesthesia are stress states that can provoke a painful sickle crisis. Currently, it is recommended that patients with SCD undergo simple transfusion to a Hgb of 10 mg/dL before elective surgery. Studies comparing aggressive transfusion (Hgb S levels <30%) versus conservative transfusion (Hgb S <60%, Hgb = 10 mg/dL) showed no benefit of the more aggressive regimen. Intraoperative overexpansion of blood volume should be avoided, particularly in patients with decreased cardiac function. Hypothermia must also be avoided in the OR to prevent sickling. After surgery, IV fluid management must ensure adequate hydration, with the avoidance of volume overload and pulmonary complications. Incentive spirometry should also be employed.

TABLE 11-2	RED FLAGS THAT REQUIRE MEDICAL ATTENTION FOR PATIENTS WITH SICKLE CELL DISEASE

Fever >101°F

Lethargy

Dehydration

Worsening pallor

Severe abdominal pain

Acute pulmonary symptoms

Neurologic symptoms

Pain associated with extremity weakness or loss of function

Acute joint swelling

Recurrent vomiting

Pain not relieved by conservative measures or home medications

Priapism lasting >3 hours

- **Dental procedures** requiring local anesthesia can be performed in the dentist's office. However, any dental procedure requiring general anesthesia warrants hospital admission.

Transfusion Therapy

- Transfusion of RBCs has been used for almost every complication of SCD, although clinical trials have not been performed supporting efficacy for each complication. Indications for transfusion include the need to improve O_2-carrying capacity (as in aplastic crisis or ACS), increase blood volume (as in splenic sequestration), or improve blood rheology (to prevent stroke recurrence, prior to surgery). Simple transfusion can be sufficient to improve O_2-carrying capacity and blood volume and is generally indicated in aplastic crisis, acute splenic and hepatic sequestration, milder cases of ACS, and prior to surgery. Partial exchange transfusion has the advantage of decreasing the percentage of Hgb S without increasing the blood volume or causing hyperviscosity. It is generally recommended for acute indications such as ACS, acute ischemic stroke, retinal artery occlusion, and multiple organ failure and may be recommended for chronic transfusion programs, in which avoiding hyperviscosity and iron overload is important. Indications for chronic transfusion, which may be either simple or exchange, are primary stroke prevention for at-risk children and secondary stroke prevention in children; of note, many clinicians apply the same principles to adults with stroke. Patients with pulmonary hypertension and recurrent ACS may also benefit from chronic transfusion. The goal of transfusion is to raise the Hgb to a level of ~10 g/dL. Levels >10 g/dL can lead to hyperviscosity and increased vaso-occlusion. Transfusion is not indicated for compensated anemia, uncomplicated acute painful crises, uncomplicated pregnancy, avascular necrosis, infection, or minor surgery without anesthesia. Transfusion is controversial for priapism and leg ulcers.
- Transfusion complications in sickle cell patients are common and include alloimmunization, iron overload, and transmission of viral illness. **Alloimmunization** in transfused sickle cell patients is due in part to minor blood-group incompatibilities (Rh, Kell, Duffy, and Kidd antigens) resulting from antigenic discrepancy in the donor (mostly Caucasian) and recipient (mostly African American) pool. Five to fifty percent of SCD patients who have received multiple transfusions develop alloimmunization, which is a risk for delayed hemolytic reactions and can make obtaining compatible blood difficult. **Hyperviscosity syndrome** is characterized by a post-transfusion elevation in blood pressure and congestive heart failure, mental status change, or stroke. Treatment is exchange transfusion.
- **Iron overload** and its complications of end-organ damage become a problem in those patients who are chronically transfused. Chelation is recommended when the total-body iron level is elevated, as measured by serum ferritin levels or, more reliably, serial liver biopsy. Chelation therapy with deferoxamine (Desferal), which requires subcutaneous overnight infusion, is an extremely time-consuming and inconvenient therapy for the patient, in addition to being very expensive. This is one of the motivating factors for a reduction in the number of transfusions and the use of exchange transfusion in patients with SCD. Oral iron chelators, such as deferasirox (Exjade), are now available, although not all patients can afford or tolerate this drug. Patients with iron overload on chelation therapy are at increased risk for infection with *Yersinia enterocolitica*.

Hydroxyurea

Hydroxyurea is a cytotoxic drug that has been shown to decrease the frequency of acute pain crisis, ACS, hospital admissions, and blood transfusions and to decrease mortality in adults with Hgb SS. It is generally indicated in patients with more severe manifestations of SCD. The mechanism by which hydroxyurea influences sickle cells and vaso-occlusion is likely multifactorial, including increases in Hgb F synthesis, improved red cell deformability, modulation of sickle cell adherence properties, increased nitric oxide production, and effects on WBCs. Hydroxyurea causes a decrease in the reticulocyte, platelet, and WBC counts. The dose is titrated to achieve clinical effect with minimal toxicity. However, not all patients respond to hydroxyurea. Of note, hydroxyurea has been shown to be teratogenic in mice, and should be avoided in pregnancy. Hydroxyurea has the potential to be carcinogenic, but the exact risk is unknown.

KEY POINTS TO REMEMBER

- SCD is a group of genetic disorders characterized by the presence of Hgb S.
- Hgb S results from the substitution of valine for glutamic acid at the sixth amino acid of the beta-globin gene, which leads to the polymerization of Hgb tetramers when deoxygenated and, thus, the sickled RBC.
- Sickle cell trait is a benign carrier condition with no associated hematologic abnormalities.
- The two hallmark features of SCD are a chronic hemolytic anemia and vaso-occlusion, resulting in ischemic tissue injury.
- There is a tremendous variability in acute painful crises, even within the same patient over time.
- There is no pathognomonic clinical or lab finding for acute painful crisis, and the diagnosis is based on history and physical exam.
- The acute management of painful crises is IV fluid hydration, analgesia, and treatment of identifiable precipitating factors such as infection.
- Aplastic crisis is the transient arrest of erythropoiesis characterized by abrupt falls in Hgb and reticulocytosis. The most common causes are infections (e.g., parvovirus B19) and bone marrow necrosis.
- ACS is characterized by dyspnea, chest pain, fever, tachypnea, pulmonary infiltrates, and leukocytosis, may be indistinguishable from acute painful crisis, and is associated with a 10% mortality rate due to multisystem organ failure.
- The management of ACS is supplemental O_2, antibiotics, and partial-exchange transfusion to decrease the amount of Hgb S in the patient.
- All patients with SCD should be transfused to a Hgb of 10 mg/dL before elective surgery to decrease the risk of perioperative complications from sickling.

REFERENCES AND SUGGESTED READINGS

Beutler, E. Disorders of hemoglobin structure: sickle cell anemia and related abnormalities. In: Lichtman MA, Beutler E, Kipps TJ, et al., eds. *Williams Hematology*. 7th ed. New York: McGraw-Hill; 2006:667–700.

Bunn HF. Pathogenesis and treatment of sickle cell disease. *N Engl J Med.* 1997;337:762–769.

Gladwin MT, Sachdev V, Jison ML, et al. Pulmonary hypertension as a risk factor for death in patients with sickle cell disease. *N Engl J Med.* 2004;350:886–895.

Johnson CS. The acute chest syndrome. *Hematol Oncol Clin N Am.* 2005;19(5):857–879.

Manci EA, Culberson DE, Yang YM, et al. Causes of death in sickle cell disease: an autopsy study. *Br J Haematol.* 2003;123(2): 359–365.

National Institutes of Health. *Management of Sickle Cell Disease*. NIH publication 02-2117. Bethesda, MD: NIH.

Reid CD, Charache S, Lubin B, eds. *Management and Therapy of Sickle Cell Disease*. NIH publication 96-2117. Bethesda, MD: National Institutes of Health; 1995:1–114.

Rogers Z. Priapism in sickle cell disease. *Hematol Oncol Clin N Am*. 2005;19(5):917–928.

Stuart MJ, Nagel, RL. Sickle cell disease. *Lancet*. 2004;364:1343–1360.

Switzer J, Hess DC, Nichols FT, et al. Pathophysiology and treatment of stroke in sickle-cell disease: present and future. *Lancet Neurol*. 2006;5:501–512.

Vichinsky E, Neumayr LD, Earles AN, et al. Causes and outcomes of the acute chest syndrome in sickle cell disease. *N Engl J Med*. 2000;342;1855–1865.

Vichinsky EP, Haberkern CM, Neumayr L, et al. A comparison of conservative and aggressive transfusion regimens in the perioperative management of sickle cell disease. *N Engl J Med*. 1995;333:206–213.

Wanko S, Telen M. Transfusion management in sickle cell disease. *Hematol Oncol Clin N Am*. 2005;19(5):803–826.

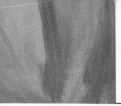

Drugs That Affect Hemostasis: Anticoagulants, Thrombolytics, and Antifibrinolytics

12

Nasreen Ilias and Mohsen Nasir

INTRODUCTION

Hemostasis is a regulatory process with two functions: (1) maintain clot-free blood flow and (2) aggressively respond to localized vascular injury with formation of a hemostatic plug. Aberrancies in this system can cause detrimental thrombus formation or the opposite, uncontrolled bleeding. When hemostasis is inappropriately or overexuberantly activated, **anticoagulants** or **thrombolytics** are used to moderate this process with a potential consequence of bleeding. **Procoagulants** are used to stop bleeding, reverse the effects of anticoagulation medications, or replenish factors required for clot formation and stabilization. An understanding of hemostasis and how various drugs disrupt coagulation is necessary to treat pathological conditions.

NORMAL HEMOSTASIS

Endothelial cells line the inner surface of blood vessels. These cells produce vasodilators that prevent platelet aggregation and block the coagulation cascade, thrombus formation, and fibrin deposition. Disruption of endothelial cells bares the subendothelial extracellular matrix (ECM), which promotes platelet adherence and activation and exposes tissue factor, a membrane-bound procoagulant factor. Tissue factor, in conjunction with secreted platelet factors, induces platelet aggregation and activates the coagulation cascade. This converts prothrombin to thrombin (factor IIa), which forms the initial hemostatic plug. Thrombin converts fibrinogen to insoluble fibrin, which forms a permanent plug.

The coagulation cascade (Fig. 12-1) is a series of enzymatic reactions with feedback promotion and inhibition that regulate and restrict the process of hemostasis to the site of vascular injury. A deficiency or decreased function of procoagulant factors or cofactors, such as vitamin K (necessary for the function of factors II, VII, IX, and X), can cause bleeding, whereas low levels or decreased function of factors involved in limiting coagulation can trigger thrombosis.

ANTICOAGULANTS: AGENTS THAT PREVENT THROMBOSIS

Antiplatelet Drugs

The adhesion of platelets (Fig. 12-2) to exposed collagen is mediated by von Willebrand factor (vWF), which links collagen fibrils to the surface of platelets. Activated platelets release factors such as thromboxane A_2 (TXA_2) and adenosine diphosphate (ADP), which bind to their respective receptors. This initiates a series of enzymatic reactions that decrease cyclic adenosine monophosphate (cAMP) levels and promote the release of the same factors

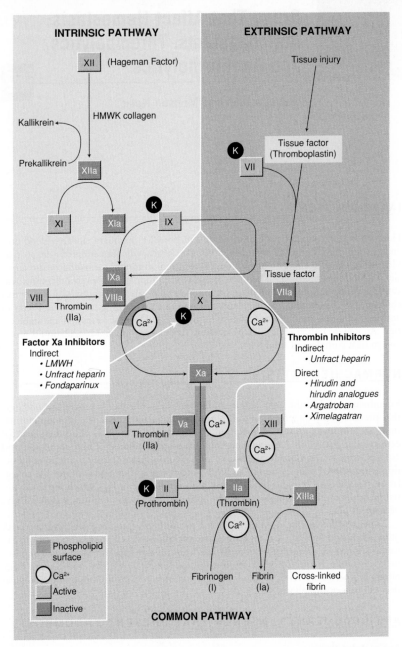

FIGURE 12-1. The coagulation cascade. The coagulation cascade is divided into two pathways, extrinsic and intrinsic, which converge at factor X, the start of the common pathway leading to thrombin formation and fibrin cross-linking. The extrinsic pathway is activated by tissue factor. Contact with subendothelial surfaces or a negatively charged surface activates factor XII (Hageman factor) and starts the intrinsic coagulation cascade. (Diagram modified from Kumar V. *Robbins & Cotran Pathologic Basis of Disease*. Philadelphia: W. B. Saunders; 2004: Fig. 4-9.)

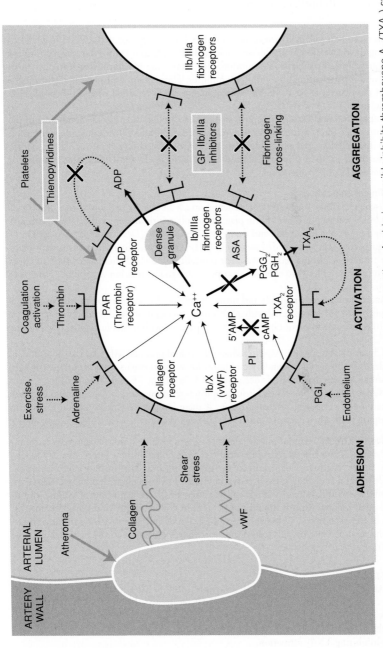

FIGURE 12-2. Mechanisms implicated in platelet adhesion, activation, and aggregation. Aspirin irreversibly inhibits thromboxane A_2 (TXA_2) synthesis, dipyridamole increases cAMP levels, clopidogrel irreversibly modifies the ADP receptor, and abciximab antagonizes the glycoprotein IIb/IIIa receptor. (Diagram from Hankey G, Eikelboom J. new drugs, old drugs antiplatelet drugs. *Med J Austral.* 2003;178[11]:568–574.)

to recruit additional platelets. Recruited platelets are connected by fibrin cross-linking of glycoprotein (GP) IIb/IIIa receptors.

Aspirin

Aspirin (acetylsalicylic acid) irreversibly inhibits cyclo-oxygenase-1 (COX-1) in platelets, blocking the conversion of arachidonic acid to TXA_2, which is involved in the recruitment and aggregation of platelets. A minimum dose of 160 mg of aspirin is required to maximally inhibit platelet function within 30 minutes. The effect of aspirin remains for the life span of the platelet (8 to 10 days). Normal hemostasis is regained when 20% of platelets have normal COX-1 activity.

Preparation and Dosage. Aspirin is absorbed through the mucous membranes of the gastrointestinal tract, achieving peak levels between 30 and 60 minutes, depending on dosage, formulation, and physiologic factors. Aspirin is hydrolyzed in the plasma, conjugated in the liver, then primarily cleared by the kidneys. In the United States, aspirin is available as 81- or 325-mg doses.

Clinical Indications

- Ischemic stroke and transient ischemic attack (TIA): In patients with a history of stroke or ischemia due to fibrin platelet emboli, aspirin therapy reduces the combined end point of TIA, stroke, and death by 13% to 18%. (*Dose: 50 to 325 mg daily.*)
- Suspected acute myocardial infarction (MI): Aspirin treatment in patients with acute coronary syndrome reduces vascular mortality by 23%. Patients are asked to chew the aspirin tablet(s) to enhance absorption due to formulation variability. (*Dose: 160 to 325 mg.*)
- Prevention of recurrent MI and unstable angina: Aspirin therapy in patients with a history of MI is associated with a 20% reduction in death and reinfarction. A 5% to 10% decrease in event rate is observed in patients with unstable angina. (*Dose: 75 to 325 mg daily.*)
- Chronic stable angina: Aspirin reduces the risk of nonfatal MI, fatal MI, and sudden death by 34%. The secondary end point for vascular events (first occurrence of MI, stroke, or vascular death) is decreased by 32%. (*Dose: 75 to 325 mg daily.*)
- Revascularization procedure: Lifelong aspirin is recommended for patients who undergo cardiac or peripheral revascularization, if there is a pre-existing condition for which aspirin is already indicated. (*Initial dose, 325 mg; maintenance dose, 160 to 325 mg daily.*)

Adverse Effects. Common side effects of aspirin include stomach pain, nausea, vomiting, dyspepsia, and risk of gastrointestinal bleeding. Some of these effects can be moderated by enteric coating, which protects the gastric mucosa. Aspirin may cause urticaria, angioedema, and bronchospasm. It is contraindicated in patients with a known allergy to nonsteroidal anti-inflammatory drugs and in patients with the syndrome of asthma, rhinitis, and nasal polyps. Aspirin should not be used in children with viral illness because of the risk of Reye syndrome. *Overdose*: The earliest sign of salicylate toxicity is tinnitus (ringing in the ears). Respiratory alkalosis occurs early but is quickly followed by metabolic acidosis. Treatment is supportive.

Dipyridamole

Dipyridamole (Aggrenox, Persantine) reversibly inhibits the uptake of adenosine into platelets and endothelial cells, increasing cAMP levels and therefore inhibiting platelet response to recruitment factors. Dipyridamole also inhibits tissue phosphodiesterase, augments the antiplatelet adhesion effects of nitric oxide, and stimulates prostacyclin release, thereby inhibiting TXA_2 formation.

Preparation and Dosage. Peak levels of dipyridamole are generally achieved 2 hours after ingestion (range, 1 to 6 hours). Metabolism occurs by liver conjugation and excretion through the gastrointestinal tract. Aggrenox is available as a capsule containing 25 mg of aspirin and 200 mg of extended-release dipyridamole. Persantine is available as 25-, 50-, and 75-mg tablets.

Clinical Indications. In patients with a history of ischemic stroke or TIA, Aggrenox reduced the risk of subsequent stroke by 22% compared to aspirin, 50 mg/day; by 24% compared to Persantine, 400 mg/day; and by 36% compared to placebo. All-cause mortality was ~11% in all three treatment groups. (*Aggrenox dose, 1 tablet twice daily; Persantine dose, 75 to 100 mg 4_ daily.*)

Adverse Effects. Aggrenox and Persantine have a gastrointestinal side-effect profile similar to that of aspirin, with twice the rate of headache and dizziness. Serious side effects include thrombocytopenia.

Clopidogrel

Clopidogrel (Plavix) irreversibly modifies the ADP receptor on platelets, inhibiting the binding of ADP to its receptor and the subsequent activation of the GPIIb/IIIa complex involved in platelet aggregation.

Preparation and Dosage. Peak levels of clopidogrel occur 1 hour after tablet ingestion. Metabolism occurs by hydrolysis and renal excretion. Plavix is available as a 75-mg tablet.

Clinical Indications

- Recent MI, recent stroke, or established peripheral vascular disease: The CAPRIE (Clopidogrel versus Aspirin in Patients at Risk of Ischemic Events) study compared a daily dose of 325 mg aspirin to 75 mg Plavix and demonstrated a relative risk reduction of 7% for fatal and nonfatal myocardial infarction, stroke, and overall event rate in the Plavix-treated group. (*Dose: 75 mg daily.*)
- Acute coronary syndrome: The CURE (Clopidogrel in Unstable Angina to Prevent Recurrent Events) study demonstrated that patients presenting with a non-ST-elevation MI within 24 hours of the onset of symptoms had a 20% relative risk reduction in cardiovascular death, MI, or stroke when treated with an oral load of Plavix in addition to standard therapies (aspirin and heparin, no GPIIb/IIIa-receptor blocker 3 days prior to randomization) compared to patients receiving only standard therapies. (*Acute MI dose, 300 mg Plavix, followed by a maintenance dose of 75 mg daily. Please note that some cardiovascular surgeons prefer to avoid Plavix loading or to allow a 5- to 7-day washout period after acute loading when a coronary bypass surgery is necessary for revascularization.*)

Adverse Effects. Plavix is associated with a higher rate of rash, diarrhea, and gastrointestinal bleeding compared to aspirin. The combination of Plavix and aspirin versus aspirin alone increases the risk of major bleeding (3.7% vs. 2.7%, respectively). There is a rare association with thrombotic thrombocytopenic purpura after short exposure (<2 weeks). Ticlopidine (Ticlid) is chemically similar to Plavix and is associated with a 0.8% risk of severe agranulocytosis. There was no difference in the incidence of agranulocytosis between the Plavix and the aspirin-treated groups.

Glycoprotein IIb/IIIa Antagonists

Abciximab (ReoPro), **tirofiban** (Aggrastat), and **eptifibatide** (Integrilin) are GPIIb/IIIa antagonists. Abciximab is the Fab fragment of the chimeric human-murine monoclonal antibody, which binds to and causes a conformational change in the GPIIb/IIIa receptor, preventing the binding of platelet "glue"—fibrinogen or vWF. Abciximab also blocks other procoagulant properties of platelets and leukocytes. Tirofiban (a nonpeptide) and eptifibatide (a cyclic heptapeptide) are reversible antagonists of the GPIIb/IIIa receptor. GPIIb/IIIa inhibitors are intended for use with aspirin and heparin.

Preparation and Dosage. Following IV bolus administration, plasma levels of abciximab decrease rapidly, with a half-life of <10 minutes. The second half-life is about 30 min, likely related to dose-dependent reversible binding of the GPIIb/IIIa receptor. Platelet function recovers over 48 hours, although abciximab remains in the circulation for 15 days. Within 30 minutes of tirofiban infusion >90% platelet inhibition is obtained. The half-life is ~2 hours, with clearance largely influenced by renal function; however, tirofiban can be dialyzed out of circulation, if needed. The pharmacokinetics of eptifibatide is essentially the same as that of tirofiban.

Clinical Indications
Abciximab:
- Adjunct to percutaneous coronary intervention (PCI): Following PCI or atherectomy, an IV abciximab bolus followed by an infusion decreased the composite of death, MI, and urgent intervention for recurrent ischemia in the first 48 hours post-procedure, a benefit that extended to 3 years. *(Dose: 0.25 mg/kg bolus followed by 0.125 µg/kg/min infusion × 12 hours.)*
- Unstable angina not responding to conventional medical therapy: The CAPTURE trial demonstrated a lower pre- and 30-day postintervention MI rate with IV abciximab. However, there was no mortality benefit at 1 or 6 months and no difference in event rate between the abciximab-treated and the placebo groups. *(Dose: 0.25mg/kg bolus followed by 10 µg/min infusion × 18 to 24 hours, continuing for 1 hour after completion of the intervention.)*

Tirofiban:
- Acute coronary syndrome and percutaneous transluminal coronary angioplasty (PTCA) or arthrectomy: Tirofiban (with heparin therapy) decreased the composite end point (death, new MI, refractory ischemia, and repeat cardiac procedure) by 32%. *(Dose: 0.4 µg/kg/min for 30 minutes, then decrease to 0.1 µg/kg/min for 48 to 108 hours or until 12 to 24 hours after coronary intervention for normal renal function.)*

Eptifibatide:
- Acute coronary syndrome and intracoronary stenting (PCI): Eptifibatide infusion, in the ESPRIT (Enhanced Suppression of the Platelet IIb/IIIa Receptor with Integrilin Therapy) study, prior to PCI decreased the composite end point of death, MI, and urgent intervention by 1% at 30 days and this benefit extended to 1 year. *(Dose: 180 µg/kg bolus, then 2 µg/kg/min for up to 72 hours or until 18 to 24 hours after PCI.)*

Adverse Effects. GPIIb/IIIa receptor blockers are associated with thrombocytopenia, which can be severe.

Anticoagulation Drugs
Anticoagulants interfere with the coagulation cascade, reducing the generation of thrombin and the buttressing effects of fibrin.

Warfarin
Warfarin (Coumadin) is an anticoagulant that acts by inhibiting the synthesis of vitamin K-dependent coagulation factors (II, VII, IX, and X, proteins C and S). Since the half-lives of proteins C and S are about one third the half-life of the other vitamin-K dependent procoagulation factors, patients are briefly hypercoagulable before anticoagulation effects take place. For this reason, patients are often bridged with heparin or Lovenox, as they become therapeutic (as measured by international normalized ratio [INR]) on warfarin.

Preparation and Dosage. The anticoagulation effects of warfarin occur within 24 hours of ingestion, peaking at 72 to 96 hours and lasting 2 to 5 days. Cytochrome P-450 is involved in the metabolism of warfarin. Drugs that affect P-450 expression will alter the metabolism of warfarin and affect INR levels. Warfarin is available in multiple-dose tablets and therapy requires periodic INR monitoring. For more detailed suggestions on dosage initiation for warfarin, visit www.WarfarinDosing.org.

Clinical Indications

- Venous thrombosis and pulmonary embolism: Current recommendation for anticoagulation in patients with an initial event and reversible risk factor for deep venous thrombosis or pulmonary embolism is 6 to 12 months. Recurrent thromboembolic disease warrants a hypercoagulable workup, and studies suggest a benefit of lifelong anticoagulation therapy. *(Goal INR: 2 to 3.)*
- Atrial fibrillation: Prospective trials of patients with atrial fibrillation show a risk reduction of 60% to 86% in systemic thromboembolism and less bleeding in the low INR range (1.4 to 3.0) compared to the high INR range (2.0 to 4.5). *(Goal INR: 2 to 3.)*
- MI: The Warfarin Re-Infarction Study (WARIS) demonstrated that patients treated with warfarin 2 to 4 weeks postinfarction with INR targets of 2.8 to 4.5 had a mortality, recurrent MI, and stroke risk reduction of 24%, 34%, and 54%, respectively. Some cardiologists would consider discontinuing anticoagulation 2 to 3 months postinfarction if wall motion abnormalities on echocardiography have resolved. *(Goal INR: 2 to 3.)*
- Mechanical and bioprosthetic valves: Anticoagulation with warfarin is generally not required in the management of bioprosthetic valves. A goal INR of 2.5 to 3.5 is generally recommended for mechanical aortic and mitral valve replacements, with the following exceptions: aortic St. Jude's and other bileaflet aortic values can be maintained with an INR of 2 to 3. A subtherapeutic INR or need to rapidly manage anticoagulation status generally is performed with IV heparin.

Adverse Effects. Warfarin is associated with a significant risk of hemorrhage, which is associated with higher INR levels. The anticoagulation effects of warfarin can be reversed within 1 to 3 days with oral or IV vitamin K (Table 12-1). Immediate reversal of anticoagulation can be achieved with administration of fresh-frozen plasma (FFP). Warfarin is contraindicated in pregnancy due to teratogenic effects and the risk of fetal hemorrhage. Warfarin-induced skin necrosis (microthrombi due to earlier deficiency of proteins C and S compared to other vitamin K factors) is a rare complication of therapy; it occurs in areas of high percentage adipose tissue and may become life-threatening.

TABLE 12-1	REVERSAL OF WARFARIN
No bleeding	
INR > 5	Hold warfarin
5 < INR < 9	Vitamin K, 1–2.5 mg PO Redose if INR high at 48 hours
INR ≥ 9	Vitamin K, 2–10 mg PO or IV Follow INR q 8 hours
Minor bleeding	Vitamin K, 1–5 mg PO or IV
Major bleeding	Vitamin K, 10 mg IV, and FFP or factor VII concentrate

FFP, fresh-frozen plasma.

TABLE 12-2   HEPARIN NOMOGRAM

PTT (Seconds)	Bolus (U)	Infusion Rate
<40	3000	↑3 U/kg/h
40–50	2000	↑2 U/kg/h
51–59	None	↑1 U/kg/h
60–94	None	No change
95–104	None	↓1 U/kg/h
105–114	Hold 30 min	↓2 U/kg/h
≥114	Hold 1 h	↓3 U/kg/h

PTT, partial thromboplastin time. Typical heparin bolus, 60 U/kg (80 U/kg for pulmonary embolus/deep venous thrombosis); maximum, 5000 U. Typical infusion, 14 U/kg/h. Monitor PTT q6h until two consecutive PTTs are therapeutic and at least once daily thereafter. Monitor CBC q48h.

Unfractionated Heparin

Unfractionated heparin is a polysaccharide that binds to anti–thrombin III (ATIII) and increases the rate of ATIII inactivation of thrombin (II) and factor Xa.

Preparation and Dosage. Heparin is administered IV or SC based on patient lean body weight and clinical context (Table 12-2). IV heparin affects are monitored by measuring the partial thromboplastin time (pTT). Discontinuation of IV heparin results in normalization of anticoagulation within 2 to 3 hours.

Clinical Indications

- Anticoagulation bridge therapy: Heparin is used as bridge therapy to initiate and discontinue anticoagulation in patients with prosthetic heart valves (to prevent valve thrombosis) and thrombotic disease. *(Dose: heparin bolus IV, followed by a drip that is titrated by goal pTT of 60 to 96.)*
- Prophylaxis: Hospitalized patients at significant risk for developing deep venous thrombosis and associated sequelae are given SC heparin to decrease the incidence of thrombotic disease. *(Dose: 5000 units heparin SC, bid to tid.)*
- Acute coronary syndrome and vascular surgery: The advantage of heparin is immediate anticoagulation. *(Dose: heparin bolus, followed by a drip that is titrated by goal pTT of 60 to 96.)*
- Invasive lines and catheters: Invasive pressure catheters and lines are flushed with heparin (to prevent catheter clotting).

Adverse Effects. Heparin is associated with a risk of bleeding. Rapid reversal of heparin can be achieved by infusion of protamine sulfate (1 mg protamine reverses 100 units of circulating heparin). Heparin-induced thrombocytopenia (HIT) is a complication that results in a rapid fall in platelet number (see Chap. 4). Suspicion of HIT should prompt discontinuation of heparin; platelet counts generally recover within 1 to 2 weeks. Warfarin should be avoided in acute HIT, unless combined with another anticoagulant while the INR is subtherapeutic.

Low Molecular Weight Heparin

Enoxaparin (Lovenox) is a low molecular weight heparin that inhibits thrombin (factor IIa) and factor Xa.

Preparation and Dosage. Enoxaparin is administered SC. Maximum activity occurs 3 to 5 hours after SC injection and needs to be administered every 12 hours, except in patients with renal impairment, in whom once-daily dosing is sufficient for anticoagulation.

Clinical Indications

- Prophylaxis of deep venous thrombosis: Enoxaparin is used to prevent thrombosis complications in patients with orthopedic, general surgical, or medical problems requiring prolonged immobilization (walking ≤10 meters for ≤3 days). (*Dose: 40 mg SC every 24 hours or 30 mg SC every 12 hours.*)
- Prophylaxis of ischemic complications of unstable angina (*Dose: 1 mg/kg lean body weight SC every 12 hours.*)
- Treatment of deep venous thrombosis and pulmonary embolism (*Dose: 1 mg/kg lean body weight SC every 12 hours.*)

Adverse Effects. Bleeding is a complication of enoxaparin; no therapy to reverse anticoagulation is available. Thrombocytopenia occurs in about 1% of patients. A drop in platelet count to $<100,000/mm^3$ should prompt discontinuation of this medication. Patients with HIT from heparin therapy are at risk for enoxaparin-induced thrombocytopenia, thus other anticoagulation drugs are preferred in these situations. The use of enoxaparin for thromboprophylaxis in pregnant women and in patients with mechanical valves has not been properly studied.

Fondaparinux

Fondaparinux (Arixtra) binds to ATIII and selectively inhibits factor Xa.

Preparation and Dosage. A therapeutic level of fondaparinux is achieved within 2 hours of SC injection and is eliminated by renal excretion. Multiple prefilled syringe doses are available.

Clinical Indications

- Prophylaxis: Fondaparinux is indicated for deep venous thrombosis prophylaxis in patients undergoing orthopedic and general surgery procedures.
- Deep venous thrombosis and pulmonary embolism: Fondaparinux is approved as bridge therapy for anticoagulation with warfarin. (*Dose based on body weight: 5 mg [<50 kg], 7.5 mg [50 to 100 kg], and 10 mg [>100 kg] SC daily.*)

Adverse Effects. Fondaparinux carries a slightly higher risk of hemorrhage compared to Lovenox (4% vs. 3%, respectively) and similar rates of thrombocytopenia. There is no antidote for fondaparinux.

Direct Thrombin Inhibitors: Hirudin Derivatives

Lepirudin (Refludan) and **bivalirudin** (Angiomax) are recombinant hirudin polypeptides that directly inhibit thrombin. The hirudins were originally isolated from leech saliva but are now derived from recombinant DNA in yeast cells.

Preparation and Dosage. The half-life of lepirudin is 10 minutes and that of bivalirudin is 25 minutes. Metabolism occurs by catabolic hydrolysis. The half-life is prolonged in patients with creatinine clearance ≤15 mL/min. Lepirudin and bivalirudin dosages are adjusted by PTT, checked 2 hours after the start or a change in infusion rate.

Clinical Indications

Lepirudin:

- Anticoagulation in patients with HIT and associated thromboembolic disease (*Dose: 0.5 mg/kg bolus, then 0.15 mg/kg/min [up to 110 kg] continuous infusion to target PTT of 45 to 70 seconds.*)

Bivalirudin:

- Anticoagulation in patients undergoing PCI (*Dose: 0.75 mg/kg bolus prior to intervention, then 1.75 mg/kg/h for the duration of the procedure and up to 4 hours postprocedure.*)
- Anticoagulation with streptokinase thrombolysis in ST-elevation MI and known HIT (*Dose—starting 3 minutes before streptokinase: 0.25 mg/kg bolus, followed by 0.5 mg/kg/hr × 12 hours, then 0.25 mg/kg/h × 36 hours.*)

- Acute coronary syndrome *(Dose: 0.1 mg/kg bolus, followed by 0.25 mg/kg/h.)*
- Anticoagulation in patients with HIT *(Dose: 0.08 to 0.1 mg/kg/h for CrCl ≥30 mL/min or 0.04 to 0.06 mg/kg/h for CrCl <30 mL/min to target PTT of 45 to 70 seconds.)*

Adverse Effects. Antihirudin antibodies are observed in 40% of HIT patients treated with lepirudin. Back pain and nausea are common side effects of hirudin derivatives. There are reports of hypersensitivity and allergic reactions and liver function test abnormalities.

Direct Thrombin Inhibitor: Argatroban
Argatroban is a synthetic derivative of L-arginine that directly inhibits thrombin by reversibly binding to the thrombin active site.

Preparation and Dosage. Argatroban is 54% protein-bound and is metabolized by the liver. Its half-life is 39 to 51 minutes. No dosage adjustment is necessary in renal dysfunction; however, the dosage should be adjusted in hepatic impairment (0.5 μg/kg/min). The INR may be falsely elevated with therapy.

Clinical Indications
- Anticoagulation for prophylaxis or treatment of thrombosis in patients with HIT *(Dose: 0.5 to 2 μg/kg/min until PTT is 1.5× to 3× times baseline [45 to 90 seconds] but not more than 100 seconds.)*
- Anticoagulation in patients with HIT PCI). *(Dose: 350 μg/kg IV bolus over 3 to 5 minutes, then 25 μg/kg/min infusion.)*

Adverse Effects. Argatroban prolongs the INR with warfarin and should be discontinued when the INR >4 on combined therapy. Fever and diarrhea are frequent side effects. Hypotension can occur with infusion.

THROMBOLYTICS AND FIBRINOLYTICS: AGENTS THAT DISINTEGRATE CLOT

Thrombolytics and fibrinolytics convert plasminogen to the active enzyme plasmin, which digests fibrin clots.

Streptokinase
Streptokinase (Streptase) is a protein derived from beta-hemolytic streptococcus. Streptokinase binds to plasminogen and increases conversion of plasminogen to plasmin, the proteolytic enzyme that breaks down fibrin clots.

Preparation and Dosage
The dose of streptokinase used depends on the clinical context. Generally, the medication is given parenterally, either IV or via the intracoronary route. Since allergic responses to streptokinase have occurred, an intradermal test dose of 100 IU has been suggested. If no reaction occurs, than the drug may be given systemically. Streptokinase is metabolized by the liver.

Clinical Indications
- Acute MI: The Second International Study of Infarct Survival (ISIS-2) examined streptokinase ± aspirin versus placebo for treatment of MI. The investigators showed a 42% reduction in the odds of death with combined treatment versus placebo and a 25% reduction in the odds of death with streptokinase alone versus placebo. *(Dose: 1,500,000 IU IV over 60 minutes.)*
- Pulmonary embolism *(Dose: 250,000 IU IV over 30 minutes, then 100,000 IU/h over 24 hours.)*

- Deep venous thrombosis *(Dose: 250,000 IU IV over 30 minutes, then 100,000 IU over 72 hours.)*

Adverse Effects

As with other thrombolytic agents, bleeding is a side effect of streptokinase. Patients exposed to streptococci may have antibodies to this organism and thus an allergy to streptokinase. The most commonly reported reactions are fever and shivering (1% to 4%). Anaphylactic shock is a much rarer event, occurring in <0.1% of patients. Severe reactions should be managed with adrenergic, corticosteroid, and/or antihistamine agents as needed, as well as discontinuation of the medication. Certain conditions are associated with an increased risk when using the medication and should be weighed against the benefits. These include, but are not limited to, recent surgery (within 10 days), gastrointestinal bleed or trauma, systolic pressure >180 mm Hg or diastolic pressure >110 mm Hg, subacute bacterial endocarditis, pregnancy, and cerebrovascular disease.

Urokinase

Urokinase (Abbokinase) is a thrombolytic agent that is obtained from human neonatal kidney cells. Like streptokinase, it converts plasminogen to plasmin, which subsequently degrades fibrin clots.

Preparation and Dosage

Urokinase is supplied in vials containing 250,000 IU of the medication. Dosing of the medication depends on the patient's weight. The medication is primarily metabolized by the liver.

Clinical Indications

- Pulmonary embolism: A recent review examined 26 patients given urokinase via intrapulmonary artery infusion for a pulmonary embolism. The authors noted that the medication was an effective and safe treatment option for patients both with and without contraindications to systemic thrombolytic therapy. *(Dose: 4400 IU/kg bolus IV over 10 minutes, followed by 4400 IU/kg/h IV for 12 hours.)*

Adverse Effects. As with other thrombolytic agents, bleeding is a side effect of urokinase. Hypersensitivity and anaphylaxis reactions to the medication have been reported. These should be treated with adrenergic, corticosteroid, and/or antihistamine agents as needed. Contraindications to the medication are similar to those for alteplase (see below).

Alteplase

Alteplase (Activase) is a tissue plasminogen activator (tPA) prepared from recombinant DNA technology.

Preparation and Dosage

Alteplase is available in 50- or 100-mg vials and is given IV. Dosage varies depending on patient weight and clinical context, and doses >100 mg are rarely indicated. Alteplase has a very short half-life and is rapidly cleared from the plasma, primarily through the liver.

Clinical Indications

- Coronary artery thrombosis: In the setting of an acute MI, alteplase should be administered within 12 hours of the onset of symptoms. It is given IV in 3-hour (long) or 1.5-hour (accelerated) infusions. Investigators have shown alteplase to be superior to streptokinase in restoring coronary blood flow. *(Dose, acute MI [accelerated infusion]: 15-mg IV bolus, followed by 0.75 mg/kg infusion [maximum, 50 mg] for 30 minutes, then 0.5 mg/kg infusion [maximum, 35 mg] for 1 hour.)*

- Pulmonary embolism: Alteplase is indicated for patients with pulmonary embolism if they are hemodynamically unstable. It is given as a 90-minute infusion. Recent data support the use of alteplase with heparin in patients with submassive pulmonary emboli. *(Dose: 100 mg IV over 2 hours.)*
- Acute ischemic stroke: Alteplase is indicated for patients with an ischemic stroke (1) if given within 3 hours of onset of symptoms and (2) after intracranial hemorrhage has been excluded. Investigators have shown that patients receiving alteplase are 30% more likely to have decreased or no disability (vs. placebo) at 3 months. *(Dose: 0.9 mg/kg IV [maximum, 90 mg] over 60 minutes, with 10% of dose as IV bolus.)*
- Peripheral arterial disease: Alteplase can be given intra-arterially for acute arterial occlusions in patients without limb-threatening ischemia.

Adverse Effects

The most common reaction associated with alteplase use is bleeding. Allergic reactions to the medication have also been reported. Contraindications to the medication depend on the clinical context and include (but are not limited to) active internal bleeding, recent intracranial or intraspinal surgery/trauma (within 3 months), known intracranial neoplasm or arteriovenous malformation, known bleeding diathesis or INR >1.7, platelet count of <100,000/mm^3, systolic blood pressure >180 mm Hg and/or diastolic pressure >110 mm Hg, and documented allergic reaction.

Reteplase

Reteplase (Retavase) is produced in *E. coli* by recombinant DNA technology. Reteplase is a second-generation tPA that binds fibrin with less affinity than alteplase, enabling it to better penetrate clots.

Preparation and Dosage

Because reteplase has a longer half-life than alteplase, it can be given as two bolus doses instead of one. The drug is cleared from the plasma primarily by the kidneys and liver.

Clinical Indications

- Acute MI: The RAPID-2 (Second Reteplase versus Alteplase Patency Investigation during Myocardial Infarction) trial studied coronary artery perfusion 90 minutes after alteplase or reteplase administration for acute MI. Although the results demonstrated TIMI 3 flow in 60% of reteplase patients versus 45% for alteplase, reocclusion rates were similar for the two treatments. The GUSTO-III (Global Utilization of Streptokinase and t-PA for Occluded Coronary Arteries III) trial examined the efficacy and safety of alteplase versus reteplase, and neither drug was found to be superior to the other regarding 30-day mortality, hemorrhagic stroke, or bleeding complications. *(Dose: 10 units IV × 1, followed by 10 units IV 30 minutes later.)*

Adverse Effects

Bleeding is the most common side effect of reteplase. Allergic reaction to the medication can also be seen. Contraindications to reteplase are similar to those for alteplase (see above).

Tenecteplase

Tenecteplase (TNKase) is a tPA produced by recombinant DNA technology. It differs from alteplase by three amino acid substitutions, which gives the drug decreased plasma clearance and increased binding to fibrin.

Preparation and Dosage

Tenecteplase is given as a single-bolus injection over 5 seconds. Dosing depends on patient weight and should not exceed 50 mg. The drug comes in 50-mg vials. Tenecteplase has a longer half-life than alteplase and is cleared by the liver.

Clinical Indications
- Acute MI: Tenecteplase can be used as a one-time bolus for patients with acute MI. The ASSENT-2 trial compared tenecteplase and alteplase as reperfusion therapy for patients with acute MI. While the 30-day mortality was equivalent between the two drugs, the investigators showed a decreased risk of major bleeding events (4.7% vs. 5.9%) with tenecteplase. *(Dose: for weight <60 kg, 30 mg IV × 1; weight 60 to 69 kg, 35 mg IV × 1; weight 70 to 79 kg, 40 mg IV × 1; weight 80 to 89 kg, 45 mg IV × 1; weight >90 kg, 50 mg IV × 1.)*

Adverse Effects
The most common adverse reaction associated with tenecteplase is bleeding. Allergic reactions have also been reported. As with alteplase, contraindications to the medication exist, including active internal bleeding, history of cerebrovascular accident, intracranial or intraspinal surgery/trauma within 2 months, known bleeding diathesis, severe uncontrolled hypertension, and known intracranial neoplasm, arteriovenous malformation, or aneurysm.

COAGULANTS: AGENTS THAT TREAT BLEEDING

Desmopressin

Desmopressin (DDAVP) is a synthetic copy of the naturally occurring pituitary hormone vasopressin (ADH). In patients with type 1 von Willebrand disease (vWD) and mild hemophilia A, desmopressin exerts its effect by transiently increasing plasma levels of vWF and factor VIII.

Preparation and Dosage
Desmopressin can be administered intranasally, SC, IV, or orally. The dose and route of administration depend on the clinical context. The half-life of desmopressin given IV is 3 hours, and the drug is metabolized primarily by the kidney.

Clinical Indications
- Hemophilia A: Desmopressin is used in patients with hemophilia A prior to surgery or patients who have spontaneous bleeding.
- vWD (type 1): Studies have demonstrated that patients with type 1 vWD have a qualitatively normal vWF and respond to desmopressin, unlike patients with type 2 vWD, who synthesize a qualitatively abnormal vWF.
- Acute bleeding *(Dose: 0.3 μg/kg IV, once. May be repeated in 8 to 24 hours if needed.)*

Adverse Effects
Desmopressin has been associated with headaches, tachycardia, and facial flushing. Other side effects include rhinitis, stomach cramps, vulvar pain, and vomiting. In patients receiving repeated doses of the medication, tachyphylaxis can occur. Patients taking desmopressin should be educated to limit fluid intake to satisfaction of thirst only, as hyponatremia may occur via the ADH effect of the drug. Consequently, children taking this medication should have their body weight routinely monitored. Rarely, water intoxication and coma can occur.

Vitamin K

Phytonadione (vitamin K) is a fat-soluble vitamin required by the liver for synthesis of clotting factors II, VII, IX, and X. Vitamin K is derived from green, leafy vegetables and is also produced by bacteria in the digestive tract. It is given to reverse the effects of warfarin.

Preparation and Dosage

Vitamin K can be taken orally from 2.5 mg to a maximum dose of 25 mg. Alternatively, the drug can be given SC, IM, or IV at doses ranging from 1 to 10 mg. Vitamin K is metabolized in the liver and excreted in the bile.

Clinical Indications

- Anticoagulation reversal: Vitamin K can be administered to reverse the effects of warfarin. Please see section on warfarin (above) for more details.

Adverse Effects

Reactions to vitamin K include taste changes, flushing, dizziness, and hypotension. Severe anaphylaxis reactions and death have been reported following parenteral administration of the drug. Hyperbilirubinemia can be seen in infants following administration of the drug.

Aminocaproic Acid

Aminocaproic acid (Amicar) is a medication used to inhibit fibrinolysis by inhibiting PA substances. It is often used to treat excessive postoperative bleeding, as well as gingival bleeding in hemophiliacs undergoing dental work.

Preparation and Dosage

Aminocaproic acid can be administered orally or IV. The drug comes in 500- or 1000-mg tablets and 250-mg syrup or injectable vials. Aminocaproic acid is metabolized in the liver and is primarily excreted in urine.

Clinical Indications

- A recent observational study prospectively examined the use of three antifibrinolytic agents (aprotinin, aminocaproic acid, and tranexamic acid) in patients who underwent coronary artery bypass graft surgery. While aprotinin was associated with serious end-organ damage, including renal failure, heart failure, and encephalopathy, this was not seen with aminocaproic acid, which was deemed to be a safe alternative.
- Studies have shown aminocaproic acid to be safe and efficacious as an adjunctive therapy for hemophiliacs undergoing dental procedures.
- Acute bleeding *(Dose: 5 g of aminocaproic acid IV or PO over 1 hour, followed by 1 g/h IV or PO for 8 hours or until bleeding is controlled.)*

Adverse Effects

Side effects of the medication include abdominal pain, diarrhea, pruritus, headache, malaise, allergic reactions, thrombocytopenia, hypotension, convulsions, dyspnea, rash, and tinnitus. Rarely, rhabdomyolysis, and acute renal failure can occur with this medication. CPK monitoring should occur regularly in patients undergoing long-term therapy, and it should be discontinued if elevations of the enzyme are noted.

Protamine

Protamine sulfate is a parenterally administered medication used to treat heparin overdose. It exerts its effects by binding heparin and forming a stable complex, which negates the anticoagulation effects of heparin. When given alone, protamine has a mild anticoagulant effect.

Preparation and Dosage

Protamine has a rapid onset of action, and the reversal of heparin occurs within 5 minutes after administering the drug. Protamine comes in 25-mL vials that contain 250 mg of the drug.

Clinical Indications

- A retrospective study in 1999 examined the incidence of acute and subacute stent thrombosis in patients who received protamine after PCI. The authors concluded that protamine did not predispose to stent thrombosis and that it could be safely used to treat bleeding complications in patients undergoing PCI.

- Heparin reversal *(Dose: 1 mg of protamine neutralizes ~ 100 units of heparin, and it is given at a rate of 5 mg/min. Protamine is given IV over 10 minutes, and the maximum dose given should not exceed 50 mg at one time.)*

Adverse Effects
Following administration of the protamine, patients may experience hypotension and bradycardia. Other effects of the medication include nausea, vomiting, dyspnea, flushing, and fatigue. Severe reactions to protamine include anaphylaxis and anaphylactoid reactions. Some penicillins and cephalosporins have been shown to be incompatible with protamine. Protamine overdoses may cause bleeding in patients.

Humate-P

Humate-P (antihemophilic factor/vWF complex) is a product pooled from human plasma which contains factor VIII and vWF. Administration of Humate-P promotes coagulation. It is approved for the treatment of (1) bleeding in hemophilia A patients, (2) bleeding in patients with severe vWD, and (3) treatment of patients with mild to moderate vWD in whom desmopressin is ineffective.

Preparation and Dosage
Dosage of Humate-P depends on patient weight, severity of bleeding, and vWF:RCo (ristocetin cofactor) activity. Dosage is calculated as [patient's weight (kg) × desired % increase in VFW activity] ÷ 1.5. The dose can be adjusted for the extent of bleeding.

Clinical Indications
A recent retrospective review of 97 patients with vWD (types 1, 2A, 2B, and 3) showed Humate-P to have >95% efficacy in bleeding episodes.

Adverse Effects
As Humate-P is derived from human plasma, it carries a risk of transmission of infectious agents. Common side effects include flushing, chills, fever, dizziness, and headache. Although allergic reactions have been reported, severe anaphylaxis is rare.

Recombinant Coagulation Factor VIIa

Coagulation factor VIIa (NovoSeven) is a recombinant human coagulation factor approved for bleeding in patients with hemophilia A or B with inhibitors or in patients with congenital factor VII deficiency. NovoSeven works by activating the extrinsic pathway of coagulation.

Preparation and Dosage
NovoSeven is administered IV and the dosage depends on the clinical context. For hemophiliacs with bleeding episodes, 90 μg/kg is given every 2 hours until bleeding stops. In patients with congenital factor VII deficiency, NovoSeven is given at 15 at 30 μg/kg every 4 to 6 hours until cessation of bleeding.

Clinical Indications
- NovoSeven has been shown to be effective or partially effective in 85% of serious bleeding episodes.
- Another study examined the efficacy of NovoSeven in 518 serious bleeding episodes, and it was excellent or effective in 62% of muscle, 80% of ear, nose, and throat, 88% of CNS, and 76% of joint bleeding episodes.

Adverse Effects
As with any recombinant product, anaphylaxis is a potential side effect. NovoSeven is contraindicated in patients who have a known allergic reaction to mouse, hamster, or cow products. Common side effects include bleeding, fever, and hypertension. There is a slightly increased risk of thrombosis after administration of the medication.

KEY POINTS TO REMEMBER

- Aspirin irreversibly inhibits platelet aggregation for the life span of the platelet.
- Warfarin inhibits the synthesis of the vitamin K-dependent factors II, VII, IX, and X, protein C, and protein S; the INR is monitored while the patient is on warfarin.
- Unfractionated heparin acts by binding ATIII. The PTT is monitored for appropriate dosing.
- If HIT is suspected, all unfractionated heparin and low molecular weight heparin products should be discontinued.
- Alternatives to heparin in a patient with HIT include bivalirudin, lepirudin, and argatroban.
- Vitamin K is indicated for reversal of anticoagulation with warfarin.

REFERENCES AND SUGGESTED READINGS

Assessment of the Safety and Efficacy of a New Thrombolytic (ASSENT-2) Investigators, Van De Werf F, Adgey J, Ardissino D, et al. Single-bolus tenecteplase compared with front-loaded alteplase in acute myocardial infarction: the ASSENT-2 double-blind randomised trial. *Lancet.* 1999;354(9180):716–722.

Briguori C, Di Mario C, De Gregorio J, et al. Administration of protamine after coronary stent deployment. *Am Heart J.* 1999;138(1; Pt 1):64–68.

Chong BH, Chong JH. Heparin-induced thrombocytopenia. *Exp Rev Cardiovasc Ther.* 2004;2:547–559.

Cotran R, Kumar V, Collins T. Hemostasis and thrombosis. In: *Robbins Pathologic Basis of Disease.* 7th ed. Philadelphia: W. B. Saunders; 2005 [online].

Djulbegovic B, Marasa M, Pesto A, et al. Safety and efficacy of purified factor IX concentrate and antifibrinolytic agents for dental extractions in hemophilia B. *Am J Hematol.* 1996;51(2):168–170.

GUSTO Angiographic Investigators. The effects of tissue plasminogen activator, streptokinase, or both on coronary-artery patency, ventricular function, and survival after acute myocardial infarction. *N Engl J Med.* 1993;329:1615–1622.

GUSTO Investigators. An international randomized trial comparing four thrombolytic strategies for acute myocardial infarction. The GUSTO investigators. *N Engl J Med.* 1993;329:673–682.

Hankey G, Eikelboom J. New drugs, old drugs antiplatelet drugs. *Med J Austral.* 2003;178 (11):568–574.

ISIS-2 (Second International Study of Infarct Survival) Collaborative Group. Randomised trial of intravenous streptokinase, oral aspirin, both, or neither among 17,187 cases of suspected acute myocardial infarction: ISIS-2. *Lancet.* 198;2(8607):349–360.

Konstantinides S, Geibel A, Heusel G, et al. Management Strategies and Prognosis of Pulmonary Embolism-3 Trial Investigators. Heparin plus alteplase compared with heparin alone in patients with submassive pulmonary embolism. *N Engl J Med.* 2002;347(15):1143–1150.

Lillicrap D, Poon M-C, Walker I, et al. Efficacy and safety of the factor VIII/von Willebrand factor concentrate, Haemate-P/Humate-P: ristocetin cofactor unit dosing in patients with von Willebrand disease. *Thromb Haemost.* 2002;87:224–230.

Lusher J, et al. Clinical experience with recombinant Factor VIIa. *Blood Coag Fibrinolys.* 1998;9:119–128.

Mangano DT, Tudor IC, Dietzel C, Multicenter Study of Perioperative Ischemia Research Group, Ischemia Research and Education Foundation. The risk associated with aprotinin in cardiac surgery. *N Engl J Med.* 2006;354(4):353–365.

Mannucci, PM. Treatment of von Willebrand's disease. *N Engl J Med.* 2004;351:683–694.

McCotter CJ, Chiang KS, Fearrington EL. Intrapulmonary artery infusion of urokinase for treatment of massive pulmonary embolism: a review of 26 patients with and without contraindications to systemic thrombolytic therapy. *Clin Cardiol.* 1999;22(10): 661–664.

National Institute of Neurological Disorders and Stroke rt-PA Stroke Study Group. Tissue plasminogen activator for acute ischemic stroke. *N Engl J Med.* 1995;333(24): 1581–1587.

Physicians' Desk Reference. 61st ed. Montvale, NJ: Thomson PDR; 2007.

Scharrer I. Recombinant factor VIIa for patients with inhibitors to factor VIII or IX or factor VII deficiency. *Haemophilia.* 1999;5(4):253–259.

Weaver D. Results of the RAPID 1 and RAPID 2 thrombolytic trials in acute myocardial infarction. *Eur Heart J.* 1996;17 (Suppl E):14–20.

Plasma Cell Disorders

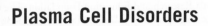

Philip E. Lammers and Tanya M. Wildes

INTRODUCTION TO PLASMA CELL DISORDERS

Background

Plasma cell disorders encompass a group of syndromes characterized by malignant plasma cells that produce a monoclonal protein. The range and severity of diseases are quite broad and include multiple myeloma (MM), monoclonal gammopathy of undetermined significance (MGUS), Waldenström macroglobinemia (WM), and amyloidosis. The monoclonal protein (M protein) varies by disease entity; MM generally produces IgG and IgA, whereas WM usually produces IgM gammopathy.

Epidemiology

The incidence of each entity varies tremendously. For instance, in one study the prevalence of MGUS was found to be 3.2% among those older than 50 years and 5.3% among those older than 70 years . In comparison, ~4 of 100,000 people in the United States are diagnosed with MM each year.

MULTIPLE MYELOMA

Pathophysiology

The pathophysiology of MM begins with the production of an M protein by clonal plasma cells. Approximately 50% of patients have cytogenetic abnormalities that involve translocations joining the immunoglobulin heavy-chain locus on chromosome 14q32 and one of five partner chromosomes: 11q13, 4p16.3, 6p21, 16q23, and 20q11. Myeloma cells produce lytic lesions through interactions with bone marrow stromal cells, increased osteoclast activity, and inhibition of osteoblast activity.

Clinical Presentation

Patients with MM often present with complaints such as fatigue, nausea, and weight loss. They may also complain of bone pain, have abnormal bleeding, or develop recurrent bacterial infections.

On evaluation, patients can be found to have anemia, hypercalcemia, and renal failure. Due to hyperviscous blood, a patient can have thrombotic complications such as stroke, a transient ischemic attack, or deep venous thrombosis (DVT). MM can be associated with plasmacytomas that invade vertebrae or other structures. Lytic bone lesions caused by plasma cell infiltration and plasmacytomas can result in vertebral fractures or neurological emergencies such as cord compression. Diffuse osteopenia or osteolytic lesions occur in ~85% of patients with MM.

Management

Diagnosis

The International Myeloma Working Group developed diagnostic criteria for MM, most recently refined in 2003. The three criteria are:

- presence of a serum or urinary monoclonal protein (M protein);
- presence of clonal plasma cells in the bone marrow or a plasmacytoma; and
- presence of end-organ damage thought to be related to the disease such as hypercalcemia, lytic bone lesions, anemia, or renal failure.

Workup

All patients suspected of MM should undergo an extensive diagnostic workup beginning with a full history and physical. Initial laboratory workup should include a CBC, serum electrolytes, BUN, serum creatinine, serum calcium, albumin, and quantitative immunoglobulins. β2-Microglobulin is an important prognostic indicator and should be checked on each patient at time of diagnosis. A serum protein electrophoresis (SPEP), urine protein electrophoresis (UPEP), and immunofixation should be performed. An M protein is detectable in the serum of >90% of patients. In about one half of patients, the M protein is an IgG, and in 20% of patients it is IgA. A 24-hour urine collection may be done to quantitate urinary light-chain excretion. The serum-free light-chain assay allows for quantitation of free light chains in the serum. C-Reactive protein can be used as a surrogate marker for IL-6, which is a prime stimulator of myeloma cell growth. Lactate dehydrogenase should also be checked as a measure of tumor burden.

Diagnostic Tests

A skeletal survey to assess for lytic lesions should be performed on all patients. A unilateral bone marrow aspirate and biopsy should be done as well. Cytogenetics and FISH should be performed on the bone marrow aspirate, as certain translocations have prognostic significance.

Prognosis

International Staging System. Staging can be done with one of two systems. The International Staging System for myeloma was developed in 2005 and consists of three stages. It is based on a patient database of more than 10,000 patients and carries prognostic value. Median survivals are 62, 44, and 29 months for stages I, II, and III, respectively.

- Stage I: β2-Microglobulin <3.5 mg/L and serum albumin >3.5 g/dL
- Stage II: Neither stage I nor stage III
- Stage III: β2-Microglobulin >5.5 mg/L

Durie-Salmon Staging System. The older staging system is called the Durie-Salmon Criteria and also consists of three stages. This system was developed based on total tumor cell mass but has not been shown to correlate definitively with prognosis.

- Stage I. All of the following must be present: hemoglobin >10 g/dL, normal serum calcium, normal bone x-rays or a solitary bone plasmacytoma only, urine monoclonal protein excretion <4 g/day, IgG <5 g/dL, IgA <3 g/dL, and Bence Jones protein <4 g/24 h.
- Stage II. Neither stage I nor stage III.
- Stage III. One or more of the following must be present: hemoglobin <8.5 g/dL, serum calcium >12 mg/dL, advanced lytic bone lesions, urine monoclonal protein excretion >12 g/day, IgG level >7 g/dL, IgA level >5 g/dL, and Bence Jones protein >12 g/24 h.

- In addition to stages I–III, it also includes an element of renal function: category A includes those with serum creatinine <2 mg/dL, and category B includes those with serum creatinine >2 mg/dL.

Cytogenetics. Cytogenetics can yield important prognostic information. Deletion of chromosome 13 and translocation of chromosomes 4 and 14 are associated with a poor prognosis. Alternatively, translocation between 11 and 14 seems to be associated with improved survival. However, it should be noted that there are no current recommendations to use cytogenetic data to direct patient management.

Treatment

Management of patients with MM depends on the stage at presentation. Patients with stage I MM or those with so-called smoldering MM (M protein <3 g/dL and <10% plasma cells in bone marrow, but asymptomatic and without bony lesions, kidney involvement, etc.) can be managed with watchful waiting. These patients can often do well for months or years before progression. They should initially be observed at 3- to 6-month intervals.

Initial Therapy. Patients with stage II or stage III disease on presentation should undergo evaluation for future stem cell transplant. Advanced age and multiple comorbidities may preclude stem cell transplantation and therefore affect initial induction chemotherapy options. Patients expected to advance to stem cell transplantation should not be exposed to alkylating agents prior to harvest of the stem cells. Those deemed to be transplant candidates generally undergo initial induction therapy soon after diagnosis. There are multiple induction regimens to choose from, but the standard agents used are currently thalidomide and dexamethasone. The combination of these agents was shown to be superior to dexamethasone alone, with response rates of 63 % versus 41% in the two arms; however, toxicity (DVT, neuropathy, rash) was significantly higher in the combination arm, including a 17% DVT rate versus 3% in the dexamethasone-only group.

Those patients deemed to be poor stem cell transplant candidates due to poor performance status or advanced age may be treated with melphalan (an alkylating agent), prednisone, and thalidomide (MPT) or melphalan and prednisone alone (MP).

Stem Cell Transplant. After induction of chemotherapy, patients deemed suitable for stem cell transplant should proceed to harvesting of stem cells. Currently, autologous stem cell transplant is considered the standard of care for MM patients. Response rates approach 90%, with one third of patients experiencing a complete response. Allogeneic transplants are also occasionally performed, although they are generally reserved for young patients with a matched sibling donor who have failed autologous transplant.

Therapy for Relapsed Myeloma. Second-line agents for relapsed disease are numerous and include bortezomib, a proteasome inhibitor, and lenalidomide, an immunomodulatory agent like thalidomide. Bortezomib has shown success in treating relapsed myeloma and has also shown promise as an initial agent in induction. Its mechanism of action is not completely known, but it is thought to have direct cytotoxic effects, to impact the microenvironment of the bone marrow, and to stimulate apoptosis. Lenalidomide alone or in combination with dexamethasone is approved for relapsed myeloma, and studies regarding its use as up-front therapy are ongoing. There are multiple other options for salvage chemotherapy, but no therapy can provide a cure.

Adjunctive Therapy. Adjunctive therapy can be a very important part of MM treatment. Patients with bony pain due to bony lesions can benefit from low-dose radiation therapy. The use of bisphosphonates has been shown to decrease bony pain and improve quality of life. Erythropoietin therapy should be considered in those with renal involvement and anemia. Monitoring for infections is very important and patients with life-threatening infections may need intravenous IgG. In addition, all patients should be vaccinated against *Streptococcus pneumoniae*. Patients on thalidomide or lenalidomide and dexamethasone should be on prophylactic anticoagulation because of increased risk of thrombotic events.

Follow-up
Follow-up after initial therapy should be done by following the M-protein level and other markers of disease progression including the CBC and serum creatinine. Skeletal surveys are not used to follow disease progression as lesions may not show healing on x-rays.

SOLITARY PLASMACYTOMAS

Introduction

Solitary plasmacytomas are collections of plasma cells in tissues classified as either solitary plasmacytomas of bone or extramedullary plasmacytomas. By definition, they are present without evidence of MM; therefore, careful workup to rule out MM should be performed. Plasmacytomas in the bone are more common than in extramedullary sites. The axillary skeleton is most often involved, and the thoracic spine is the most common site. Extramedullary plasmacytomas occur most often in the head and neck area of the upper respiratory tract.

Presentation

Solitary plasmacytomas of bone often present with bony pain, pathological fracture, or cord compression.

Natural History

It is estimated that 50% to 60% of patients who originally present with plasmacytomas of bone will eventually progress to MM. This is in contrast to extramedullary plasmacytomas, in which only 10% to 15% of patients will progress to MM.

Management

Workup
Imaging with MRI is indicated to characterize the lesion and to evaluate for other bony involvement.

Treatment
Radiation therapy is the treatment of choice for these isolated tumors; however, in cases of fracture or cord compression, surgery may be performed to stabilize the spine and to remove the tumor. There have been no data indicating that adjuvant chemotherapy lessens the risk of progression.

Follow-up
Patients should be followed every 3 months after therapy for the first year to evaluate for signs of progression to MM.

MONOCLONAL GAMMOPATHY OF UNDETERMINED SIGNIFICANCE

Introduction

MGUS is characterized by the presence of an M-protein level <3 g/dL, <10% plasma cells in the marrow, and no clinical symptoms of MM or other plasma cell disorders. It is a very common entity, often found incidentally during evaluation of total serum protein elevation or proteinuria.

Pathophysiology and Natural History

The pathophysiology is the same as that in MM; in fact, MGUS will progress to a malignant plasma cell disorder at a rate of 1% per year. A monoclonal gammopathy has been associated with disease processes such as HIV, chronic hepatitis C infection, and rheumatoid arthritis. In these instances, treatment of the offending disease often will result in resolution of the monoclonal protein spike. It is rare, however, for MGUS to disappear on its own.

Clinical Presentation

By definition, patients with MGUS have no symptoms due to the syndrome itself. If the patient has bony pain or anemia, for example, then the patient either has another plasma cell disorder or has another unrelated disease process accounting for the symptoms.

Management

Diagnosis

The diagnosis of MGUS is made on the basis of SPEP and UPEP with the demonstration of lab criteria as stated above. The initial workup for MGUS should be the same as in MM to rule out the more serious disease. Clinicians should perform a complete history and physical. Lab and imaging should include a CBC, BUN, and serum creatinine, serum electrolytes, serum calcium, albumin, and serum free light chains. A bone marrow aspirate should be performed to evaluate the amount of plasma cell infiltration. A skeletal survey is generally performed to rule out lytic lesions but is not recommended if the M-protein level is <1.5 g/dL. Notably, β2-microglobulin has not been shown to predict the risk of progression to MM, so it is not recommended in the initial workup.

Staging/Prognosis

There is no staging system in MGUS. The rate of progression from MGUS to a malignant plasma cell disorder is ~1% per year. The risk of progression is not related to the duration of the MGUS or the age of the patient. The amount of M protein appears to predict progression; for example, a patient with an M-protein level of 2.5 g/dL has a greater risk than a patient with 1.5 g/dL M protein. In addition, it appears that the amount of plasma cell infiltration in the bone marrow and the presence of abnormal free light-chain ratios may be indicative of a higher risk of progression to a malignant plasma cell disorder.

Treatment/ Follow-up

There is currently no treatment indicated for MGUS. As it is generally a slowly progressing disorder, the vast majority of patients will not progress to a malignant disease. Generally, it is accepted practice to follow these patients annually with an evaluation that includes SPEP, UPEP, CBC, and serum creatinine. Of course, if patients develop symptoms concerning for a malignant plasma cell disease, they should undergo an extensive evaluation.

WALDENSTRÖM MACROGLOBINEMIA

Introduction

WM is a rare malignant lymphoproliferative disorder characterized by the production of IgM paraprotein. It is also known as lymphoplasmacytic lymphoma, and patients with the disorder have excess lymphoplasmacytoid cells in the bone marrow.

Clinical Presentation

Patients generally present with vague complaints such as weakness, fatigue, and neuropathy; anemia is often present. Markedly elevated levels of IgM can result in a hyperviscosity syndrome characterized by confusion, ataxia, and blurred vision. Symptoms of hyperviscosity can be mitigated quickly with plasmapheresis. In contrast to MM, visceral organ involvement to the liver or spleen may occur. There has been an association noted between WM and hepatitis C, so it is recommended to check a hepatitis panel.

Treatment/Prognosis

Treatment of WM includes alkylating agents, nucleoside analogues, and rituximab, a monoclonal antibody directed against B lymphocytes. No treatment has been shown to offer a cure, and the median survival from time of diagnosis is ~5 years.

AMYLOIDOSIS

Introduction

Amyloidosis is characterized by the tissue deposition of amyloid protein in a beta-pleated sheet configuration that is resistant to proteolysis. It is a rare disorder, affecting 5.1 to 12.8 per million people each year.

Causes

Primary amyloidosis is a plasma cell dyscrasia where the amyloid protein consists of monoclonal immunoglobulin fragments; it may coexist with a diagnosis of MM. Secondary amyloidosis occurs in the setting of an underlying chronic inflammatory condition or a familial syndrome. Manifestations of amyloidosis include nephrotic syndrome, congestive heart failure, peripheral and autonomic neuropathy, and skin manifestations.

Presentation

Symptoms of primary amyloidosis are nonspecific and include weight loss, fatigue, and lightheadedness. Neuropathy may be present. Physical examination may reveal macroglossia, periorbital ecchymosis, hepatomegaly, or edema. Laboratory evaluation may demonstrate renal insufficiency or hypoalbuminemia reflective of nephrotic syndrome. A paraprotein may be identified on serum protein electrophoresis and urine protein electrophoresis. The serum free light-chain assay may demonstrate a clonal light chain in the serum despite a negative SPEP.

Management

The diagnosis of amyloidosis may be confirmed on biopsy of the abdominal fat pad. If this is negative but amyloidosis remains in the differential diagnosis, bone marrow biopsy or biopsy of another organ such as the myocardium or kidney may be required. Workup should also include complete blood counts, complete metabolic profile, electrocardiogram, echocardiogram, and a 24-hour urine collection for protein and creatinine clearance. Treatment in primary amyloidosis is directed at the underlying plasma cell dyscrasia. Melphalan and dexamethasone, thalidomide, and high-dose melphalan followed by autologous stem cell transplant have been utilized. Amyloidosis is invariably fatal, with a median survival of 1 to 2 years.

KEY POINTS TO REMEMBER

- MM is a malignant plasma cell disorder that is diagnosed by the presence of all of the following: an M protein on SPEP or UPEP, clonal cells in the bone marrow or a plasmacytoma, and end-organ damage.
- β2-Microglobulin is an important prognostic indicator in MM and is included in the International Myeloma Working Group staging criteria.
- Although there is no cure for MM, autologous stem cell transplant currently offers the best chance for a complete response.
- Bortezomib is a proteosome inhibitor that has been shown to have a good result as a second-line agent, and may be considered for first-line treatment in the future.
- MGUS is an indolent disorder often found incidentally on routine lab work. It has a 1% rate of progression to a plasma cell malignancy each year.
- Amyloidosis results from deposition of light chains within tissues. Treatment is directed at the underlying plasma cell disorder.

REFERENCES AND SUGGESTED READINGS

Blade J. Monoclonal gammopathy of undetermined significance. *N Engl J Med.* 2006;355(26):2765–2770.

Gertz MA, Giampaolo M, Treon S. Amyloidosis and Waldenstrom's macroglobinemia. *Hematol Am Soc.* 2004;257–282.

Kyle RA, Rajkumar SV. Multiple myeloma. *N Engl J Med.* 2004;351(18):1860–1873.

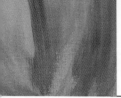

Introduction and Approach to Oncology

14

Prapti Patel and Tanya M. Wildes

APPROACH TO THE PATIENT WITH CANCER

There have been enormous advances in our understanding of the biology of cancer over the past 30 years. This has led to advances in treatment, including targeted therapies, that have improved survival. Yet a new diagnosis of cancer raises emotional and spiritual issues in a manner that few other diagnoses do, giving the medical oncologist a unique role in caring for the patient. The coordination of the oncologist with the referring physician needs to be individualized in the best interest of the patient. A trusting relationship with both the patient and the referring physician is important in coordinating the patient's care. Listening and taking the time to explain terminology, prognosis, and treatment options are key components to the relationship between the oncologist and the patient. Given that most advanced cancers cannot be cured, the oncologist's knowledge of and experience with the behavior of advanced malignancies combined with the use of complex medical regimens often lead to the oncologist's serving as the primary care physician during active treatment. Oncologists also are central in providing palliative care for symptom relief as well as assisting in the role of end-of-life discussions and care.

EPIDEMIOLOGY

Currently, cancer is the second most common cause of death and accounts for one in every four deaths in the United States. The lifetime risk of developing cancer in the United States is one in two for men and one in three for women.

Incidence and Prevalence

It is important to make a distinction between cancer incidence and prevalence. The **cancer incidence rate** is the number of newly diagnosed cancers in a set population in a finite amount of time. It is usually expressed as number of new cancer diagnoses per 100,000 people in 1 year. **Cancer prevalence** is the number or percentage of people alive with a cancer diagnosis on any given date. This includes new cases and existing cases and is therefore a function of incidence and survival.

Most Common Cancers/Causes of Cancer Death

According to the American Cancer Society, the most common sites of new cancer cases for men are prostate (29%), lung/bronchus (15%), and colorectal (10%). For women, breast cancer is the most common (26%), followed by lung/bronchus (15%) and colorectal (11%). These statistics do not include squamous and basal cell skin cancers or in situ carcinomas. The highest number of cancer deaths is due to lung cancer (31% in men and 26% in women). This is followed by prostate cancer (9%) and colorectal cancer (9%) in men and breast cancer (15%) and colorectal cancer (10%) in women.

Cancer Trends

Relative 5-year survival rate for all cancers diagnosed between 1996 and 2002 is 66%, which is up from 51% in 1975 to1977. This reflects progress in diagnosing certain cancers at an earlier stage and improvements in treatment. Along with the increase in survival rates, there has been an increase in the incidence of certain cancers. The reason for this is multi-factorial, including earlier detection of certain cancers, the increasing sensitivity of diagnostic tests, immunosuppression, and the aging of the population. Examples of the widespread use of basic diagnostic tests include mammograms, Pap smears, and prostate specific antigen to diagnose breast, cervical, and prostate cancer, respectively. Also, as the number of immunosuppressed patients increases, either from HIV or from bone marrow or solid organ transplant, the incidence of lymphoma increases. The body's major defense against malignancy is the immune system's ability to detect and destroy abnormal-appearing cells. If this function is impaired by drugs or infection, malignant cells have the potential to divide and metastasize. Most important to note among cancer trends is the increasing incidence of cancer. This is likely due to the increasing age of the population as a whole. As the therapies for common illnesses such as congestive heart failure and diabetes improve, the population as a whole is living longer. Since increased age confers an increased risk of cancer, the incidence of cancer has increased.

Cancer Statistics

Median Survival/Overall Survival/Relative Five-Year Survival

When a patient is diagnosed with cancer, one of the first questions an oncologist will be asked is: "How long do I have?" It is not an oncologist's place to assign a life expectancy to any single patient. Each clinical scenario is different; to speculate on life expectancy can have serious emotional ramifications. Survival is described in three broad terms: relative 5-year survival, median survival, and overall survival. These statistics are based on observational studies. **Relative 5-year survival rates** compare the survival among cancer patients with survival among the general population. It is calculated by dividing the percentage observed 5-year survival for cancer patients by the 5-year survival for people in the general population who are matched in age, gender, and race. It is also adjusted for comorbidities. This statistic is used in monitoring the progress of cancer detection and treatment. **Overall survival** is the percentage of subjects in a study that have survived a given amount of time. The **median survival** is more indicative of prognosis and is the statistic that is most commonly quoted to cancer patients. According to the National Cancer Institute, median survival is the time from diagnosis or treatment at which half of the patients with a given disease are found to be alive. In a clinical trial, the median survival time is one way to measure how effective a treatment is.

MANAGEMENT

Approach to Diagnosing a Malignancy

The treatment of a malignancy requires a *diagnosis based on tissue pathology.* In only rare emergent situations is treatment started without a diagnosis. Consultation from the surgical, medical, and radiologic oncology team members is essential. These oncology professionals are crucial to include in cases in which prompt therapy should be delivered to the patient to reduce the risk of morbidity or mortality in certain oncologic emergencies.

Pathology

Light microscopy is central to diagnosis. It delineates the microscopic structure of the malignancy, such as nuclear-to-cytoplasm ratio in leukemia, invasion into the microvasculature, or extent of glandular crowding in adenocarcinoma. Additional studies, including immunohistochemical staining, flow cytometry, cytogenetics, and molecular studies for gene rearrangements can corroborate a suspected diagnosis and assist in further subclassification.

Immunohistochemical staining identifies proteins on the cell membrane surface via an antigen-antibody complex. Antibodies to specific proteins are tagged with fluorescent markers (in direct immunohistochemical staining) and mixed with the biopsy specimen. If the specimen contains that particular protein, it will be tagged with the antibody and seen under fluorescent microscopy. In indirect staining, the specimen is mixed with a predetermined untagged antibody. Then a tagged IgG antibody is added and binds the antigen-antibody complexes. Immunohistochemistry is often used to identify certain receptors, such as CD20 in lymphoma, or protein markers, such as carcinoembryonic antigen (CEA) in colon cancer.

Flow cytometry characterizes cells suspended in liquid as they flow in a narrow stream and pass through a beam of laser light; it is most frequently applied in hematologic malignancies where certain antigen profiles are diagnostic (e.g., CD5/CD23 coexpression in chronic lymphocytic leukemia). In **cytogenetic testing**, chromosomes from blood, bone marrow, or solid tissue can be isolated to identify deletions, translocations, trisomies, or insertions into the genome. In this process, chromosomes of 20 cells are suspended in metaphase. The bands within the chromosomes are studied to identify any of the aforementioned abnormalities. Now cytogenetic testing has been taken one step further with the advent of **FISH** (fluorescence in situ hybridization). The DNA from the biopsy specimen is isolated and mixed with a known fluorescently labeled probe, such as 9;22 rearrangement for chronic myeloid leukemia. If the DNA contains that translocation, the probe will bind and light up under fluorescent microscopy. The advantage of this test is that it can identify subtle changes in the chromosome. However, it can only identify one abnormality (unlike cytogenetic testing) so the investigator must know which abnormality to look for.

Tumor Stage and Grade

Staging describes the extent of the disease in an individual patient. Staging is essential to the treatment of cancer in that it enables the oncologist to provide optimal treatment strategies and discuss outcomes or prognosis. In research studies, staging is used for comparison between cancer trials. Many tumors are associated with several staging systems. The most common staging system uses the **TNM classification system** developed by the American Joint Committee on Cancer. "T" represents the primary tumor characteristics. "N" represents the presence of nodal sites of disease. "M" represents metastatic or distant organ sites of spread. It is recommended that the reader consult an up-to-date staging manual when evaluating a patient because of frequent revisions for each individual malignancy. Clinical staging uses radiographic data to describe the extent of gross disease. Pathologic staging can identify microscopic foci of distant disease that may not be described on clinical staging exams.

The **grade** of a tumor is a pathologic description of the cellular characteristics of any given malignancy. A *low-grade malignancy* retains many of the characteristics of the originating cell type. Low-grade malignancies tend to be associated with a less aggressive cell type and more favorable prognosis. A *high-grade malignancy* is characterized by the loss of the characteristics of the originating cell type and evidence of higher mitotic activity. High-grade malignancies are often associated with a poorer prognosis, given the more aggressive behavior of the cells.

Performance Status

Performance status describes the functional abilities of the oncology patient. It is frequently used to provide a standardized assessment of patients considered for inclusion in protocols or to characterize patients at diagnosis or during treatment or follow-up. The initial performance status score predicts survival. The Karnofsky Performance Status and the

TABLE 14-1	KARNOFSKY AND EASTERN COOPERATIVE ONCOLOGY GROUP (ECOG) PERFORMANCE STATUS SCALES

The **Karnofsky scale** runs in increments of 10 from 0 (death) to 100 (no impairment) and can be divided into three broad ranges.

100–80: Normal activity without the need for special assistance and no or minimal symptoms of disease

50–70: Unable to work but able to live at home and capable of self-care, although varying levels of assistance may be required

10–40: Incapable of self-care, requiring acute or chronic care in a hospital or institutional setting, with rapidly progressive disease process

0: Death

The **ECOG scale** runs in increments of 1 from 0 (no impairment) to 5 (death).

0: Full activity, without symptoms
1: Ambulatory, able to carry out light activity, minimal symptoms
2: Unable to work, ambulatory for >50% of daytime activity
3: In bed or chair for >50% of daytime activity, limited self-care
4: Completely disabled, confined to bed or chair, unable to do any self-care
5: Death

Eastern Cooperative Oncology Group (ECOG) performance status scale (Table 14-1) are two of the most frequently used scales.

Imaging Modalities

- CT (computed tomography) allows cross-sectional imaging of the patient. Additional applications of CT include three-dimensional reconstructions and CT angiography. Intravenous radiocontrast medium is frequently utilized to enhance the sensitivity of the imaging. Risks of radiocontrast media include allergic reaction and nephrotoxicity.
- MRI (magnetic resonance imaging) is widely used in imaging the brain for either primary CNS tumors or metastases. MRI also has an emerging role in evaluation of breast cancer with breast MRI. MRI of the liver has a role in hepatocellular carcinoma as well as evaluation of solitary liver metastases in colon cancer. Absolute contraindications to MRI scanning include pacemakers, aneurysm clips, certain metallic cardiac prosthetic valves, and intraocular metal fragments.
- PET (positron emission tomography) is a functional imaging modality that images the distribution of intravenously administered radiolabeled tracers. 18-Flurodeoxyglucose (FDG) is the most widely utilized metabolic tracer. PET is most sensitive in aggressive and metabolically active tumors such as melanoma, head and neck, breast, lung, esophageal, cervical, and colorectal cancer, as well as aggressive subtypes of lymphoma. FDG-PET has a lower sensitivity in slower-growing tumors such as low-grade lymphomas, neuroendocrine tumors, and bronchioalveolar cell lung carcinoma. PET scans can be performed with concurrent CT (PET-CT) to merge both functional and anatomic imaging.
- Radionuclide bone scans are frequently used to detect bone metastases. They are less sensitive to purely osteolytic lesions, such as in multiple myeloma.
- Skeletal survey includes plain x-rays of the skull, spine, pelvis, and extremities. It is utilized in multiple myeloma to survey for osteolytic bone lesions.

TABLE 14-2 SENSITIVITY OF MALIGNANT TUMORS TO RADIATION

Very Responsive	Moderately Responsive	Poorly Responsive
Hodgkin lymphoma	Head and neck cancer	Melanoma
Non-Hodgkin lymphoma	Breast cancer	Glioblastoma
Seminoma, dysgerminoma	Prostate cancer	Renal cancer
Neuroblastoma	Cervical cancer	Pancreatic cancer
Small-cell cancers	Esophageal cancer	Sarcoma
Retinoblastoma	Rectal cancer	
	Lung cancer	

Approach to Oncology Treatment

The majority of adult solid malignancies are best managed through a multidisciplinary approach involving surgeons, radiation oncologists, and medical oncologists. There are often multiple different treatment options, and patients should be an active part of the decision-making process. An important element in the treatment of cancer patients is to *define the goals of treatment,* addressing potential for cure, prolongation of survival, or improvement in quality of life. Treatment recommendations should be carefully tailored to the individual patient, taking into account comorbid conditions, performance status, and other psychosocial issues.

Surgical Approach to Cancer

Surgery still remains the most effective modality for curing cancer confined to a local site. In many instances, the surgical removal of the primary cancer also involves the removal of a regional node-bearing area. Appropriate patients can be identified for definitive or curative surgery. The goal is for the surgeon to remove all neoplastic cells, including the resection of a complete margin of normal tissue around the primary tumor. Depending on the tumor, patients with a solitary or limited number of metastases to sites such as the brain, liver, and lung can be cured by the surgical resection of the metastatic disease. Cytoreductive surgery or tumor debulking can facilitate subsequent radiation and/or chemotherapy in some malignancies such as ovarian cancer. Surgery may also be necessary in the palliative setting to relieve symptoms, such as the relief of an intestinal obstruction from colon cancer.

Radiation Therapy

Radiation therapy is the treatment of choice for some cancers. The use of this treatment modality is based on the responsiveness of a cancer to ionizing radiation. Some cancers are extremely sensitive, including lymphomas and seminomas, whereas others are relatively resistant (Table 14-2). Radiation therapy can be the sole curative local modality in malignancies such as cervical cancer and prostate cancer. It is also useful in the adjuvant setting to increase the likelihood of local or regional control after surgery. Radiation therapy also plays a key role in the palliation of symptoms from primary or metastatic tumor masses, including spinal cord compression and bone metastases. For more information regarding radiation therapy, see Chapter 17.

Systemic Therapy

- In contrast to surgery or radiation therapy, which has only local effects on the tumor, the role of systemic therapy is geared at treating both the local tumor and potential or actual areas of metastatic disease throughout the body. Before the initiation of chemotherapy, the **goal of treatment** must be clearly defined and discussed with the patient. Not all patients are candidates for chemotherapy. Potential risks and benefits must be considered when deciding to treat a patient with cytotoxic agents. The performance status and overall nutritional state of the cancer patient is extremely important when making the decision to use chemotherapy. Performance status scores of 3 to 4 on the ECOG scale are usually not candidates for systemic therapy unless they have previously untreated tumors known to be especially responsive to chemotherapy.

- **Adjuvant therapy** refers to the use of systemic therapy following complete surgical resection to improve both disease-free and overall survival. The goal is to eliminate undetected local and micrometastatic foci of tumor. There is no way to measure or follow response to therapy, and thus duration of treatment is determined empirically by clinical trials. Cancers for which adjuvant chemotherapy has proved to benefit survival include colorectal, breast, lung, ovarian cancers, and osteosarcoma. Similarly, adjuvant hormonal therapy is effective in improving survival in breast cancer patients who are estrogen receptor positive.

- **Neoadjuvant therapy** refers to systemic therapy that is administered before surgery. The goal of neoadjuvant therapy is to decrease the tumor burden for the definitive surgical procedure, thus minimizing complications and making organ preservation more feasible. In addition, the clinician can monitor the tumor response to a systemic agent for effectiveness. Neoadjuvant chemotherapy is used in breast, esophageal, rectal, lung, and bladder cancers, as well as osteosarcomas.

- **Combined modality therapy** refers to the combination of chemotherapy and radiotherapy used to treat bulky disease. The goal of combined modality therapy may be to decrease the size of the tumor for either a curative or a salvage surgical procedure. Combined modality therapy improves survival for some patients with locally advanced lung, esophageal, head and neck, pancreatic, and cervical cancers. The combination can also be curative and organ-preserving in certain tumors such as laryngeal and anal cancers.

- **Induction chemotherapy** is used as the initial treatment of a malignancy to achieve complete remission or significant cytoreduction. It is commonly used in the treatment of acute leukemias and lymphomas. **Consolidation chemotherapy** is given after a patient is in remission to prolong the duration of remission and overall survival in patients with acute leukemias. **Maintenance chemotherapy** is the use of prolonged, low-dose chemotherapy to prolong the duration of remission and achieve a cure in those patients; it is currently only utilized in certain leukemias. **Salvage chemotherapy** is given with the intent to control disease or palliate symptoms after the failure of initial treatments.

- **High-dose chemotherapy** is typically used in the treatment of hematologic malignancies. The high doses of chemotherapy are used to ablate the bone marrow requiring rescue with **allogeneic** or **autologous** bone marrow or stem cell replacement to repopulate the marrow. Allogeneic transplants have been curative in selected patients with chronic myelogenous leukemia and acute leukemias. Autologous stem cell transplants have been most successful for aggressive lymphomas and multiple myeloma. The use of bone marrow transplant in solid organ malignancies remains controversial.

- **Immunotherapy** refers to the use of pharmacologic agents that are intrinsic to the immune system. High concentrations of these biologic response modifiers stimulate the immune system to kill cancer cells. Examples include interferon-alpha, interleukin-2, and monoclonal antibodies. Toxicities can range from fevers and flulike symptoms to anaphylaxis and adult respiratory distress syndrome–like manifestations. Tumor vaccines and gene therapies remain experimental.

- **Targeted therapies** interfere with specific pathways needed for the growth and survival of cancer cells. These therapies may include monoclonal antibodies or small molecule inhibitors which target specific receptors or kinases such as the epidermal growth factors receptor, the vascular endothelial growth factor receptor, and the bcr-abl tyrosine kinase.

Response to Therapy

In general, responses to therapy are measured by objective changes in tumor size and increases in disease-free and overall survival. The RECIST (Response Criteria in Solid

Tumors) is a widely utilized tool for describing change in solid tumor size in response to therapy. Other response criteria are utilized in hematologic malignancies. The single most important indicator of the effectiveness of chemotherapy is the complete response rate. No patient with advanced cancer can be cured without attaining a complete remission.

- A **complete response** is defined as the disappearance of disease on imaging studies of at least 1 month's duration.
- A **partial response** is a decrease of 50% or more in the sum of the products of the biperpendicular diameters of the measurable disease (as measured by radiology or physical exam), with no new sites of disease for at least 1 month's duration. For example, if the oncologist is following a lung lesion measuring 3×2 cm and a liver lesion measuring 4×5 cm, then the sum of the products of the biperpendicular diameters in this example is $(3 \times 2) + (4 \times 5)$, which is 26. To document a partial response in this example, on follow-up measurements, the sum should be ≤ 13.
- **Progression** of a tumor is defined as a $>25\%$ increase in the product of the biperpendicular diameters in one or more sites, the appearance of new lesions, or the death of the patient as a result of the tumor. Chemotherapy is discontinued in the setting of progression, and the patient is re-evaluated.
- The term **stable disease** is used when the measurable disease does not meet the criteria for complete response, partial response, or progression. Stable disease represents a difficult challenge to oncologists. If therapy is tolerated with no significant side effects, it is often continued, provided it is recognized that progressive disease will eventually occur.

Goals of Care

Prognosis

An individual's **prognosis** is based on staging, comorbidities, performance status, and response to treatment. Although it is possible to predict curability or median survival, long-term follow-up is essential to get a more accurate sense of prognosis for any given patient. Even when the overall prognosis is poor, an honest and compassionate discussion with the patient and family members is essential. This is a key role of the medical oncologist. Up-front and honest answers to even the most difficult questions allow the patient and family to set realistic goals that will help guide future health care decisions. See Table 14–3 for a list of potentially curable malignancies.

TABLE 14-3	CANCERS CURABLE OR OCCASIONALLY CURABLE WITH CHEMOTHERAPY ALONE

Curable with chemotherapy alone

- Gestational choriocarcinoma
- Hodgkin lymphoma
- Germ cell cancer of the testis
- Acute lymphoid leukemia
- Non-Hodgkin lymphoma (some subtypes)
- Hairy cell leukemia

Occasionally curable with chemotherapy alone

- Acute myeloid leukemia
- Ovarian cancer
- Small-cell lung cancer

Palliative Care

Palliative care of cancer patients entails the management of all of the symptoms related to the cancer itself and the toxicities of treatment. It also includes the multidisciplinary care of psychosocial issues, with the primary goal of optimizing the quality of life and minimizing the morbidity and symptoms related to cancer and its treatments. Prolongation of survival is a secondary goal, which may or may not be achieved, but cure is not the primary intent in palliative care. Chemotherapy, hormonal therapy, radiation, and surgery are still useful in palliation. Patient selection for interventions is crucial. For patients with advanced cancer and poor performance status, aggressive treatment may be detrimental rather than beneficial.

Hospice

Hospice is a philosophy of care based on a coordinated program of support services for terminally ill patients and their families. Palliative care is provided with the aim to improve quality of life and allow a comfortable death. Any patient with a limited life expectancy (≤6 months) may be eligible for hospice care. The interdisciplinary hospice team consists of nurses trained in pain and symptom management, physicians, home health aides, social workers, chaplains, and volunteers. Care is generally given in the home but may be imparted in nursing homes or hospitals if necessary. Medicare hospice benefits also include complete coverage for all medications pertaining to the hospice diagnosis, durable medical equipment, and oxygen. Most hospice agencies provide 24-hour on-call service, brief respite care, and bereavement counseling for up to 1 year after the patient dies.

COMMON PRESENTATIONS

Lymphadenopathy

Lymphadenopathy may cause a patient to seek medical attention or may be found incidentally on physical examination or imaging. The differential diagnosis is broad, including infectious etiologies, autoimmune, sarcoidosis, drug hypersensitivity, benign or clonal lymphoproliferative disorders, and malignancy. Malignant causes of lymphadenopathy include lymphoma and metastatic solid tumors. Features that suggest a malignant etiology of lymphadenopathy include lymph nodes >2 cm in size, lymph nodes that are hard or fixed to adjacent structures, and supraclavicular or epitrochlear lymphadenopathy. Lymphadenopathy may be localized or generalized, and the differential diagnosis varies depending on the location and distribution of the enlarged lymph nodes. When biopsy is indicated, an open biopsy is preferred over a core biopsy or aspiration as it allows for evaluation of the lymph node architecture, which is often necessary for classification of lymphoma.

Solitary Pulmonary Nodule

A solitary pulmonary nodule is a round opacity <3 cm in diameter without any associated lymphadenopathy, infiltrate, or atelectasis. The broad differential diagnosis includes malignancy, benign neoplasms such as hamartomas, infectious etiologies including granulomas, and noninfectious inflammatory disorders such as sarcoidosis and vasculitides. See Chapter 19 for discussion of the appropriate evaluation of a solitary pulmonary nodule.

Brain Mass

The differential diagnosis for a brain mass includes metastatic disease, primary brain tumors, CNS lymphoma, hamartoma, AV malformation, demyelination, cerebral infarction or bleeding, and infection. Brain metastases are the most common intracranial tumors in adults, accounting for 50% of all brain tumors. This is due to the blood-brain barrier, which prevents penetration of chemotherapeutic agents into the CNS, thus providing a sanctuary site for metastatic tumor cells. The incidence of brain metastases is increasing, perhaps due to the increasing sensitivity of MRI. Lung, kidney, colorectal, and breast carcinomas and melanoma frequently metastasize to the brain. Cancer of the prostate, esophagus, and oropharynx and nonmelanoma skin cancers rarely metastasize to the brain. Signs and symptoms of a brain mass include headache, focal neurological deficits, altered mental status, seizures, and stroke. The imaging study of choice is a contrast-enhanced MRI, which will delineate the location, presence of other lesions, margins of the lesion, and presence of vasogenic edema. Brain metastases are usually located in the gray and white matter junction and have a large amount of vasogenic edema. A brain biopsy should be preformed whenever the diagnosis is in doubt. This is particularly important in patients who have a single lesion or have a cancer that rarely metastasizes to the brain. Often, a brain lesion is the primary presentation of a malignancy. Evaluation for a source of a metastatic focus, particularly lung and breast cancer, should precede biopsy. Basic initial workup includes CT of the chest, colonoscopy, comprehensive skin exam, and mammogram.

Liver Metastases

The differential diagnosis of a focal liver lesion includes primary malignant liver tumors (such as hepatocellular carcinoma, cholangiocarcinoma, lymphoma, and sarcoma), metastatic liver lesions, benign hepatic cysts, cavernous hemangioma, hepatic adenoma, and abscesses. Before proceeding to diagnostic testing, it is important to assess the clinical scenario. For example, is this an incidental finding? Does the patient have any risk factors such as hepatitis C/cirrhosis, oral contraceptive use, travel history, history of malignancy, or constitutional symptoms? Diagnostic modalities include liver ultrasound, triphasic CT of the liver, and MRI of the liver. If there is a likelihood of malignancy, a fine-needle biopsy can be done. It is important to note that if a patient has a remote history of cancer, one cannot assume that a new liver lesion is due to metastases. It must be definitively diagnosed, as a second unrelated malignancy cannot be ruled out.

Bone Lesions

Bone lesions can be the initial presentation of metastatic cancer or can present later in advanced malignancy. Bone metastases are most commonly due to multiple myeloma, breast cancer, or prostate cancer. They are classified as osteolytic or osteoblastic lesions. **Osteolytic** lesions refer to the destruction of normal bone, whereas **osteoblastic** lesions are the result of deposition of new bone. Multiple myeloma lesions are purely osteolytic. Metastases from prostate cancer are usually osteoblastic. Breast cancer metastases are usually a combination of both. Bone is a preferential site for metastasis because tumor cells express and produce various chemokines and adhesive molecules that bind corresponding molecules on the stromal cells of the bone. For example, expression of RANKL (receptor activator of nuclear factor kappa B ligand) in bone facilitates development of metastasis by binding RANK (receptor activator of nuclear factor kappa B) on the surface of tumor cells. Also, tumor cells can express bone sialoprotein and bind collagen type I in the extracellular matrix in the bone, thus becoming more adhesive. Signs and symptoms of bone involvement include focal pain, pathologic fractures, hypercalcemia, and cord compression. Diagnosis is usually made by radiological testing, including plain films, which diagnose osteolytic lesions, and bone scans, which detect osteoblastic lesions only. Treatment includes systemic chemotherapy and hormone therapy. Local radiation can be used to palliate symptoms and prevent pathological fractures. Bisphosphonates are used to treat hypercalcemia, treat bone pain, prevent fractures, and prevent further destruction of the normal bone.

KEY POINTS TO REMEMBER

- A tissue diagnosis of a cancer is usually required before an oncology consult is appropriate.
- The oncologist often becomes a primary care giver to the patient during active treatment.
- Mutual goal setting between the patient and the physician is an important part of the care of the oncology patient and should be reassessed frequently.
- Patients should be offered enrollment in clinical trials whenever possible, but respecting the patient's wishes regarding this is the first principle.
- The philosophy behind hospice is to provide patients who have a limited life expectancy the care and support needed to improve their quality of life and ensure a comfortable death.

REFERENCES AND SUGGESTED READINGS

Brown JR, Skarin AT. Clinical mimics of lymphoma. *Oncologist.* 2004;9:406–416.
Jaffe CC. Measures of response: RECIST, WHO, and new alternatives. *J Clin Oncol.* 2006;24:3245–3251.
Torigian DA, Huang SS, Houseni M, et al. Functional imaging of cancer with emphasis on molecular techniques. *CA Cancer J Clin.* 2007;57:206–224.
Winer-Muram HT. The solitary pulmonary nodule. *Radiology.* 2006;239(1):34–49.

Cancer Biology

15

Priya K. Gopalan

INTRODUCTION

Our understanding of the biology of cancer has expanded considerably over the last few decades. With the completion of the human genome project and the advent of array-based screening techniques, we are beginning to understand the molecular mechanisms by which cells transform into malignant cells, proliferate, and metastasize. Our current understanding of all these facets of cancer biology is too detailed to review comprehensively here. In this chapter, we try to highlight general mechanisms of tumorigenesis and metastasis.

TUMORIGENESIS

Tumorigenesis is the production of tumors by uncontrolled cellular proliferation. This tissue grows more rapidly than normal, continues to grow after the stimuli that initiated the new growth cease, and survives longer than the parent cells.

In order to transform into a cancer cell, a cell must be able to escape mechanisms in place to control cell proliferation, differentiation, and/or apoptosis (programmed cell death). Hanahan and Weinberg proposed that all tumor cells must first acquire six essential characteristics: self-sufficiency in growth signals, insensitivity to antigrowth signals, evasion of apoptosis, limitless replication potential, angiogenesis, and tissue invasion and metastasis. In addition, they must also be able to evade DNA repair mechanisms and the immune system.

- **Self-sufficiency in growth signals**. Tumor cells can generate their own growth signals (autocrine production), stimulate the release of growth factors bound to the extracellular matrix, amplify their response to growth signals, or proliferate independently of growth signals (constitutive activation of signaling pathways).
- **Insensitivity to antigrowth signals**. Growth inhibitors can act by forcing cells into the quiescent (G0) state in the cell cycle or by blocking progression from G1 to S phase. For example, transforming growth factor beta (TGFβ) is a soluble signaling molecule that acts as an antigrowth factor. It prevents the inactivation of Rb, a gene that is critical for controlling progression from G1 into S phase. Tumor cells can evade regulation by TGFβ by downregulating TGFβ receptors, displaying mutant receptors, or inactivating downstream signaling proteins.
- **Evasion of apoptosis**. There are several tumor suppressor genes promoting apoptosis, including p53 and PTEN, which are inactivated in tumors.
- **Limitless replication potential**. Senescence, which limits the number of times a cell can replicate, can be avoided in cancer cells by overexpression of telomerase. This enzyme maintains telomeres, which are highly repetitive sequences at the ends of chromosomes that stabilize the chromosome. In normal cells, a section of telomeres

is lost during each replicative cycle, until ultimately the telomere is too small and the cell is no longer able to replicate. By maintaining telomere length, a tumor cell has limitless replication potential. Another mechanism that provides tumors with extensive, although not limitless, replication potential is the creation of cancer stem cells. These are cells that are mutated either from normal stem cells or from committed progenitor cells that are capable of self-renewal, development into multiple lineages, and extensive proliferation. Cancer stem cells have been identified in leukemia (chronic myeloid leukemia, acute myeloid leukemia [AML], and possibly acute lymphocytic leukemia), central nervous system cancers, and breast cancer. Most cancer stem cells appear to be quiescent, rendering them insensitive to most nonsurgical therapies.

- **Angiogenesis.** Tumors cannot grow larger than 0.4 to 2 mm in diameter without access to blood vessels. Therefore, there must be growth of new blood vessels from pre-existing vessels, termed angiogenesis, in concert with tumor growth. The growth of new blood vessels, often induced by hypoxia, requires upregulation of proangiogenic factors, such as vascular-endothelial growth factor (VEGF) and fibroblast growth factor (FGF)-1 and -2, with simultaneous inhibition of antiangiogenic factors such as angiopoietin-1 and thrombospondin-1, either directly or through mutation of regulating tumor suppressor genes or oncogenes. The importance of VEGF in angiogenesis is evident by the efficacy of anti-VEGF agents, such as bevacizumab, in many cancers.
- **Tissue invasion and metastasis.** This property is discussed in more detail below.
- **Evasion of repair mechanisms.** This property is discussed in more detail below.
- **Evasion of the immune system.** Cells must escape the immune response, particularly cytotoxic T lymphocytes and natural killer cells in the circulation, by either preventing immune recognition or inducing immune tolerance. Escape from immune recognition is mediated by downregulating mechanisms necessary for antigen presentation. Examples include downregulation of MHC molecules and inhibition of costimulatory molecules on tumor cells. Generation of immune tolerance involves altering the complex cellular and cytokine network of antigen presentation. Examples include production of inhibitory cytokines, suppression of stimulatory cytokines, and induction of formation of T-regulatory cells.

Tumorigenesis can be thought of as a continuum of the changes in cell characteristics described above, which transforms a cell population from benign to malignant. Recent studies have suggested that several sequential events may be required for malignant transformation. These events may involve mutations in multiple genes with different roles in normal cell function. Colon cancer demonstrates such a progression, from normal colonic epithelium to increasingly dysplastic adenomas and then frank malignancy, usually progressing over many years. The genetic mutations underlying this phenotypic progression occur sequentially. Fearon and Vogelstein formulated a model of tumor progression in colon cancer, correlating molecular with phenotypic changes. In their model, there is first a sporadic or inherited mutation in one copy of APC, a gene involved in proliferation and differentiation, without any change in phenotype. Subsequent deletion of the other copy of APC, however, leads to aberrant crypt foci. Mutation of K-ras, a gene promoting proliferation that is mutated in 50% of colorectal cancers, then leads to the development of a dysplastic adenoma. Finally, functional loss of both p53 alleles causes loss of both cell cycle arrest and apoptosis, leading to malignancy.

GENETIC CHANGES

There are two main categories of genes that are involved in the initiation of most cancers: oncogenes and tumor suppressor genes. These genes often have physiologic roles in normal cells. However, mutations that cause oncogene gain of function or tumor suppressor gene loss of function promote uncontrolled tumor growth.

Oncogenes

Proto-oncogenes are genes that usually promote controlled growth and proliferation in normal cells. When mutated or overexpressed, they promote tumorigenesis and are termed "oncogenes." The first oncogene identified was in Rous sarcoma virus, a retrovirus that causes sarcoma in chickens upon infection. The transforming retrovirus contains a nucleotide sequence derived from integration of the host proto-oncogene, c-src, into the viral genome and is converted to a viral oncogene, v-src, with transforming activity. Other oncogenes include K-ras, c-myc, abl, bcl-2, VEGFR, and EGFR. Their activation represents a gain-of-function mutation. Their mutations are dominant, with mutation of only one allele necessary to convert the proto-oncogene to the activated oncogene. For example, in colon cancer, ~50% of tumors carry a single mutant K-ras allele that promotes uncontrolled proliferation.

Tumor Suppressor Genes

These genes are typically inactivated by a loss-of-function mutation. They are recessive at the cellular level and require loss or inactivation of both copies of the allele for transformation. Examples include PTEN, p53, Rb, BRCA-1, BRCA-2, MSH-2, MLH-1, and APC. For example, loss of function of both Rb alleles allows unchecked progression through the cell cycle. Most inherited cancer syndromes are caused by the transmission of inactivating mutations in tumor suppressor genes, such as PTEN (Cowden syndrome) and p53 (Li-Fraumeni).

Functions of Oncogenes and Tumor Suppressor Genes in Normal Cells

- **Growth factors.** Platelet-derived growth factor (PDGF) and epidermal growth factor are examples of proto-oncogenes that are growth factors. When the genes are activated by mutation or amplification, there is increased secretion of growth factors, resulting in enhanced ligand activation and cell signaling.
- **Receptor tyrosine kinases.** Receptors such as Her-2/neu, VEGFR, and EGFR are proto-oncogenes that can cause constitutive activation and cell signaling when mutated.
- **Intracellular signaling molecules.** Proto-oncogenes and tumor suppressor genes are involved in many intracellular signaling pathways. K-Ras, a GTPase, is a proto-oncogene that is upstream of the Raf-MEK-Erk pathway. PTEN, a tumor suppressor gene, negatively regulates the PI3K-Akt-mTOR pathway.
- **Nuclear transcription factors.** Transcription factors include c-myc (a proto-oncogene) and Rb (a tumor suppressor gene). Abnormalities in these genes can lead to enhanced transcription.
- **Cell cycle regulation.** The cell cycle is carefully regulated, with multiple genes involved. Many of these genes are associated with cyclins and cyclin-dependent kinases. Two such genes involved in cell cycle regulation are the tumor suppressor genes Rb and p53. Rb can bind transcription factor E2F and inhibit transcription of many target genes, including initiation factors that are involved in DNA replication. This effectively arrests the cell in G1 phase. p53 can also induce cell cycle arrest in the G1 phase, following DNA damage. It is discussed in more detail below. Loss of function of these tumor suppressor genes results in dysregulated cell cycling.
- **DNA repair.** Normally, a cell with a mutated DNA sequence will undergo either DNA repair or apoptosis if the damage is irreparable. Defective DNA repair mechanisms allow mutations in oncogenes or tumor suppressor genes to propagate, increasing the chance of malignant transformation. Patients with inherited deficiencies in

DNA repair genes have a greater susceptibility to cancers. For example, patients with mutations in BRCA-1 or BRCA-2, genes involved in DNA double-strand break (dsb) repair, have an increased risk of breast and ovarian cancers. As another example, the DNA mismatch repair (MMR) genes, MLH1 and MSH2, are mutated in hereditary nonpolyposis colorectal cancer. This deficiency leads to microsatellite instability, which are short regions of DNA repeats that are gained or lost. The MMR repair defect then leads to an accumulation of mutations in other genes such as p53 and APC, which ultimately leads to colon cancer.

- **Apoptosis.** Apoptosis is crucial for normal cell regulation. p53 and PTEN are two tumor suppressor genes that also play a role in apoptosis. p53 can initiate apoptosis by targeting several key apoptotic genes, including Fas and Bax. Bcl-2 functions as a proto-oncogene and prevents apoptosis when overexpressed, as is seen in some lymphoid malignancies.

Causes of Genetic Changes

- **Inherited defects.** These are traditionally mutations in one copy of a tumor suppressor gene that increase the susceptibility to cancers. There is usually enough function by the remaining allele to prevent loss of function. Examples include Ret, which increases the risk of multiple endocrine neoplasia syndromes, and BRCA-1. Mutated BRCA-1 is identified in ≤3% of women with breast cancer, but it increases their cumulative risk of breast cancer to 54% and that of ovarian cancer to 30% by age 60.
- **Exogenous damage.** Chemicals, radiation, and substances such as asbestos fibers can cause damage to DNA. Cancer was first linked to chemical exposure with the documentation of increased scrotal cancer in chimney sweeps. Ames et al. then discovered that mutagenic chemicals, such as mitomycin C, can be carcinogenic, underscoring the relationship between DNA damage and carcinogenesis. Radiation can mutate DNA through cross-linking and lead to cancers such as thyroid carcinoma (ionizing radiation) and basal cell carcinoma (UV radiation).
- **Viruses.** Both DNA viruses and retroviruses can lead to tumorigenesis. Viruses can either aberrantly express their own viral form of an oncogene (transduction) or drive aberrant expression of a cellular proto-oncogene (proviral insertion). Specific viruses are often associated with specific tumors. Examples include human papillomavirus in cervical cancer, Epstein-Barr virus in Burkitt lymphoma and nasopharyngeal carcinoma, hepatitis B and C virus in hepatocellular carcinoma, and human T cell leukemia virus (HTLV)-1 and -2 in T cell leukemia.
- **Errors during replication (point mutations and deletions, cytogenetic abnormalities).** Point mutations and deletions in proto-oncogenes and tumor suppressor genes can lead to their activation. Cytogenetic abnormalities include amplification (e.g., Her-2/neu in breast cancer and EGFR in colon cancer), deletions, and translocations. Perhaps the best-studied translocation is t(9;22) in chronic myeloid leukemia, which forms the bcr-abl fusion oncogene. Other examples include t(15;17) in APL, which forms the PML-RARα fusion oncogene and t(8;21) in AML M2, which forms the fusion oncogene, AML1-ETO.

p53

The tumor suppressor p53 is the most frequently mutated gene in human cancer and therefore warrants further discussion. Inactivating mutations have been found in more than 50% of all cancers. Patients with Li-Fraumeni syndrome have germline mutations in the p53 gene and are at a high risk for early-onset cancers of multiple tissues types, including breast, bone, soft tissue, head and neck, and brain and, less commonly, lung, stomach, colon, and blood (leukemia). p53 is a tumor suppressor gene that is involved in the normal cellular response to stresses such as DNA damage, hypoxia, and oncogene activation.

It is a transcription factor that primarily activates genes responsible for cell cycle arrest and apoptosis. Normally, p53 upregulates expression of proapoptotic genes, such as Bax, in response to DNA damage. The majority of p53 mutations (~75%) are missense mutations, usually within the DNA-binding domain. The missense mutations in p53 cause an abnormal tertiary structure of the protein that can no longer bind DNA, which is critical for its role as a transcription factor. p53 mutation may play a role in the timing of malignant transformation. p53 alterations (mutations or epigenetic inactivation) are early events in lung, esophageal, head and neck, breast, cervical, bladder, and stomach cancers but late events in brain, thyroid, prostate, and ovarian cancers. There is no consistent pattern in p53 alteration in colon, bladder, and liver cancers.

EPIGENETIC CHANGES

Epigenetic changes are inheritable changes in the pattern of gene expression mediated by mechanisms other than changes in the primary nucleotide sequence of a gene. They lead to suppression of gene expression and often affect tumor suppressor genes in cancer. There are two main types of epigenetic regulation: DNA methylation and histone modification. MicroRNAs (miRNAs), although not categorized as epigenetic regulators, are discussed in this section because they, too, mediate changes in gene expression, rather than the primary nucleotide sequence.

DNA Methylation

DNA methylation of cytosines in CG dinucleotide sequences, mediated by DNA methyltransferases, generally leads to repression of a transcriptional promoter and, thus, transcriptional silencing. In normal physiology, it plays a critical role in embryogenesis and gametogenesis. However, in cancer, abnormal DNA methylation can lead to inactivation of tumor suppressor genes. For example, hypermethylation of the promoter for MLH1, a gene involved in DNA mismatch repair, has been implicated in the pathogenesis of hereditary nonpolyposis colorectal cancer. DNA methylation is also important in hematologic malignancies. Two DNA methyltransferase inhibitors, 5-azacytadine and decitabine (2'-deoxy-5-azacytidine), are approved therapy for the treatment of myelodysplastic syndrome and also have activity in acute leukemia.

Histone Deacetylation

Histone deacetylation (HDAC) is another type of epigenetic modification, which leads to silencing of gene expression. Deacetylation of histones causes them to wrap more tightly around DNA, which blocks access of transcription factors to DNA, thus blocking transcription. HDAC inhibitors can reactivate silenced genes. The HDAC inhibitor Vorinostat was recently approved for treatment of cutaneous T cell lymphoma. Many others are in development.

MicroRNAs

miRNAs are small, noncoding RNAs that bind mRNA and negatively regulate their expression by mediating their degradation or translational repression. Hence, they act as tumor suppressors. For example, miR-15a and miR-16-1 negatively regulate bcl-2, an antiapoptotic gene. These miRNAs are often deleted or downregulated in B-cell CLL, which would allow unregulated expression of bcl-2.

TUMOR METASTASIS

One of the hallmarks of cancer is the ability to invade surrounding tissues and metastasize, or spread. Most solid tumors progress in an orderly manner, from localized to locally advanced to metastatic sites. The timing of metastasis is dependent on tumor type. For example, head and neck cancers initially spread to regional lymph nodes and only later to distant sites, while breast cancer can spread early to distant sites.

The sites of metastasis also vary by tumor type. Populations of metastatic cells with enhanced preference for a specific organ can by isolated by serially selecting cells from these organs. These cells have been used in gene expression profiling studies to detect molecules that are important in metastasis. Genes suppressing metastasis have also been identified using this method.

The exact mechanism of metastasis is not known, but in order for a tumor cell to metastasize, it must acquire several additional properties, detailed below.

- **Detachment from the primary tumor.** Detachment is dependent on cell-to-cell adhesion. Decreased expression of cell-cell adhesion molecules, such as E-cadherin, can lead to detachment of individual cells from the primary tumor. In addition, increased expression of proteases, such as matrix metalloproteases, helps cleave cell-cell adhesions.
- **Invasion, migration, and intravasation.** Invasion is also facilitated by proteases and changes in expression of cell adhesion molecules. Migration is mediated by motility factors such as hepatocyte growth factor. Migration of carcinomas is also aided by epithelial-to-mesenchymal transition, by which epithelial cells lose cell-cell contacts that anchor them (especially E-cadherin-mediated adhesion) and acquire a mesenchymal cell phenotype that promotes motility and invasion. Epithelial-to-mesenchymal transition is probably mediated by various growth factors, including TGFβ, FGF, hepatocyte growth factor, insulinlike growth factor, and epidermal growth factor. Motility and intravasation are also enabled by changes in expression of cell-to-matrix adhesion molecules, such as integrins and members of the immunoglobulin superfamily (cell adhesion molecules), and proteases that degrade the extracellular matrix.
- **Survival in the vasculature or lymphatic system.** Tumor cells must evade the immune system, as described above. In addition, they must be able to survive in the absence of adhesions to the extracellular matrix. In normal cells, the absence of such adhesions leads to apoptosis. However, malignant cells are able to survive independently of interactions with the extracellular matrix.
- **Arrest at the metastatic site and extravasation.** The anatomy of blood and lymphatic drainage is an important determinant of the site of metastasis. Chemokines also play an important role in organ-specific metastasis. For example, breast cancer cells have high expression of the chemokine receptor, CXCR4, while its ligand, CXCL12, is highly expressed in organs to which it most commonly metastasizes: lung, liver, bone, and regional lymph nodes. Once at the target organ site, cells must arrest in the vasculature and extravasate, which again involves alterations in expression of cell adhesion molecules and proteases.
- **Survival in the metastatic microenvironment.** Once they have reached the target organ, tumor cells must have an adhesive substrate on which they can attach and grow. In addition, either they or the target organ must secrete the growth factors, including angiogenic factors, necessary for their proliferation and survival.

FUTURE

With our current understanding of tumor biology and with the tools of genomic and gene expression profiling, we are now finally beginning to categorize cancers into individual molecular subtypes. This molecular characterization will eventually allow us to predict prognosis and response to specific therapies. As we learn more about the molecular pathogenesis of different types of cancers, we will eventually be able to truly personalize patients' treatment to their individual cancer.

KEY POINTS TO REMEMBER

- Typically, multiple sequential mutational events (genetic or epigenetic) occur in tumor formation.
- Oncogenes and tumor suppressor genes function in normal cells but lead to unregulated proliferation and survival when mutated.
- Cell cycle regulators, apoptotic genes, and DNA repair mechanisms must be disabled in order to propagate mutations.
- Tumor metastasis is a complex process involving cell adhesion molecules, proteases, and chemokines. Organ-specific metastasis is due in part to the microenvironment that is favorable for growth of the tumor cell.

REFERENCES AND SUGGESTED READINGS

Ames BN, Cathcart R, Schwiers E, et al. Uric acid provides an antioxidant defense in humans against oxidant- and radical-caused aging and cancer: a hypothesis. *Proc Natl Acad Sci USA.* 1981;78:6858–6862.

Chambers AF, Groom AC, MacDonald IC. Dissemination and growth of cancer cells in metastatic sites. *Natl Rev Cancer.* 2002;2:563–572.

Christofori G. New signals from the invasive front. *Nature.* 2006;441:444–449.

Duvic M, Vu J. Vorinostat: a new oral histone deacetylase inhibitor approved for cutaneous T-cell lymphoma. *Expert Opin Invest Drugs.* 2007;16(7):1111–1120.

Easton DF, Ford D, Bishop DT. Breast and ovarian cancer incidence in BRCA1-mutation carriers. Breast Cancer Linkage Consortium. *Am J Hum Genet.* 1995;56(1):265–271.

Egeblad M, Werb Z. New functions for the matrix metalloproteinases in cancer progression. *Natl Rev Cancer.* 2002;2(3):161–174.

Esquela-Kerscher A, Slack FJ. Oncomirs—microRNAs with a role in cancer. *Natl Rev Cancer.* 2006;6(4):259–269.

Fearon ER, Vogelstein B. A genetic model for colorectal tumorigenesis. *Cell.* 1990; 61(5):759–767.

Greenblatt MS, Bennett WP, Hollstein M, et al. Mutations in the p53 tumor suppressor gene: clues to cancer etiology and molecular pathogenesis. *Cancer Res.* 1994;54:4855–4878.

Hahn WC, Weinberg RA. Rules for making human tumor cells. *N Engl J Med.* 2002; 347(20):1593–1603.

Hanahan D, Folkman J. Patterns and emerging mechanisms of the angiogenic switch during tumorigenesis. *Cell.* 1996;86(3):353–364.

Hanahan D, Weinberg RA. The hallmarks of cancer. *Cell.* 2000;100(1):57–70.

Herman JG, Baylin SB. Gene silencing in cancer in association with promoter hypermethylation. *N Engl J Med.* 2003;349(21):2042–2054.

Herman JG, Umar A, Polyak K, et al. Incidence and functional consequences of hMLH1 promoter hypermethylation in colorectal carcinoma. *Proc Natl Acad Sci USA.* 1998;95(12):6870–6875.

Joerger AC, Fersht AR. Structure-function-rescue: the diverse nature of common p53 cancer mutants. *Oncogene.* 2007;26:2226–2242.

Jones PA, Baylin SB. The epigenomics of cancer. *Cell.* 2007;128(4):683–692.

Jordan CT, Guzman ML, Noble M. Cancer stem cells. *N Engl J Med.* 2006;355: 1253–1261.

Kinzler KW, Vogelstein B. Lessons from hereditary colorectal cancer. *Cell.* 1996;87(2): 159–170.

Marchion D, Munster P. Development of histone deacetylase inhibitors for cancer treatment. *Expert Rev Anticancer Ther.* 2007;7(4):583–598.

Momparler RL. Cancer epigenetics. *Oncogene.* 2003;22:6479–6483.

Muller A, Homey B, Soto H, et al. Involvement of chemokine receptors in breast cancer metastasis. *Nature.* 2001;410(6824):50–56.

Newman B, Mu H, Butler LM, et al. Frequency of breast cancer attributable to BRCA1 in a population-based series of American women. *JAMA.* 1998;279(12):915–921.

Petitjean A, Achatz MIW, Borresen-Dale AL, et al. TP53 mutations in human cancers: functional selection and impact on cancer prognosis and outcomes. *Oncogene.* 2007;26:2157–2165.

Renan MJ. How many mutations are required for tumorigenesis? Implications from human cancer data. *Mol Carcinogen.* 1993;7:139–146.

Steeg PS. Metastasis suppressors alter the signal transduction of cancer cells. *Natl Rev Cancer.* 2003;3(1):55–63.

Tannock IF, Hill RP. *The Basic Science of Oncology.* 4th ed. Chicago: McGraw-Hill Medical; 2005.

Thiery JP. Epithelial-mesenchymal transitions in tumour progression. *Natl Rev Cancer.* 2002;2(6):442–454.

Vousden KH, Lu X. Live or let die: the cell's response to p53. *Natl Rev Cancer.* 2002;2(8):594–604.

Weiss L. Comments on hematogenous metastatic patterns in humans as revealed by autopsy. *Clin Exp Metastasis.* 1992;10:191–199.

Zou W. Immunosuppressive networks in the tumour environment and their therapeutic relevance. *Natl Rev Cancer.* 2005;5(4):263–274.

Chemotherapy

Kristan M. Augustin and Lindsay M. Hladnik

16

INTRODUCTION

The management of malignancy with chemotherapy is the specific specialty of medical and hematology oncologists. Most cancers are treated with multiple therapies, including surgery, radiation, chemotherapy, and/or biologic or targeted therapies, and therefore require collaboration by specialists in each of these areas of expertise. The appropriate and safe use of chemotherapy requires an understanding of various factors including, but not limited to, principles of the cell cycle and tumor growth kinetics; the timing of chemotherapy administration; chemotherapy response assessment; the pharmacology of chemotherapy agents including mechanisms of action, pharmacokinetic/pharmacodynamic properties, and adverse effects; and mechanisms of drug resistance. The prescribing and administration of these agents should therefore only be by those specifically trained and experienced in doing so. The intent of this chapter is to provide a brief overview of some of the general principles of chemotherapy, various classes of chemotherapy agents, their respective mechanisms of action, and selected adverse effects. See Table 16-1 for chemotherapy agent classification, mechanisms of action, selected toxicities, and other pertinent information relating to these agents.

Endocrine-related tumors are often affected by hormone therapy (e.g., antiestrogens in breast cancer, thyroid hormone to suppress thyroid cancer, and antiandrogens to inhibit prostate cancer). These agents are not discussed here, and the reader is referred to Chapters 18, 25, and 26 regarding those tumors. In addition, please see Chapter 34 for nonchemotherapeutic medication and symptomatic and supportive treatment of the cancer patient.

GENERAL PRINCIPLES

Most chemotherapy agents are toxic to cells of the human body. The justification for using substances that are toxic to normal cells is that malignant cells are preferentially sensitive to the effects of chemotherapy. A balance must be struck between toxicity to malignant cells that are intended to be killed and benign, normal tissues that are intended to be spared but are often harmed as "innocent bystanders." This concept is the therapeutic index, which is the ratio of toxicity to tumor cells to that of normal cells. The therapeutic index is quite narrow for many antineoplastic agents. Traditional chemotherapeutic agents interfere with normal cell processes, typically DNA synthesis or repair. However, it should be appreciated that these agents may act in methods other than simple cell killing (e.g., as initiators of apoptosis or maturation agents). Several newer agents have been developed that depart from the traditional concept of cell killing as their primary action. These agents are targeted to specific receptors in the cancer cell, often in signal transduction pathways

TABLE 16-1   PHARMACOLOGIC AGENTS IN ONCOLOGY

Drug Classification/ Subclassification/ Agents	Mechanism of Action	Selected Toxicities	Other Pertinent Information
Antimetabolites	Interfere with normal synthesis pathways of tumor cells; often inhibit DNA or RNA synthesis; S phase specific		
Pyrimidine antagonists			
5-Azacitidine	Hypomethylation of DNA	Myelosuppression, N/V, diarrhea, fever, renal tubular acidosis, elevated LFTs, alopecia, fatigue	
Capecitabine	Inhibits thymidylate synthase	Palmar-plantar erythrodysesthesia, diarrhea, stomatitis, N/V, fatigue, fever, abdominal pain, anorexia, myelosuppression, elevated bilirubin	
Cytarabine		Myelosuppression, fever, cerebral and cerebellar toxicity, N/V diarrhea, mucositis, conjunctivitis, rash, alopecia, abnormal LFTs, flu-like syndrome	May be given intrathecally. High-dose regimens are toxic to the cerebellum and need to be monitored closely. Conjunctivitis associated with high-dose cytarabine may be prevented with prophylactic corticosteroid eye drops.
Decitabine	Hypomethylation of DNA	Myelosuppression, edema, fever, headache, N/V, diarrhea, constipation, anorexia, elevated LFTs, cough	

Floxuridine	Inhibits thymidylate synthase	Myelosuppression, diarrhea, stomatitis, peptic ulcer disease
5-Fluorouracil	Inhibits thymidylate synthase	Myelosuppression, N/V, mucositis, diarrhea, palmar-plantar erythrodysesthesia
Gemcitabine		Myelosuppression, N/V, diarrhea, constipation, stomatitis, elevated LFTs, flulike syndrome, alopecia, rash, hemolytic uremic syndrome, pain, dyspnea
Purine antagonists		
Cladribine	Inhibits ribonucleotide reductase and DNA synthesis and repair	Myelosuppression, opportunistic infections, fever, fatigue
Clofarabine	Inhibits ribonucleotide reductase and DNA polymerase	Myelosuppression, opportunistic infections, N/V, diarrhea, constipation, headache, fatigue, cardiotoxicity, dyspnea, renal tubular acidosis, elevated LFTs, rash
Fludarabine	Inhibits ribonucleotide reductase, DNA polymerase, primase, and ligase I	Myelosuppression, opportunistic infections, neurotoxicity
6-Mercaptopurine	Inhibits purine synthesis	Myelosuppression, elevated LFTs
Pentostatin	Inhibits adenosine deaminase	Myelosuppression, fever, acute renal failure, elevated LFTs
6-Thioguanine	Inhibits purine synthesis	Myelosuppression

(continued)

TABLE 16-1   PHARMACOLOGIC AGENTS IN ONCOLOGY (Continued)

Drug Classification/ Subclassification/ Agents	Mechanism of Action	Selected Toxicities	Other Pertinent Information
Folate antagonists	Inhibit dihydrofolate reductase, which inhibits synthesis of thymidylate and purines		
Methotrexate	S phase specific	Myelosuppression, stomatitis, N/V, diarrhea, nephrotoxicity, abnormal LFTs, neurotoxicity	May be given intrathecally. Leucovorin administration and following methotrexate levels should be considered with high-dose therapy.
Pemetrexed	G_1-S phase specific	Myelosuppression, rash, chest pain, fatigue, N/V, neuropathy, nephrotoxicity, dyspnea	Rash may be painful and generalized. Premedicate with corticosteroids. Supplement with folic acid and vitamin B_{12}.
Trimetrexate	S phase specific	Myelosuppression, stomatitis, elevated LFTs, rash, peripheral neuropathy	
Microtubule agents	Bind to tubulin and inhibit microtubule assembly; M and S phase specific		
Vinblastine		Myelosuppression, stomatitis, alopecia, SIADH	
Vincristine		Peripheral neuropathy, constipation, paralytic ileus, alopecia	
Vinorelbine		Myelosuppression, peripheral neuropathy, constipation, stomatitis, fatigue, elevated LFTs	

Taxanes

Bind to microtubules and prevent their disassembly; G_2 phase specific

	Mechanism	Toxicities	Notes
Docetaxel		Myelosuppression, hypersensitivity reaction, peripheral neuropathy, elevated LFTs, rash, alopecia, stomatitis, fluid retention	Hypersensitivity reaction (dyspnea, fluid retention, tachycardia, flushing, hypotension, chest pain), due to docetaxel or its vehicle, Polysorbate 80, occurs in 2% of patients despite premedication with dexamethasone.
Paclitaxel		Myelosuppression, hypersensitivity reaction, peripheral neuropathy, hypotension, bradycardia, alopecia, elevated LFTs	Hypersensitivity reaction due to paclitaxel or its vehicle, Cremophor EL. Premedicate with corticosteroids and H1- and H2-blockers.
Topoisomerase inhibitors			
Topoisomerase I inhibitors	Active in the unwinding of DNA, causing DNA strand breaks; S phase specific		
Irinotecan		Acute and delayed diarrhea, abdominal pain/cramping, N/V, myelosuppression, dyspnea, alopecia, elevated transaminases, fatigue, fever, weakness	Acute diarrhea may be treated with atropine and delayed diarrhea may be treated with loperamide.
Topotecan		Myelosuppression, N/V, diarrhea, alopecia, rash, elevated transaminases, fatigue, headache, fever, stomatitis, dyspnea, weakness	

(continued)

TABLE 16-1 PHARMACOLOGIC AGENTS IN ONCOLOGY *(Continued)*

Drug Classification/ Subclassification/ Agents	Mechanism of Action	Selected Toxicities	Other Pertinent Information
Topoisomerase II inhibitors	Inhibit the ability to restore the structure of cleaved DNA, resulting in double-strand breaks; S and G_2 phase specific		
Etoposide		Myelosuppression, N/V, mucositis, anorexia, diarrhea, hypotension, disorientation, alopecia	Etoposide formulation contains ethanol, 30.3% (v/v).
Teniposide		Myelosuppression, N/V, mucositis, diarrhea, anorexia, alopecia, hypotension	
Antitumor antibiotics			
Anthracyclines	Inhibit topoisomerase II, produce free radicals, and intercalate adjacent DNA base pairs		
Daunorubicin		Myelosuppression, cardiotoxicity, mucositis, alopecia	Recommended lifetime cumulative dose is 400–600 mg/m².
Doxorubicin		Myelosuppression, cardiotoxicity, mucositis, N/V, diarrhea, alopecia	Recommended lifetime cumulative dose is 450–550 mg/m².
Epirubicin		Myelosuppression, cardiotoxicity, mucositis, N/V, diarrhea, alopecia	Recommended lifetime cumulative dose is 750–900 mg/m².

Drug	Mechanism	Toxicities	Comments
Idarubicin		Myelosuppression, cardiotoxicity, mucositis, N/V, diarrhea, alopecia, elevated LFTs	Recommended lifetime cumulative dose is unknown.
Mitoxantrone		Myelosuppression, elevated LFTs, alopecia, mucositis, N/V, anorexia, cardiotoxicity, diarrhea	
Other antitumor antibiotics			
Bleomycin	Inhibits DNA synthesis; S and G_2 phase specific	Pulmonary fibrosis, stomatitis, fever, skin changes, hypersensitivity reactions, Raynaud phenomenon	A test dose is recommended.
Dactinomycin	Intercalates into DNA resulting in inhibition of DNA and RNA synthesis	Myelosuppression, pulmonary fibrosis, elevated LFTs, alopecia, N/V, mucositis, diarrhea, fatigue	
Mitomycin C	Produces DNA crosslinks; non-cell cycle specific, but maximal effects in late G and early S phases	Myelosuppression, hemolytic uremic syndrome, acute bronchospasm, alopecia, congestive heart failure, nail banding, fever	May be given intravesically.
Covalent DNA-binding agents			
Alkylating agents	Produce DNA-DNA cross-links; non-cell cycle specific		
Busulfan		Myelosuppression, N/V, diarrhea, constipation, anorexia, VOD, pulmonary fibrosis, seizures	Seizure prophylaxis should be used with high-dose regimens.

(continued)

TABLE 16-1 PHARMACOLOGIC AGENTS IN ONCOLOGY *(Continued)*

Drug Classification/ Subclassification/ Agents	Mechanism of Action	Selected Toxicities	Other Pertinent Information
Carmustine		Myelosuppression, N/V, elevated LFTs, VOD, alopecia, renal insufficiency	Diluent for intravenous preparation contains ethanol.
Chlorambucil		Myelosuppression, pulmonary fibrosis, rash, elevated LFTs	
Cyclophosphamide		Myelosuppression, N/V, hemorrhagic cystitis, SIADH, alopecia, cardiomyopathy, VOD, secondary malignancies, facial flushing, headache	The inactive metabolite, acrolein, may cause direct bladder toxicity resulting in hemorrhagic cystitis. Prevent this with brisk hydration and Mesna.
Dacarbazine		Myelosuppression, N/V	
Ifosfamide		Myelosuppression, N/V, hemorrhagic cystitis, nephrotoxicity, SIADH, alopecia, neurotoxicity (somnolence, confusion, and hallucinations)	The inactive metabolite, acrolein, may cause direct bladder toxicity resulting in hemorrhagic cystitis. Prevent this with brisk hydration and Mesna.
Lomustine		Myelosuppression, N/V	
Mechlorethamine		Myelosuppression, N/V, diarrhea, mucositis, alopecia	
Melphalan		Myelosuppression, N/V, diarrhea, mucositis, alopecia	
Procarbazine		Myelosuppression, N/V, neurotoxicity, hallucinations	

Streptozocin		N/V, elevated LFTs, nephrotoxicity, hypoalbuminemia	
Temozolomide		Myelosuppression, peripheral edema, headache, fever, fatigue, seizures, N/V, diarrhea	
Thiotepa		Myelosuppression, alopecia, rash	Cystitis may occur when given intravesically.
Platinum agents	Produce DNA-DNA adducts and crosslinks resulting in inhibition of DNA replication and synthesis; non-cell cycle specific		
Carboplatin		Nephrotoxicity, myelosuppression, peripheral neuropathy, hypomagnesemia, hypokalemia, hypocalcemia, hypophosphatemia, N/V, diarrhea, mucositis, alopecia	
Cisplatin		Nephrotoxicity, myelosuppression, peripheral neuropathy, hypomagnesemia, hypokalemia, hypocalcemia, hypophosphatemia, N/V, diarrhea, ototoxicity	
Oxaliplatin		Myelosuppression, peripheral neuropathy, fatigue, N/V, diarrhea, constipation, anorexia, fever, elevated LFTs, alopecia	May induce acute and delayed N/V, which can be severe

(continued)

TABLE 16-1 PHARMACOLOGIC AGENTS IN ONCOLOGY *(Continued)*

Drug Classification/ Subclassification/ Agents	Mechanism of Action	Selected Toxicities	Other Pertinent Information
Differentiating agents			
Arsenic trioxide	Apoptosis of leukemia cells	QT prolongation, tachycardia, fatigue, fever, electrolyte abnormalities, N/V, leukocytosis, APL differentiation syndrome, dyspnea	
Tretinoin	Terminal differentiation and apoptotic cell death	Headache, fever, weakness, fatigue, N/V, bleeding, leukocytosis, dyspnea, elevated cholesterol and triglycerides, APL differentiation syndrome	
Other agents			
Bortezomib	26S proteasome inhibitor (enzyme complex that regulates cellular protein homeostasis)	Peripheral neuropathy, edema, hypotension, myelosuppression, fever, rash, N/V, diarrhea, constipation, infection, CHF, QT prolongation, pulmonary toxicities, elevated LFTs	Monitor for drug interactions, as it undergoes hepatic metabolism via CYP450.
Hydroxyurea	Inhibits ribonucleotide reductase and DNA synthesis; S phase specific	Myelosuppression	
L-Asparaginase	Inhibits protein synthesis by converting asparagine to aspartic acid and ammonia; G_1 phase specific	Fever, chills, hyperglycemia, acute pancreatitis, hypofibrinogenemia, elevated LFTs, hypersensitivity reactions, nephrotoxicity	A test dose is recommended.

Targeted therapies		
Monoclonal antibodies (MAbs)	May affect cellular signaling pathways by inhibiting ligand-receptor interactions, may stimulate host defense mechanisms causing antitumor activity, or may be combined with protein toxins or cytotoxic agents that disrupt protein synthesis	
Alemtuzumab	Binds to CD52 resulting in complement-mediated and/or antibody-dependent cell-mediated cytotoxicity	Hypo-/hypertension, peripheral edema, tachycardia, fever, fatigue, rash, N/V, diarrhea, myelosuppression, rigors, myalgias, infection, serious and potentially fatal infusion-related reactions	Prophylactic therapy against *Pneumocystis carinii* pneumonia and herpes viruses needed. Premedicate. Dose escalation is required at initiation and after therapy interruption for $\geq$7 days.
Bevacizumab	Binds to and neutralizes VEGF	Hypertension, N/V, diarrhea, constipation, leukopenia, proteinuria, nephrotic syndrome, GI perforations, intra-abdominal abscesses, impaired wound healing, hemorrhage, thromboembolic events, CHF, infusion reactions, reversible posterior leukoencephalopathy	

(continued)

TABLE 16-1 PHARMACOLOGIC AGENTS IN ONCOLOGY (Continued)

Drug Classification/ Subclassification/ Agents	Mechanism of Action	Selected Toxicities	Other Pertinent Information
Cetuximab	Binds to EGFR and inhibits ligand binding	Dermatologic toxicities, hypomagnesemia, N/V, diarrhea, constipation, infusion reactions, peripheral edema, cardiopulmonary arrest (in combination with radiation therapy), elevated LFTs, interstitial lung disease, photosensitivity	Risk of infusion-related reactions. Premedications and monitoring during infusion and for at least 1 hour after infusion is complete are required.
Denileukin diftitox	Recombinant fusion protein (diphtheria toxin + IL-2), which delivers a cytotoxic dose of diphtheria toxin after interacting with IL-2 receptors on malignant cells	Vascular leak syndrome, flulike illness, rash, N/V, diarrhea, myelosuppression, elevated LFTs, hypersensitivity reactions, infection, loss of visual acuity or color	Serum albumin levels should be ≥3 g/dL before and during therapy.
Gemtuzumab	MAb against CD33 conjugated to a cytotoxic antibiotic (calicheamicin). When the antibody-antigen complex is internalized, calicheamicin is released intracellularly, resulting in double-strand breaks in DNA.	Infusion-related reactions (may be severe and potentially fatal), N/V, peripheral edema, tachycardia, rash, diarrhea, constipation, myelosuppression, elevated LFTs, weakness, infection, VOD, tumor lysis syndrome	Premedications are required.

Rituximab	Binds to CD20; induces complement-dependent cytotoxicity and ADCC	Cytokine release syndrome, rash, nausea, myelosuppression, infection, tumor lysis syndrome, severe and potentially fatal mucocutaneous reactions, infusion reactions (may be severe or fatal)	Premedications and infusion rate titration are required.
Trastuzumab	Binds to the HER2 coreceptor protein and inhibits HER-family receptor dimerization, inhibiting signal transduction; induces ADCC vs. cells that overproduce HER2; internalizes the HER2 receptor; downregulates surface HER2	Infusion-related reactions, diarrhea, CHF, left ventricular dysfunction, cardiomyopathy, myelosuppression, severe hypersensitivity reactions, pulmonary events	
Tyrosine kinase inhibitors (TKIs)	Inhibit signal transduction within cellular signaling cascades affecting DNA synthesis, cell growth, proliferation, migration, angiogenesis, and apoptosis		
Dasatinib	Multitargeted TKI; inhibits BCR-ABL tyrosine kinase; targets most imatinib-resistant BCR-ABL mutations except the T315I and F317V mutants	Myelosuppression, fluid retention/edema, N/V, diarrhea, constipation, mucositis, rash, QTc prolongation, arrhythmia, elevated LFTs, arthralgia/myalgia, neuropathy, infection, CHF, alopecia, photosensitivity	Monitor for drug interactions (via CYP450). Antacids, H2-blockers, and proton pump inhibitors may decrease dasatinib absorption.

(continued)

TABLE 16-1 PHARMACOLOGIC AGENTS IN ONCOLOGY (Continued)

Drug Classification/ Subclassification/ Agents	Mechanism of Action	Selected Toxicities	Other Pertinent Information
Erlotinib	EGFR TKI	Edema, fatigue, dermatologic toxicities, GI toxicities, hyperbilirubinemia, pulmonary toxicities, infection, MI, cerebrovascular events, pancreatitis	Monitor for drug interactions (via CYP450). Administer on an EMPTY stomach at least 1 hour before or 2 hours after meals.
Imatinib	BCR-ABL TKI; inhibitory effects on other receptor tyrosine kinases (SCF/c-KIT, PDGFRα, PDGFRβ)	N/V, diarrhea, dyspepsia, rash, fluid retention/edema, hepatotoxicity, hemorrhage, myelosuppression, arthralgia/myalgia, LV dysfunction, CHF, photosensitivity, Stevens-Johnson syndrome	Monitor for drug interactions (via CYP450).
Lapatinib	EGFR and HER2 TKI	In combination with capecitabine: GI toxicities, dermatologic toxicities, fatigue, decrease in LVEF, QT prolongation, abnormal LFTs, myelosuppression	Monitor for drug interactions (via CYP450). Administer at least 1 hour before or 1 hour after meals; once-daily dosing only.
Sorafenib	Raf kinase TKI; effects on other receptor tyrosine kinases (VEGFR 2, VEGFR 3, PDGFRβ, Flt-3, c-KIT)	Rash, hand-foot syndrome, N/V, diarrhea, constipation, hypertension, fatigue, neuropathy, alopecia, pruritus, dry skin, hypophosphatemia, elevated amylase/lipase, myelosuppression, cardiac ischemia/ infarction, wound healing complications	Monitor for drug interactions (via CYP450). Administer on an EMPTY stomach at least 1 hour before or 2 hours after meals.

| Sunitinib | VEGF TKI; effects on other receptor tyrosine kinases (SCF/c-KIT, PDGFRα, PDGFRβ, Flt-3) | Hypertension, edema, fatigue, rash, hyperpigmentation, dry skin, hair color changes, hand-foot syndrome, alopecia, N/V, diarrhea, mucositis, constipation, increased amylase/lipase, myelosuppression, increased LFTs, arthralgia/myalgia, decreased left ventricular ejection fraction, deep vein thrombosis, pulmonary embolism, MI, peripheral neuropathy, hemorrhagic events, adrenal function abnormalities | Monitor for drug interactions (via CYP450). Avoid grapefruit juice, as it increases sunitinib concentrations. |

ADCC, antibody-dependent cell-mediated cytotoxicity; APL, acute promyelocytic leukemia; BCR-ABL, breakpoint cluster region-Abelson; CHF, congestive heart failure; CYP450, cytochrome P450; EGFR, epidermal growth factor receptor; Flt-3, FMS-like tyrosine kinase 3; HER2/neu, human epidermal growth factor receptor 2; LFTs, liver function tests; LVEF, left ventricular ejection fraction; MI, myocardial infarction/ischemia; N/V, nausea/vomiting; PDGFR, platelet-derived growth factor receptor; SCF/c-KIT, stem cell factor; SIADH, syndrome of inappropriate secretion of antidiuretic hormone; VEGF, vascular endothelial growth factor; VOD, veno-occlusive disease.

that regulate tumor cell growth, proliferation, migration, angiogenesis, and apoptosis. Recent advances in cancer have led to the identification of several of these specific molecular targets for drug therapy. Please refer to Chapter 15 for additional information.

Cell Cycle

The growth and division of cells can be conceptualized by the cell cycle. There are several phases to the life cycle of the dividing cell, including the growth (G) phase, the synthesis (S) phase, and a mitosis (M) phase. There also is a "rest" phase, or G_0, in which cells are not actively participating in the cell cycle. Cells can then undergo terminal differentiation or re-enter the cell cycle. One of the factors that influences the development of chemotherapy regimens is the point at which the chemotherapy agent works in the cell cycle. Many chemotherapeutic agents are cell cycle specific (e.g., they have activity only in certain parts of the cell cycle). Those that are non-cell cycle specific may cause damage to a cell in any part of the cell cycle.

KEY POINTS TO REMEMBER

- Cytotoxic chemotherapeutic agents typically have a narrow therapeutic index, which may contribute to selected toxicities observed.
- Chemotherapy agents should typically be prescribed only by clinicians experienced in their use.
- The use of chemotherapy requires close and careful monitoring.

REFERENCES AND SUGGESTED READINGS

DeVita VT, Rosenberg SA, Hellman S, eds. *Cancer: Principles and Practice of Oncology.* 7th ed. Philadelphia: Lippincott Williams & Wilkins; 2005.

Kasper DL, et al. *Harrison's Principles of Internal Medicine.* 16th ed. New York: McGraw-Hill; 2005.

Pazdur R, Coia LR, Hoskins WJ, et al., eds. *Cancer Management: A Multidisciplinary Approach* [book online]. Manhasset, NY: CMP Healthcare Media; 2005. Available at: http://www.cancernetwork.com/handbook/contents.htm. Accessed August 8, 2007.

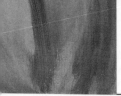

Introduction to Radiation Oncology

Parag J. Parikh and Imran Zoberi

17

INTRODUCTION

Radiation oncology unifies the study of cancer with the therapeutic use of radiation. The radiation oncologist is the medical specialist who decides when and how best to use radiation. Under the supervision of the radiation oncologist, an array of nonmedical specialists, including physicists, dosimetrists, and technicians, assist in the planning and delivery of radiation to patients. This chapter introduces some of the basic principles of radiation oncology, some common treatment strategies, and an overview of the common toxicities that may be encountered in the inpatient setting.

PHYSICAL AND BIOLOGIC PRINCIPLES

- **Ionizing radiation** is energy that causes the ejection of an orbital electron. It may be either electromagnetic (photons or gamma rays) or particulate (electrons, protons, or other atomic particles). The energy of photons that can be generated in the clinic has increased over the years, which allows more doses to be delivered to internal malignancies while respecting the tolerance of the skin to radiation. **Radiation dose** is measured as energy per unit mass, where 1 joule (J)/kg is 1 gray (Gy). The previously used term, **rad,** is equal to 1 centigray (cGy).
- Radiation causes DNA damage in both normal tissues and tumor cells. In general, cells are most susceptible in the G1, G2, and M phases of the cell cycle. Susceptible cells may enter apoptotic cell death by a variety of mechanisms or undergo necrosis. Hypoxic cells are thought to be less susceptible to radiation than well-oxygenated cells, owing to preferential free radical formation. Fractionated radiotherapy (radiation given in multiple small doses over a given period instead of a single large dose) allows normal tissue to repair sublethal damage and repopulate while the tumor cells re-sort themselves in the cell cycle and become better oxygenated. A great deal of current research involves the cell cycle–signaling pathways involved in each aspect of the damage, repair, and reoxygenation pathways.

RADIATION TREATMENT GOALS AND METHODS

- Radiation can be given by directing x-rays from a treatment machine to the patient (**external beam radiotherapy**) or by placing a radioactive source in close proximity to the patient (**brachytherapy**). Brachytherapy is most often used in gynecologic cancers, prostate cancer, and head and neck cancer. Sometimes both techniques are used to provide the optimal dose distribution.

- Radiation can be given for curative or palliative intent and commonly is the definitive treatment. Often, it is combined with chemotherapy and surgery in the complete cancer care of the patient. It can be given before (neoadjuvant) or after (adjuvant) the definitive therapy. Many solid tumors are treated with radiation and chemotherapy at the same time (concurrent chemoradiation).
- Accurate tumor **localization** is essential for optimum delivery of radiation. This can be done clinically (e.g., in palliative cases and gynecologic cancers) or using radiographic studies. Clinical localizations are done on patients receiving whole-brain radiotherapy and some patients with bone metastases. This approach is quick and allows the patient to start treatment immediately but does not allow for conformal delivery of radiation. To plan most radiotherapy, the patient needs to have a **simulation** ("sim") in which he or she is brought to the radiation oncology department to make a treatment plan. This plan will aid in delivering the maximal dose of radiation to tumor tissue while attempting to avoid healthy tissue. Either two-dimensional (2D; fluoroscopy, plain x-rays) or three-dimensional (3D; CT scanners) methods can be used to generate images for treatment planning. These are sometimes merged with other radiologic modalities such as magnetic resonance imaging, ultrasonography, angiography, or positron emission tomography (PET) scanning to better delineate tumor localization. Often, specialized immobilization devices are constructed for the patient during simulation to reduce intertreatment variation in patient position. After the simulation, the radiation oncologist develops a treatment plan. Because the time between the initial consultation and the first treatment is often 2 to 3 weeks, patients are best served by early radiation oncology consultation.
- In general, for external-beam radiotherapy, a patient will be placed on a flat, mobile treatment table each day during the course of radiation therapy. Marks on the patient's skin and any immobilization devices are used to obtain accurate and precise patient positioning. Each treatment may last 10 to 30 minutes. The total course of radiation therapy can vary from 1 day (prostate brachytherapy) to several weeks (fractionated external-beam radiotherapy). Most fractionated treatment is given once a day, 5 days per week, although some treatments are given more frequently.

INDICATIONS FOR URGENT RADIATION THERAPY

Urgent radiation therapy is useful in certain oncologic emergencies. **Spinal cord compression** is the only true radiation oncology emergency and is described further in Chapter 35. It is imperative that radiation oncology and surgical services are consulted early and that an MRI of the entire spine is obtained as soon as possible. **Brain metastases** can be treated with radiation therapy, with timing based on symptoms and performance status. **Uncontrolled bleeding** of tumors (commonly breast, gynecologic, lung, colon, or bladder) often responds well to radiation therapy. **Superior vena cava (SVC) syndrome**, in which the SVC is compressed by tumor (typically small-cell lung cancer), can be palliated by radiation, with resolution after weeks of therapy. Although SVC syndrome by itself is rarely fatal, these tumors frequently encase other critical structures of the mediastinum.

LATE EFFECTS AND TISSUE TOLERANCE

Radiation therapy balances side effects to normal tissue with the need to deliver adequate doses to the tumor. Side effects are considered to be either **late** (months to years after completion of radiation therapy) or **acute** (during radiation therapy). The radiation tolerance of normal tissue varies from patient to patient and depends on dose, fractionation scheme,

TABLE 17-1	NORMAL TISSUE TOLERANCE TO THERAPEUTIC IRRADIATION: DOSE (GY) THAT TYPICALLY CAUSES A 5% INCIDENCE OF LATE COMPLICATIONS IN 5 YEARS			

| | Fraction of Organ Irradiated | | | |
	$^1/_3$	$^2/_3$	$^3/_3$	End point
Kidney	50	30	23	Clinical nephritis
Brain	60	50	45	Necrosis/infarction
Lung	45	30	17.5	Pneumonitis
Heart	60	45	40	Pericarditis
Esophagus	60	58	55	Clinical stricture/perforation
Stomach	60	55	50	Ulceration/perforation
Small intestine	50	Unknown	40	Obstruction/perforation/fistula
Colon	55	Unknown	45	Obstruction/perforation/ fistula/ulceration
Rectum	75	65	60	Severe proctitis/necrosis/fistula
Liver	50	35	30	Liver failure
Spinal cord	5 cm[a]	10 cm[a]	20 cm[a]	
	50	50	47	Myelitis/necrosis

[a]As the spinal cord is an organ in a series, doses of radiation to the spinal cord are for lengths of the spinal cord and not for fraction of organ irradiated. These doses are those required to cause toxicity to the stated length of spinal cord.

Adapted from Emami B, Lyman J, Brown A, et al. Tolerance of normal tissue to therapeutic irradiation. *Int J Radiat Oncol Biol Phys.* 1991;21:109–122, and Chao KS, Perez C, Brady L. *Radiation Oncology: Management Decisions.* Philadelphia: Lippincott-Raven; 1999:24.

and exposed tissue volume. The most common fractionation scheme is 1.8 to 2 Gy/day. Based on animal experiments and the best available human data, the concept of the $TD_{x/y}$ was developed, which is the x% cumulative incidence of a certain complication in y years. Table 17-1 lists the doses at which one can expect 5% of patients to develop a late complication in 5 years as a function of the volume of the organ treated. These data represent only general parameters, and a radiation oncologist may elect to exceed these dose levels or be more conservative based on individual patient considerations.

COMMON TREATMENT GUIDELINES AND ASSOCIATED ACUTE EFFECTS

The following is a brief description of current "off-protocol" treatment regimens. It must be emphasized that many patients are treated according to research protocols, which vary considerably. Acute toxicities of radiation therapy typically result from direct tissue damage within the radiation path. Most radiation-alone acute effects can be managed on an outpatient basis. However, with concurrent chemoradiation, acute effects increase substantially and may require inpatient management. This is especially seen with head and neck, lung, and gastrointestinal cancers.

Palliative Therapy

Palliative treatment of brain and bone metastases is given at doses of 20 to 40 Gy over 1 to 3 weeks. This is a larger fraction size than used in most curative treatments, because there is less concern about late effects and a greater interest in minimizing treatment time for patient convenience.

Bone Metastases

Bone metastases can be treated with 6- to 8-Gy single doses, or with 42 Gy in fractions of 200 cGy/day, depending on the number and location of lesions and the patient's life expectancy. For patients with multiple bone metastases, an infusion of radioactive strontium, samarium, or yttrium can be used to decrease pain.

Lung Cancer

Medically inoperable stage I and II lung cancer and stage III non-small-cell lung cancer are often treated with definitive radiotherapy, typically to a dose of 60 to 70 Gy. Recently, extracranial stereotactic radiation therapy, involving very precise immobilization and delivery of a few fractions of large doses of radiation therapy (i.e., 20 Gy × 3 fractions), has been shown to be promising for medically inoperable stage I and II lung cancer patients. In many patients, the mediastinum is irradiated, which can result in the acute toxicity of esophagitis. The resultant odynophagia can lead to dehydration or significant weight loss, which may require inpatient management. Shortly after the completion of radiotherapy, radiation pneumonitis or, very rarely, radiation pericarditis may occur. Antiinflammatory steroid therapy is the mainstay of treatment for both of these conditions. 3D conformal radiation therapy, involving treatment planning based on CT scans, is being investigated as a method to increase dose to tumor while avoiding normal lung. Radiation therapy is used as adjuvant treatment in select cases of locally advanced non-small-cell lung cancer treated with definitive surgery. Both chemotherapy and radiation therapy play a central role in the definitive management of limited-stage small-cell lung cancer.

Esophageal Cancer

Radiation therapy with concurrent chemotherapy is used either as definitive treatment for esophageal/gastroesophageal junction tumors or as neoadjuvant treatment. Esophagitis is the major acute toxicity.

Central Nervous System Cancer

After maximal safe surgical resection, primary brain tumors may be treated to 50 to 60 Gy, depending on the area of the brain involved. Brain metastases are normally treated to 20 to 30 Gy. Radiosurgery, either by linear accelerator or by gamma knife, can be used for patients with few metastatic lesions that are <4 cm in size. Radiosurgery involves a single day of treatment. Mild mental deterioration is seen in children and the elderly. Neurologic changes requiring hospitalization are generally due to tumor progression, not toxicity from radiosurgery.

Head and Neck Cancer

In general, early-stage head and neck cancers are treated equally well with surgery or radiation. Advanced head and neck cancers require surgery and postoperative radiation, radiotherapy alone, or chemoradiation. Doses are typically 60 to 70 Gy. Multiple treatments per day (hyperfractionation) are often used. Side effects include xerostomia, odynophagia, dysphagia, and hoarseness. Acute toxicity often results in dehydration, which may require administration of IV fluids or placement of a gastric tube for nutritional support. Chemotherapy has been shown to improve outcome in the definitive radiotherapy of advanced head and neck cancers at the cost of 1% to 3% treatment-associated mortality and 20% to 30% risk of hospitalization for esophagitis. Treatment-associated deaths are rare with radiotherapy alone, and the frequency of hospitalization for acute toxicity is generally ≤10%.

Breast Cancer

Radiation is used in breast conservation therapy as well as postmastectomy patients with large initial tumors, positive lymph nodes, or positive resection margins. The dose to the breast is normally 54 to 60 Gy. For early-stage breast conservation therapy, partial breast radiation therapy is being investigated as a shorter-course, lower-volume alternative to whole-breast radiation. Acute side effects are usually limited to skin reactions, but pneumonitis, lymphoedema, and carditis can occur as late reactions. Hospitalization is a distinctly rare event for any acute radiotherapy effect in the breast.

Prostate Cancer

Prostate cancer can be treated with either external-beam radiation therapy or prostate brachytherapy ("seeds"). External beam radiation consists of 70 to 80 Gy. The most common side effects are urethritis and cystitis, which are managed on an outpatient basis in the vast majority of patients. Rates of impotence and cure are similar among external-beam radiation therapy, brachytherapy, and radical prostatectomy.

Colon/Rectal Cancer

Radiation is not often used in colon cancers, except in those that are locally advanced (often fixed or perforated) and require preoperative radiation therapy. The confines of the pelvis make surgical resection of rectal cancer more challenging than that of colon cancer. Preoperative radiation therapy is used in most cases to facilitate surgical resection, for sphincter preservation, and to treat the poorly accessible presacral lymph nodes. Rectal cancer doses are 20 to 50 Gy, depending on the size of the lesion and whether radiation is given before or after surgery. Radiation therapy–induced proctitis is generally quite mild unless concurrent chemotherapy (generally 5-fluorouracil) is administered, in which case proctitis can be severe enough to cause dehydration leading to hospitalization. Patients may need nutritional support.

Anal Cancer

Most anal malignancies can be managed with definitive radiotherapy plus adjuvant chemotherapy, with surgery reserved for salvage. Although generally of squamous histology, anal cancers respond well to low doses of radiotherapy. Typical curative doses are 30 to 54 Gy, classically given with concurrent mitomycin-C and 5-fluorouracil. Acute toxicities are mainly myelosuppression caused by mitomycin-C, proctitis, cystitis, hemorrhoid exacerbation, and skin reaction in the perineum.

Pediatric Cancer

Radiation is used in many pediatric tumors. Total-body irradiation and irradiation of sanctuary sites are used in leukemia, and many lymphoma protocols involve local irradiation. Many sarcomas are treated with radiation after or instead of surgery. Most CNS tumors are treated in part with radiation. Treatment varies by site, and long-term effects on development limit dose.

Lymphoma

Lymphomas are very radioresponsive, and doses from 20 to 45 Gy are used, depending on the type of lymphoma and chemotherapy regimen. Treatment is normally very well tolerated, with some cytopenia and fatigue with larger fields and some nausea/vomiting when the abdomen is treated.

Total-Body Irradiation

Total-body irradiation is used as part of the preparative scheme for peripheral blood stem cell transplant protocols. Treatment with 550 cGy in a single fraction is very common, although fractionated total-body irradiation is also used in certain protocols. This is normally well tolerated, except for self-limiting parotitis and nausea and vomiting.

Gynecologic Cancer

Cervical and uterine corpus cancers are often treated with radiation therapy. Most advanced cervical cancers are treated with definitive radiotherapy, and numerous phase III trials have demonstrated equivalent survival outcome between radical hysterectomy and radiotherapy for early cervical cancer. Radiation is generally used as adjuvant therapy in uterine corpus tumors. Radiotherapy for most gynecologic malignancies uses **brachytherapy,** because it better delivers the dose to the at-risk tissues, while sparing the bladder and rectum. Doses are anywhere from 50 to 85 Gy. Patients can develop proctitis, enteritis, and urethritis/cystitis, depending on the dose and tumor location. As with other sites, the frequency of admission for acute toxicity increases with concurrent chemoradiation.

KEY POINTS TO REMEMBER

- Consult a radiation oncology specialist before starting therapeutic chemotherapy or surgery to allow for optimum multidisciplinary management of the malignancy. Evaluating patients in their presenting state is very valuable to the radiation oncologist.
- When radiation toxicity is in the differential diagnosis, consult a radiation oncologist, who can help with diagnosis and treatment.
- The only true radiation oncology emergency is spinal cord compression, although there are other "urgent" indications for radiation therapy.
- Consider urgent radiation oncology consults when faced with SVC syndrome, new brain metastases, or uncontrolled bleeding.

REFERENCES AND SUGGESTED READINGS

Gunderson L, Tepper J, eds. *Clinical Radiation Oncology.* Philadelphia: Churchill Livingstone; 2000.

Perez C, Brady L, eds. *Principles and Practices of Radiation Oncology.* 3rd ed. Philadelphia: Lippincott-Raven; 1997.

Rubin P, ed. *Clinical Oncology for Medical Students and Physicians: A Multidisciplinary Approach.* 7th ed. Philadelphia: W. B. Saunders; 1993.

Breast Cancer

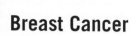

Caron Rigden and Mariana Chavez-MacGregor

INTRODUCTION

Other than skin cancer, breast cancer is the most common cancer diagnosed in women in North America. Breast cancer is second only to lung cancer as the leading cause of cancer deaths among women. Although the incidence of breast cancer has continued to rise in the United States over recent decades, the mortality appears to be declining, suggesting a benefit from screening as well as improved medical therapy.

Epidemiology

The American Cancer Society estimates that in 2007, a total of 180,510 (2030 men; 178,480 women) new breast cancers will be diagnosed, and 40,910 deaths will occur secondary to the disease. Although most breast cancers occur in women, ~1% of new cases annually occur in men. The lifetime risk of developing breast cancer in women (assuming a life expectancy of 85 years) is approximately one in eight women. The median age at diagnosis is in the seventh decade of life.

CAUSES

Risk Factors

- Identifiable risk factors for breast cancer include a history of breast cancer, female gender, increasing age, early menarche, late menopause, nulliparity, older age at first live childbirth, family history of breast cancer, genetic mutations such as BRCA1 and BRCA2, prolonged hormone replacement therapy, previous exposure to therapeutic chest wall irradiation, and benign proliferative breast disease such as atypical lobular or ductal hyperplasia.
- With regard to behavioral activities, such as weight and diet, controversy exists whether or not there is a clear association of high-fat and low-fiber diets and obesity with increased breast cancer risk. It appears that regular physical activity has been shown to correlate with a reduced risk of breast cancer. More than minimal alcohol intake (such as one to two drinks per day) has been associated with an increased risk. Cigarette smoking is a controversial risk factor, with some studies showing a correlation with risk while other studies do not.
- While the majority of breast cancers are sporadic, **inherited breast cancer** is now well documented. Mutations in BRCA1 and BRCA2, which are inherited in an autosomal dominant fashion, are responsible for ~90% of hereditary breast cancer diagnoses. Approximately 5% to 10% of all women with breast cancer have a germline mutation of the gene BRCA1 or BRCA2. BRCA1 (chromosome 17q21) and BRCA2 (chromosome 13q12-13) are associated with autosomal dominance inheritance

pattern, younger age at diagnosis, bilateral disease, multiple affected family members, and an association with other cancers, especially ovarian. Specific mutations of BRCA1 and BRCA2 are also more common in women of Ashkenazi Jewish descent. The estimated lifetime risk of developing breast cancer in women with BRCA1 or BRCA2 mutation is 40% to 85%, and the risk of bilateral breast cancer is 20% to 40%. Mutation of either gene also confers a 20% to 40% increased lifetime risk for developing ovarian cancer. Other, less common but established hereditary causes for breast cancer include Li-Fraumeni syndrome (p53 gene mutations), Cowden syndrome or multiple hamartoma syndrome (PTEN gene mutations), and Peutz-Jeghers syndrome (STK11 gene mutations).

Indications for Genetic Testing

Several indications for genetic testing for breast and ovarian cancer exist: two or more family members with breast and/or ovarian cancer at <50 years of age, breast cancer or ovarian cancer at a very young age, known BRCA1 and BRCA2 mutations in a family member, personal history of both breast and ovarian cancer, Ashkenazi Jewish ancestry plus a family member younger than 50 years with breast cancer, and a personal history of ovarian cancer. All patients should undergo genetics counseling before undergoing genetics testing.

Screening

- Monthly breast self-exam is frequently advocated as a screening tool for breast cancer, but there is little evidence showing its effectiveness in reducing mortality rates in breast cancer. Only 15% of all breast cancers are detected in a clinical breast exam. For the **average-risk patient**, both the National Cancer Institute and the American Cancer Society recommend a screening mammogram every 1 to 2 years beginning at the age of 40 and then annually in women >50 years of age. Mammography is the only screening modality that is proven to decrease mortality. Regular mammographic screening results in the early diagnosis of breast cancer and a 25% to 30% decrease in mortality in women ages 50 to 69. The benefit of screening in women older than 70 years has not been clearly established.
- Women with families at **high risk** for breast cancer, especially with BRCA1 and BRCA2 mutation, are often advised to undergo mammographic screening from the age of 25, or 5 years earlier than the earliest age at which another family member was diagnosed with breast cancer.
- MRI has also been found to be superior to mammogram and ultrasound in young women and in women with BRCA1 and BRCA2 mutations, where mammography is less sensitive and multicentric disease is more common.

Pathologic Subtypes

- Most invasive breast cancers are **adenocarcinomas**, which can be quite heterogeneous in histologic appearance. Infiltrating (invasive) ductal carcinoma accounts for ~80% of all breast cancers and originates from the cells lining the ducts of the breast. Infiltrating ductal carcinomas metastasize predominantly to the bones, liver, lungs, and brain. Lobular carcinomas make up 10% of malignant breast cancers and originate from the terminal ducts of the breast lobules. Lobular carcinomas are associated with bilateral tumors in up to 20% of cases, tend to be associated with multicentric disease within the same breast, and have a predilection to metastasize to the meninges, serosal surfaces, and mediastinal and retroperitoneal lymph nodes. Less common subtypes of ductal carcinomas include mucinous, medullary, and tubular, which carry a more favorable prognosis.

- Noninvasive carcinomas, which are characterized pathologically by the lack of penetration through the basement membrane into the surrounding stroma, include **ductal carcinoma in situ** (DCIS) and **lobular carcinoma in situ** (LCIS), which is not a true cancer but, instead, a marker for breast cancer risk. DCIS is most often identified with an abnormal mammogram showing clustered microcalcifications with or without a palpable mass. LCIS, on the other hand, is not detected on physical examination or mammography. LCIS is always an incidental finding in breast biopsies performed for another reason.

- **Paget disease** of the nipple is a specialized form of ductal carcinoma that arises from the main excretory ducts in the breasts and involves the skin of the nipple and areola. **Inflammatory carcinomas** involve the lymphatic structures in the dermis and infiltrate widely throughout the breast tissue. Inflammatory carcinomas are not a special morphologic pattern but are clinically diagnosed based on swelling, erythema, and tenderness in the involved breast and are associated with more aggressive disease.

PRESENTATION

History

Today, a majority of breast cancers are diagnosed as the result of an abnormal mammogram; however, any woman who presents with a new breast mass should have a complete history and physical examination. Symptoms related to the new mass, including duration, tenderness, relationship to menstrual cycle, presence of nipple changes, and discharge, should be elicited. An increased concern about malignancy arises if nipple discharge is unilateral, spontaneous, or bloody, especially in a postmenopausal woman. A negative family history does not exclude malignancy, given that most women who develop breast cancer do not have a family history. Patients should be asked a detailed history concerning any prior breast biopsies and family history of breast, ovarian, and other malignancies, as well as any personal history of breast cancer or other malignancies. A full gynecologic history should be taken, including age at menarche, age at menopause, use of oral contraceptives or exogenous hormone replacement therapy (type and duration), age at first live birth, and number of pregnancies.

Physical Examination

The physical characteristics of a breast mass can be helpful in determining a diagnosis. One should begin with a careful inspection for breast symmetry, contours, and retraction of the skin. Other changes in the skin can include erythema, thickening, and a peau d'orange appearance. Close inspection of the nipple can reveal rashes, ulceration, thickening, or discharge that may help identify an underlying malignancy or Paget disease of the breast. The characteristics of any nodules in the breast should be noted, including the location, size, shape, consistency, demarcation, tenderness, and mobility. A complete exam for lymphadenopathy includes evaluation for axillary, supraclavicular, and infraclavicular lymph nodes. The final element of the breast examination is compression of the areola to try to elicit any nipple discharge. A nonmilky or bloody unilateral nipple discharge suggests underlying breast pathology and should be evaluated further. The most common source of nipple discharge is an intraductal papilloma, which is a benign lesion.

Differential Diagnosis

The individual risk of a primary breast cancer can be characterized as high or low based on the patient's age, presenting symptoms, history of breast pathology, and family history. For example, a new breast mass in a woman >40 years old should be considered malignant until proven otherwise, whereas in women <35 years old with a similar lesion, cancer is possible but uncommon. The differential diagnosis of a breast mass can be broad, including malignancies, such as primary breast cancer, lymphoma, and sarcoma, and benign breast lesions, such as cysts, fibroadenomas, and fat necrosis. Skin conditions, such as sebaceous cysts, abscesses, or thrombophlebitis, may present with a palpable mass. The history and physical exam will help aid in the differential diagnosis, but ultimately a biopsy is confirmatory.

MANAGEMENT

Diagnosis

Laboratory Evaluation
- Laboratory tests do not directly aid in the staging of breast cancer but can allow the clinician to focus on possible metastatic sights of disease. Routine laboratory studies obtained are complete blood count (bone marrow infiltration), liver function tests (liver metastasis), and alkaline phosphatase (bone metastasis). Abnormal blood tests can also give the physician an objective marker to assess for clinical response after therapy in patients without identifiable measurable disease.
- **Tumors markers (CEA, CA15-3, CA27-29)**, although not specific, may be elevated in patients with breast cancer. Tumor markers are not accurate for screening or diagnostic purposes, thus they are not indicated in the initial assessment of breast cancer. In the metastatic setting, however, tumor markers may be elevated and the trend of elevation can assist in monitoring for response to therapy.

Diagnostic Evaluation and Biopsy
- Any distinct mass should be considered for biopsy, even if the mammogram is negative. A solid mass is best evaluated with **diagnostic mammography**. Mammography allows the physician to assess the radiologic characteristics of the mass and the remainder of breast tissue in the ipsilateral and contralateral breast. Ultrasound can be useful to determine whether a lesion is cystic or solid. Aspiration of a cystic mass may be helpful. Cytology may reveal malignant cells, but the absence of malignant cells does not rule out a malignant lesion.
- After radiologic evaluation to determine the location and characteristics of the mass, a biopsy can be obtained using several different methods. **Fine-needle aspiration** (FNA) is a simple method for obtaining material for cytologic exam that can be performed in the clinician's office. False-negative rates for FNA can be as high as 10% even among the most experienced technicians. FNA also cannot distinguish in situ disease from invasive carcinoma. If a negative result is obtained from FNA, a core-needle or excisional biopsy should be done to obtain appropriate tissue for pathologic review. The majority of these biopsies can also be performed in the outpatient setting. If the biopsy reveals only normal breast tissue, then further surgical biopsy is recommended if the lesion is suspicious for cancer. Needle localization or stereotactic biopsies may be helpful in this situation. **Excisional biopsy** is the **gold standard**, allowing complete histologic characterization with regard to biomarkers as well as tumor grade. Excisional biopsy also may serve as the definitive lumpectomy.

Radiographic Studies
Radiographic studies are based on the history, physical examination, and laboratory studies. Chest radiographs are recommended by the National Comprehensive Cancer Network (NCCN) practice guidelines; however, routine bone scans, computed tomography (CT), and brain imaging with CT or MRI are optional.

Staging

A simplified version of the American Joint Committee on Cancer staging system is provided in Table 18-1.

TABLE 18-1	TNM CLASSIFICATION AND AMERICAN JOINT COMMITTEE ON CANCER (AJCC) STAGING FOR BREAST CANCER

Primary tumor (T)

Tis:	Carcinoma in situ
T1:	Tumor ≤2 cm in greatest dimension
T2:	Tumor >2 cm but not >5 cm in greatest dimension
T3:	Tumor >5 cm in greatest dimension
T4:	Tumor of any size with direct extension to the chest wall or skin including peau d'orange, skin ulceration, satellite skin nodules in the same breast, and inflammatory carcinoma

Axillary nodal status (N)

N0:	No axillary nodal involvement
N1:	Ipsilateral movable axillary nodal involvement
N2:	Ipsilateral, fixed, or matted axillary nodal involvement; or ipsilateral internal mammary nodal involvement in the absence of axillary nodal involvement
N3:	Ipsilateral infraclavicular nodal involvement with or without axillary nodal involvement; or ipsilateral internal mammary nodal involvement in the presence of axillary nodal involvement; or ipsilateral supraclavicular nodal involvement with or without axillary or internal mammary involvement

Distant metastatic disease (M)

M0:	No distant sites of disease detected
M1:	Distant metastasis

AJCC stage

Stage I:	T1	N0	M0
Stage IIA:	T0	N1	M0
	T1	N1	M0
	T2	N0	M0
Stage IIB:	T2	N1	M0
	T3	N0	M0
Stage IIIA:	T0	N2	M0
	T1–2	N2	M0
	T3	N1–2	M0
Stage IIIB:	T4	Any N	M0
Stage IIIC:	Any T	N3	M0
Stage IV:	Any T	Any N	M1

Adapted from American Joint Committee on Cancer. *AJCC Cancer Staging Manual.* 6th ed. New York: Springer-Verlag; 2002.

Prognosis

The most reliable and reproducible prognostic indicator is the involvement of axillary lymph nodes. Tumors <1 cm without nodal involvement have a good prognosis. Tumors with a poorly differentiated histology and a high nuclear grade have a worse prognosis. Estrogen receptor (ER)- and progesterone (PR)-positive tumors tend to have a better prognosis, whereas human epidermal growth factor receptor 2 (Her-2) overexpression is associated with a poor prognosis. Infiltrating ductal carcinomas and lobular carcinomas have a similar prognosis. Inflammatory breast cancer has a poor prognosis.

Treatment

The treatment of breast cancer utilizes a multidisciplinary approach, including local-regional treatment with surgery ± radiation therapy and treatment of systemic disease with cytotoxic chemotherapy, hormonal therapy, biologic therapy, or a combination of these. The need for and decision to utilize the various local or systemic therapies are based on a number of prognostic and predictive factors. These factors include tumor histology, tumor size, number of lymph nodes involved, clinical and pathologic characteristics of the tumor such as grade, tumor hormone receptor status, tumor Her-2 status, patient's age, patient's comorbidities, and menopausal status, as well as presence of metastatic disease. In addition to the various prognostic and predictive factors, a patient's preference is also a major component of the decision-making process, especially when more than one option may provide similar benefits.

In terms of treatment, breast cancer can be divided into four general categories.

- Pure noninvasive carcinoma, DCIS, and LCIS (stage 0)
- Early-stage breast cancer that is operable (clinical stage I, stage II, and some stage IIIA tumors)
- Locally advanced inoperable local-regional invasive carcinoma (clinical stage IIIB, stage IIIC, and some stage IIIA)
- Metastatic carcinoma (stage IV)

Carcinoma In Situ

- **Lobular carcinoma in situ** (LCIS) is not detected on physical examination and is always an incidental finding on breast biopsies performed for another reason. The term LCIS is a misleading one, as it is not a premalignant lesion. It is a marker that identifies women at an increased risk (21% over 15 years) for the development of invasive breast cancer that may occur equally in either breast. Of note, the majority of subsequent cancers are infiltrating ductal rather than lobular carcinomas.
- LCIS can be managed by **observation alone** after biopsy. There is no evidence that re-excision after the initial biopsy to obtain histologically negative surgical margins is required. The increased risk of breast cancer persists beyond 20 years, so careful observation and diagnostic mammography should be performed indefinitely in these women. Bilateral prophylactic mastectomies are an alternate option for women who are uncomfortable with the increased risk of developing breast cancer, for patients with a strong family history of breast cancer, or for patients with known BRCA1/BRCA2 mutations. Radiation therapy has no role in the management of LCIS. According to results from the NSABP-P1 study, **tamoxifen** (20 mg daily), when taken for 5 years, is associated with a 56% decrease in the risk of all breast cancer events in women with LCIS. Recent results from the NSABP Study of Tamoxifen and Raloxifene (STAR) trial have also shown raloxifene to be as effective as tamoxifen in reducing the risk of invasive cancer in postmenopausal patients with LCIS.
- **Ductal carcinoma in situ** (DCIS), also known as intraductal carcinoma, is being encountered more frequently with the increased use of screening mammography.

These lesions are most often identified on mammography as clustered microcalcifications with or without a palpable mass. **Surgical treatments** for DCIS range from local excision to total mastectomy. Total mastectomy results in a 98% long-term disease-free survival (DFS) rate for noninvasive cancer; however, it is now generally accepted that a lumpectomy followed by radiation therapy to the breast represents the optimal treatment option, as no difference in mortality has been found between lumpectomy and mastectomy. Local **chest wall irradiation** reduces the rate of ipsilateral breast tumor recurrences by >50% compared to lumpectomy alone. Contraindications for breast conserving surgery followed by radiation include (1) inability to completely excise the underlying disease to negative surgical margins, (2) multifocal disease, and (3) patient contraindication to receive radiation. Routine axillary nodal dissection is not recommended based on a low (<5%) incidence of axillary nodal metastases in patients with DCIS. According to the NSABP-B24 trial, **tamoxifen** given after surgery and radiation has been demonstrated to reduce the rate of all breast cancer events (noninvasive or invasive ipsilateral tumors and new contralateral tumors) by up to 40%.

Early Breast Cancer
- **Surgery.** The surgical options for the management of breast cancer include **breast-conserving therapy** (BCT) followed by radiation therapy, **mastectomy with breast reconstruction**, and **modified radical mastectomy alone**. Randomized clinical trials have proven that overall survival (OS) is equivalent between BCT followed by radiation therapy and mastectomy in women with early breast cancer. The selection of a surgical approach depends on the location and size of the tumor, other abnormalities present on the mammogram, the breast size, and the patient's attitude toward breast preservation. Multicentric disease (two or more primary tumors in separate quadrants), extensive malignant-appearing microcalcifications on imaging, pregnancy, and previous breast or mantle irradiation are absolute contraindications for BCT. Relative contraindications for BCT include tumors >5 cm and active connective tissue disease involving the skin, such as scleroderma.
  - The presence of metastases to the axillary lymph nodes remains the most important prognostic factor in patients with breast cancer; therefore, **axillary lymph node dissection** remains an important part of the surgical approach. In an effort to decrease the morbidity associated with axillary lymph node dissection (especially lymphedema and pain), while maintaining accurate staging, a **sentinel lymph node** (SLN) **biopsy** can be obtained. The SLN (the first node in the lymphatic chain that receives lymphatic flow from the entire breast) is at the highest risk for harboring occult metastatic disease in breast cancer patients. Vital blue dye and/or technetium-labeled sulfur are injected in and around the tumor or biopsy site. The surgeon maps the dye or radioactive compound drainage to the axilla and identifies the SLN, which is then biopsied. The SLN can be identified in >90% of patients with breast cancer, with false-negative rates ranging from 0% to 10%. No further axillary node dissection is needed if the SLN biopsy is negative. If the SLN is positive for malignancy, further treatment options include a full axillary dissection, axillary radiation, and no further surgery and adjuvant chemotherapy. SLN biopsies are only performed on women without palpable, clinically suspicious, axillary lymph nodes on physical examination.
- **Radiation therapy.** Radiation therapy to the intact breast after BCT is the standard treatment based on several randomized trials that have shown higher local recurrence rates with BCT alone compared to BCT with radiation therapy. Radiation treatments are administered daily to the intact breast over a 5- to 6-week period to a total dose of 45 to 50 Gy. A radiation boost to the tumor bed is often administered.

Patients with positive axillary nodes may benefit from regional nodal irradiation in addition to irradiation of the intact breast. Postmastectomy, adjuvant chest wall and axillary radiation is considered for the following: positive surgical margins, primary tumors >5 cm, and involvement of four or more lymph nodes. Radiation therapy can decrease the rates of local recurrence even among patients who receive adjuvant chemotherapy. Anthracycline chemotherapy has radiation-sensitizing effects and should not be given concurrently with radiation. Typically, adjuvant radiation is given following the completion of adjuvant chemotherapy.

- **Adjuvant chemotherapy.** Adjuvant systemic therapy with cytotoxic chemotherapy, hormonal therapy, and trastuzumab has demonstrated significant improvement in DFS and OS in both premenopausal and postmenopausal women, with or without lymph node metastases. Candidates for adjuvant systemic therapy with chemotherapy, hormonal therapy, and trastuzumab depend on the prognostic factors of the tumors, such as the size, nodal involvement, and grade, as well as the biomarker status (ER/PR and Her-2).

  - Chemotherapy in the adjuvant setting has demonstrated reductions in the risk of recurrence and mortality rates of 25% and 15%, respectively, regardless of age, menopausal or hormonal status, or axillary lymph node involvement. Chemotherapy is recommended for most patients with node-positive disease. Adjuvant chemotherapy in node-negative patients is usually recommended if the tumor is >1 cm. Multiple adjuvant chemotherapy regimens exist (Table 18-2). Current literature supports that four to six courses of treatment provide optimal benefit. The current standard of practice is to initiate adjuvant chemotherapy 4 to 5 weeks after surgery, before the initiation of radiation.

  - Prior to the advent of taxanes, anthracycline-based regimens, such as AC, and CMF-type regimens were the most widely used. Whether anthracycline-containing regimens are superior to CMF-containing regimens has been the subject of

TABLE 18-2	OVERVIEW OF COMMON NON-TRASTUZUMAB-CONTAINING AND TRASTUZUMAB-CONTAINING ADJUVANT CHEMOTHERAPY REGIMENS FOR BREAST CANCER

Non-trastuzumab-containing
  Fluorouracil/Adriamycin/cyclophosphamide (FAC) × 6 cycles
  Fluorouracil/epirubicin/cyclophosphamide (FEC) × 6 cycles
  Adriamycin/cyclophosphamide (AC) × 4 cycles
  Paclitaxel/carboplatin (TC) × 4 cycles
  Cyclophosphamide/methotrexate/fluorouracil (CMF) × 6 cycles
  Adriamycin (A) × 4 cycles → paclitaxel (T) × 4 cycles → cyclophosphamide (C) × 4 cycles
  Adriamycin/cyclophosphamide (AC) × 4 cycles → paclitaxel (T) × 4 cycles (q21 days or dose-dense q14 days with growth factor support

Trastuzumab-containing
  AC × 4 cycles → paclitaxel/trastuzumab (TH) (paclitaxel × 4 cycles; trastuzumab for 52 weeks)
  Docetaxel/carboplatin/trastuzumab (TCH) (docetaxel and carboplatin × 6 cycles; trastuzumab for 52 weeks)
  AC × 4 cycles → docetaxel/trastuzumab (docetaxel × 4 cycles; trastuzumab for 52 weeks)

ongoing debate. In the EBCTCG overview, a modest but statistically significant survival benefit for anthracyclines was suggested. Also, data are available suggesting a possible improved response with anthracycline-containing regimens for Her-2-positive patients. For node-positive breast cancer, the addition of a taxane to anthracycline-containing chemotherapy improves DFS and OS. Dose-dense chemotherapy for node-positive patients with Adriamycin and cyclophosphamide followed by paclitaxel with growth factor support has also improved DFS and OS. In addition to the various prognostic and predictive factors that play a role in determining whether or not adjuvant chemotherapy is chosen and which specific regiment to use, existing comorbid conditions should be considered in the decision to offer adjuvant chemotherapy, as adverse effects related to chemotherapeutic drugs may influence the overall benefits.

- **Adjuvant hormonal therapy.** Patients with invasive breast cancer that is ER or PR positive should be considered for adjuvant hormonal therapy regardless of the patient's age, menopausal status, or lymph node status or whether or not adjuvant chemotherapy is to be administered. Adjuvant hormonal therapy should not be recommended in patients whose breast cancers are ER negative or PR negative because clinical trials have not shown any benefit in DFS or OS.

- **Tamoxifen,** a selective estrogen receptor modulator, inhibits the growth of breast cancer cells by competitive antagonism of estrogen at the ER. Tamoxifen is a well-established form of hormonal therapy for both premenopausal and postmenopausal women. In women with ER-positive early breast cancer, adjuvant tamoxifen decreased the risk of recurrence by 42% and the risk of death by 22% irrespective of the use of chemotherapy, age, menopausal status, or axillary lymph node status. Tamoxifen also decreases the incidence of breast cancer in the contralateral breast by ~50%. Prospective randomized trials have demonstrated that the optimal duration of tamoxifen is 5 years and that longer treatment may trend toward a detrimental effect. In patients receiving both tamoxifen and chemotherapy, chemotherapy should be given first.

- An alternative option for adjuvant hormonal therapy in postmenopausal women is **aromatase inhibitors.** In postmenopausal women the primary source of estrogen is the peripheral conversion of androgens to estrogen by the enzyme aromatase. Several studies have utilized aromatase inhibitors in the treatment of postmenopausal women with early-stage breast cancer. These studies have utilized aromatase inhibitors either as up-front initial therapy, as sequential therapy following 2 to 3 years of tamoxifen, or as extended therapy following 5 years of tamoxifen. Two up-front studies, ATAC and BIG I-98, have compared anastrozole versus tamoxifen and letrozole versus tamoxifen, respectively. Both studies have shown an improved DFS with the aromatase inhibitor compared to tamoxifen when used in the up-front setting. Several trials have also studied the use of sequential aromatase inhibitors following either 2 to 3 years of tamoxifen or 5 years of tamoxifen. The NCIC MA 17 trial showed an improved DFS with continuation of letrozole versus placebo following 5 years of tamoxifen. The Intergroup Exemestane Study showed an improved DFS as well as a trend toward improved OS with switching to exemestane following 2 to 3 years of tamoxifen versus continuation of tamoxifen. Given the available data, aromatase inhibitors are now largely used as the treatment of choice for postmenopausal women with hormone receptor-positive early breast cancer.

- Tamoxifen and aromatase inhibitors have different side-effect profiles. Both cause hot flashes and night sweats and may cause vaginal dryness. Aromatase inhibitors are more commonly associated with musculoskeletal symptoms, osteoporosis, and an increased rate of bone fracture, while tamoxifen is associated with an increased risk of uterine cancer and deep vein thromboses.

- For premenopausal ER-positive women, alternative strategies of hormonal therapy besides tamoxifen include surgical oophorectomy, radiation-induced ovarian ablation, and chemical suppression of ovarian function with luteinizing hormone-releasing hormone (LHRH) agonists, such as goserelin. Aromatase inhibitors are contraindicated in premenopausal women with functioning ovaries due to insufficient blockage of ovarian estrogen.
- **Adjuvant trastuzumab.** Trastuzumab is a humanized, monoclonal antibody with specificity for the extracellular domain of Her-2/neu. Recent data from five randomized trials have shown that the addition of 1 year of trastuzumab to anthracycline- and taxane-containing adjuvant chemotherapy regimens provides substantial benefit for women with Her-2-positive breast cancer, in terms of both disease recurrence and survival. An ~50% reduction in the risk of recurrence was seen across the trials, and in the B-31/NCCTG N9831 trial a 33% reduction in the risk of death was reported. Thus, 1 year of adjuvant trastuzumab in combination with anthracycline- and/or taxane-containing chemotherapy regimens should be offered to all Her-2-positive patients.
- **Neoadjuvant therapy.** Preoperative or neoadjuvant therapy with the use of hormonal or chemotherapeutic agents has been shown to be effective in downsizing the dimensions of the primary tumor, thus allowing for BCT. Results of randomized trials suggest that this strategy is safe and is equivalent to postoperative adjuvant chemotherapy with the same regimen for operable stage I and II breast cancers. Between 10% and 15% of patients have a complete pathologic response in the primary tumor after three or four cycles of an anthracycline-containing regimen, and 20% to 30% of patients with biopsy-proven lymph node metastases before neoadjuvant chemotherapy have pathologically negative lymph nodes after neoadjuvant chemotherapy. In a postmenopausal, hormone receptor-positive patient, the use of a hormonal agent, such as an aromatase inhibitor, can be used to shrink the primary tumor. In women with residual malignancy found at the time of surgery, additional hormone therapy or chemotherapy is often recommended.

Locally Advanced Breast Cancer

- Locally advanced breast cancer includes those subsets of patients with tumors >5 cm, inflammatory breast tumors, and any tumor with fixed or matted axillary lymphadenopathy or internal mammary lymph node involvement. Patients with locally advanced breast cancer need to be evaluated in order to determine whether or not an initial surgically approach is likely to achieve pathological negative margins and provide long-term local control. Patients who present with clinical stage IIIA (except T3N1M0), IIIB, or IIIC are considered to have inoperable breast cancer at presentation; therefore, anthracycline-based chemotherapy is the initial therapeutic strategy. **Neoadjuvant chemotherapy** is effective in this patient population and may allow for tumor shrinkage to adequately perform surgical resection with clear margins. Total mastectomy with lymph node dissection with or without reconstruction or lumpectomy with axillary dissection is recommended for local control. Given the high risk of recurrence, all patients need radiation therapy after surgery. Adjuvant systemic therapy with cytotoxic chemotherapy, hormonal therapy, and trastuzumab therapy, if indicated, is considered standard.
- Advanced breast cancer is associated with a poor prognosis and a high rate of local and distant recurrences, leading to a treatment approach similar to that for metastatic disease.

Metastatic Breast Cancer (MBC)

- The primary goals of treatment for patients with metastatic disease are to prolong survival and palliate symptoms related to the disease; therefore, minimally toxic therapy is preferred. The management of MBC depends on the site and extent of metastases, hormone receptor status, and HER2/neu overexpression. Patients with MBC can be divided into two groups for treatment decisions: patients with local disease only and patients with systemic metastatic disease. Patients who had mastectomy or BCT and present with local recurrence should undergo local resection with mastectomy (if obtaining clear surgical margins seems plausible) and radiation therapy. Unresectable chest wall recurrences should be treated with radiation therapy if the patient has not previously received this modality of treatment. After local control, patients should be considered for systemic chemotherapy or endocrine therapy.

- Some other important decisions regarding treatment are made based on risk categories. Patients in the low-risk group include patients with a long disease-free interval; hormone receptor-positive tumors; and bone, soft tissue, or limited visceral organ involvement. High-risk patients include those with rapidly progressive disease or extensive visceral involvement, as well as patients whose disease becomes refractory to hormonal therapy.

- MBC treatment should be multidisciplinary, and support groups tend to be very helpful. At some point in the clinical course, the disease burden from MBC may interfere with the patient's ability to tolerate further treatment options, and supportive or palliative care should be offered to the patient and family. Failure to achieve response to three sequential chemotherapy regimens or an Eastern Cooperative Oncology Group (ECOG) performance status of ≥3 is believed to be an indication for supportive therapy only.

- Hormonal therapy. In low-risk patients with advanced or MBC and ER-positive disease, hormonal therapy can achieve initial response rates as high as 60% to 70%. ER-negative tumors exhibit no clinical benefit from first-line hormonal therapy. In postmenopausal women with ER-positive tumors, who are more than 1 year past previous antiestrogen therapy or are naïve to hormonal therapy, an aromatase inhibitor or tamoxifen should be used. In patients who are within 1 year of antiestrogen exposure, aromatase inhibitors are currently preferred as first-line agents. The current treatment recommendation in premenopausal ER-positive women with locally advanced or MBC is the combination of an LHRH agonist and tamoxifen. This combination has demonstrated an improvement in time to disease progression and survival compared with an LHRH agonist alone. Surgical or radiotherapeutic oophorectomy should also be considered.

  - Patients who have a clinical response after initiation of a hormonal therapy may benefit from second- and third-line hormonal therapies when the cancer begins to progress. Other hormonal therapies to consider in postmenopausal women (or in premenopausal women after oophorectomy) include the different aromatase inhibitors (anastrozole and letrozole) or a steroidal aromatase inactivator (exemestane), fulvestrant, tamoxifen or toremifene, megestrol acetate, fluoxymesterone, or high doses of ethinyl estradiol. Subsequent response rates with second- and third-line agents become lower but remain as high as 20% to 40%. With each subsequent hormonal therapy, the duration of a clinical response becomes shorter, and ultimately, the disease will become refractory to hormone treatment. Second- and third-line hormonal therapy should be chosen based on the adverse side-effect profile of each drug. Systemic chemotherapy can be recommended in patients whose disease becomes refractory to multiple lines of hormonal therapy.

- Treatment of bone metastases. Although patients with bone-only metastatic disease have a better prognosis than those with visceral metastases, bone metastases can lead to serious complications such as pain, fractures, spinal cord compression, and hypercalcemia. Traditionally, treatment of symptomatic bone metastases has been with analgesics, localized radiation, or surgery. Although improvements in pain and quality of life have been achieved with the use of these therapeutic options, their use for the prevention of progression of bone lytic metastases has been ineffective.

Bisphosphonates, either alone or in addition to chemotherapy, have shown a reduction in bone pain and in progression of lytic bone metastases. Pamidronate (Aredia), as an IV infusion (90 mg over 2 hours), was the first bisphosphonate to demonstrate this benefit. Zoledronate (Zometa) is an alternate IV bisphosphonate that is 1000 times more potent than pamidronate and has a much shorter infusion time (4 mg IV over 15 minutes). All patients with bone metastases (if expected survival is ≥3 months and creatinine levels are <3.0 mg/dL) should be maintained on an IV bisphosphonate every 3 to 4 weeks for the duration of their treatment, in combination with calcium citrate and vitamin D.

- **Chemotherapy.** High-risk patients with rapidly progressive disease, extensive visceral involvement, or disease that becomes refractory to hormonal therapy may benefit from chemotherapy. Combination chemotherapy generally provides higher rates of objective response and longer times to progression; however these regimens are associated with increased toxicity without adding survival benefit. Preferred first-line chemotherapies include sequential single agents and combination chemotherapy (see Table 18-2). Anthracycline-based combinations, such as CAF, FEC, AC, and EC are frequently used. Single agents with activity against MBC include anthracyclines, paclitaxel, docetaxel, capecitabine, vinorelbine, and gemcitabine. All chemotherapy regimens have similar overall response rates in MBC, and individual chemotherapy regimens are offered based on the toxicity profile and the patient's performance status. Once a patient develops progressive disease on one regimen, subsequent agents may be offered if the patient desires further treatment.
- **Immunotherapies.** Among patients with MBC, HER2/neu overexpression occurs in 25% to 30% of cases. HER2/neu overexpression is associated with relative resistance to treatment with anthracycline- or taxane-based chemotherapy. **Trastuzumab** is approved for use in combination chemotherapy as first-line therapy and as a single-agent drug in second- and third-line therapy in MBC. In the original trials the response rates using trastuzumab as a single agent in first-line therapy were 20% to 25%. There are data suggesting benefit from adding trastuzumab to paclitaxel, docetaxel, vinorelbine, and platinum compounds. The use of trastuzumab in combination with anthracyclines has been associated with severe cardiac toxicity in up to 27% of patients and it should not be used in combination with this drug class.
  - **Bevacizumab** is a humanized monoclonal antibody against vascular endothelial growth factor (VEGF). A recent trial showed that in patients with recurrent or MBC the addition of bevacizumab to chemotherapy with paclitaxel increased DFS compared with paclitaxel alone.

Follow-up

Follow-up exams should be individualized either to reflect the patient's risk of recurrence or to monitor treatment or disease progression. Posttreatment follow-up includes regular physical exam and mammography. The first mammogram in patients undergoing BCT should be after 6 months, and then yearly. No randomized trials have demonstrated a benefit from routine laboratory or radiology testing compared to a careful history and physical exam. The clinical role of tumor markers (CEA, CA 15-3, CA 27-29) is also unproven. According to the most recent NCCN guidelines, routine liver function tests, bone scans, chest x-rays, CT scans, PET scans, or ultrasound is not recommended unless clinical suspicion for recurrent/metastatic disease is suggested by the history and/or physical exam. MRI can be considered as an option for surveillance in women at high risk for bilateral disease, such as BRCA1/2 mutation carriers, or in young women with dense breasts. Patients with a uterus who are taking tamoxifen should undergo yearly gynecologic evaluation. Patients taking aromatase inhibitors should have bone health monitoring given the associated increased risk of osteopenia and osteoporosis.

SPECIAL TOPICS

Breast Cancer and Pregnancy

- Breast cancer in pregnancy is an uncommon phenomenon but one that poses dilemmas for patients and their physicians. A multidisciplinary approach is recommended for optimal clinical decision making. It has been estimated that there are ~1.3 breast cancers diagnosed per 10,000 live births. Breast cancer during pregnancy tends to present at advanced stages with lymph node involvement, sometimes because there is a delay in the diagnosis. Tumors tend to be poorly differentiated, hormone receptor negative, and Her-2 positive in 30% of cases.
- The evaluation of a pregnant patient with breast cancer should involve a multidisciplinary team, with the consultation of a maternal fetal specialist. The initial workup should document the presence of metastatic disease, as this may influence the patient's decision regarding maintenance of the pregnancy. Estimation of delivery time will help in establishing the best treatment options. Fetal growth needs to be monitored during treatment.
- Surgery remains the mainstay of treatment of breast cancer during pregnancy, and in some circumstances breast-conserving surgery is an acceptable option. Sentinel lymph node biopsy with technetium 99m is considered safe; however, isosulfan blue dye should be avoided. Indications for chemotherapy are the same as for nonpregnant patients, but it should not be given during the first trimester, to avoid teratogenesis, or after week 35, to avoid complications at the time of delivery. Chemotherapy regimens containing anthracyclines or alkylating agents are most commonly used; if taxanes are indicated, they should be used after delivery. Trastuzumab, endocrine therapy, and radiation therapy should be initiated only in the postpartum period. Decisions regarding lactation and future fertility should be addressed on a per-patient basis.

Male Breast Cancer

Male breast cancer is a rare disease, accounting for ~1% of all breast cancers. Familial cases tend to be associated with BRCA2, and 20% of patients with male breast cancer have a first-degree relative with the disease. Known risk factors are those associated with hormonal alterations in estrogen and androgen balance. Patients with Klinefelter syndrome, testicular pathology (e.g., cryptorchidism, testicular injury, orchitis, or any other form of gonadal dysfunction), and infertility have an increased risk. Obesity, increased alcohol intake, exposure to radiation, high temperatures, and exhaust fumes are also considered risk factors. Gynecomastia does not increase the risk of male breast cancer. Ninety percent of the tumors are invasive ductal carcinomas, and they are usually hormone receptor positive. At presentation patients usually have stage III or IV disease, but survival is comparable to that for female breast cancer when matched for stage and grade. The same standard treatment guidelines that are used in women should be used in men. Mastectomy is the type of surgery usually performed, followed many times by radiation therapy. Tamoxifen is the first-line therapy in ER-positive tumors. Chemotherapy should be used in all cases of hormone-refractory disease or in conjunction with hormonal therapy in patients with metastatic disease.

KEY POINTS TO REMEMBER

- Breast cancer is the most commonly diagnosed malignancy in women and follows lung cancer as the leading cause of cancer deaths among women.
- Identifiable risk factors for breast cancer include age, early menarche, late menopause, nulliparity, history of breast cancer and benign breast disease, and exogenous estrogen use, as well as other familial and environmental factors.
- ER-positive disease is associated with an improved prognosis compared to ER-negative disease.
- The biologic marker HER2 protein is seen in ~25% of invasive breast cancers and is associated with a poor prognosis. Adjuvant trastuzumab + chemotherapy decreases the recurrence risk by 50%.
- Trastuzumab should not be used in combination with anthracyclines due to a high rate of cardiac toxicity.
- The most important prognostic factor in women with breast cancer is axillary nodal status, followed by hormonal receptor status.
- BCT with radiation therapy and mastectomy demonstrate equivalent survival rates.
- SLN biopsy is useful to provide accurate surgical staging of the axilla and is associated with less lymphedema than axillary node dissection.
- Radiation is a standard adjuvant therapy after BCT. In postmastectomy patients, reasons to consider adjuvant radiation include positive surgical margins, large primary tumors, and axillary lymph node involvement.
- Adjuvant hormone therapy and/or chemotherapy are recommended in all breast cancer patients with primary tumors >1 cm and positive axillary or SLN involvement.
- In inoperable tumors, neoadjuvant chemotherapy can help reduce the tumor in order to achieve local control.
- In postmenopausal patients with MBC and hormone-positive tumors, aromatase inhibitors are considered first-line therapy.

REFERENCES AND SUGGESTED READINGS

American College of Obstetrics and Gynecology Committee on Gynecologic Practice. *Tamoxifen and Uterine Cancer. ACOG Committee Opinion.* Washington, DC: ACOG; 2006;336–1114.

Bast RC Jr, Ravdin P, Hayes DF, et al. 2000 Update of recommendations for the use of tumor markers in breast and colorectal cancer: clinical practice guidelines of the American Society of Clinical Oncology. *J Clin Oncol.* 2001;19:1865–1878.

Early Breast Cancer Trialists' Collaborative Group. Effects of chemotherapy and hormonal therapy for early breast cancer recurrence and 15-year survival: an overview of the randomized trials. *Lancet.* 2005;365:1687.

Early Breast Cancer Trialists' Collaborative Group. Effects of radiotherapy and surgery in early breast cancer: an overview of randomized trials. *N Engl J Med.* 1995;333:1444.

Early Breast Cancer Trialists' Collaborative Group. Tamoxifen for early breast cancer: an overview of the randomized trials. *Lancet.* 1998;351:1451.

Fentiman IA, Fourquet A, Hortobagyi G. Male breast cancer. *Lancet.* 2006;367:595–604.

Fisher B, et al. Fifteen year prognostic discriminants for invasive breast carcinoma: National Surgical Adjuvant Breast and Bowel Project Protocol B-06. *Cancer.* 2001;91:1679.

Fisher B, et al. Five versus more than five years of tamoxifen therapy for breast cancer patients with negative lymph nodes and estrogen receptor-positive tumors. *J Natl Cancer Inst.* 1996;88:1529.

Fisher B, et al. Tamoxifen for the prevention of breast cancer: current status of the National Surgical Adjuvant Breast and Bowel Project P-1 Study. *J Natl Cancer Inst.* 2005;97:1652.

Fisher B, et al. Tamoxifen in treatment of intraductal breast cancer: National Surgical Adjuvant Breast and Bowel Project B-24 randomized controlled trial. *Lancet.* 1999;353:1993.

Gentilini O, Cremonesi M, Triffiro G, et al. Safety of sentinel node biopsy in pregnant patients with breast cancer. *Ann Oncol.* 2004;15:1348–1351.

Goss PE, et al. Randomized trial of letrozole following tamoxifen as extended adjuvant therapy in receptor-positive breast cancer: updated findings from NCIC CTG MA.17. *J Natl Cancer Inst.* 2005;97:1262–1271.

Henderson IC, et al. Improved outcomes from adding sequential paclitaxel but not from escalating doxorubicin dose in an adjuvant chemotherapy regimen for patients with node-positive primary breast cancer. *J Clin Oncol.* 2003;21:976–983.

Howell A, et al. Results of the ATAC (Arimidex, Tamoxifen, Alone or in Combination) trial after completion of 5 years' adjuvant treatment for breast cancer. *Lancet.* 2005;65:60.

Humphrey LL, et al. Breast cancer screening: a summary of the evidence for the U.S. Preventive Services Task Force. *Ann Intern Med.* 2002;137:347.

Klijin JG, Blamey RW, Boccardo F, et al. Combined tamoxifen and LHRH agonist versus LHRH alone in premenopausal advances breast cancer: a meta-analysis of four randomized trials. *J Clin Oncol.* 2001;19:343–353.

Krag D, et al. The sentinel node in breast cancer: a multicenter validation trial. *N Engl J Med.* 1998;337:941.

Kuerer HM, et al. Incidence and impact of documented eradication of breast cancer axillary lymph node metastases before surgery in patients treated with neoadjuvant chemotherapy. *Ann Surg.* 1999;230:72.

Middleton LP, Amin M, Gwyng K, et al. Breast carcinoma in pregnant woman: assessment of clinicopathological and immunohistochemical features. *Cancer.* 2003:98:1055–1160.

Paridaens R, Therasse P, Dirix L, et al. First line hormonal treatment for metastatic breast cancer with exemestane or tamoxifen in postmenopausal patients—a randomized phase III trial of the EORTC Breast Group. *J Clin Oncol.* 2004;22:14S (abstr 515).

Piccart-Gebhart MJ. Trastuzumab after adjuvant chemotherapy in HER2-positive breast cancer. *N Engl J Med.* 2005;353:1659.

Romond EH, et al. Trastuzumab plus adjuvant chemotherapy for operable HER2-positive breast cancer. *N Engl J Med.* 2005;353:1673.

Slamon DJ, Leyland-Jones B, Shak S, et al. Use of chemotherapy plus a monoclonal antibody against HER2 for metastatic breast cancer that overexpresses HER2. *N Engl J Med.* 2001;344:783–792.

Smith IC, et al. Neoadjuvant chemotherapy in breast cancer: significantly enhanced response with docetaxel. *J Clin Oncol.* 2002;20:1456.

Thurlimann B, et al. A comparison of letrozole and tamoxifen in postmenopausal women with early breast cancer. *N Engl J Med.* 2005;353:2757.

Van der Hage JA, et al. Preoperative chemotherapy in primary operable breast cancer: results from the European Organization for Research and Treatment of Cancer Trial 10902. *J Clin Oncol.* 2001;19:4224.

Vogel VC, et al. Effects of tamoxifen versus raloxifene on the risk of developing invasive breast cancer and other disease outcomes: the NSABP study of tamoxifen and raloxifene (STAR) P-2 trial. *JAMA.* 2006;295:2727–2741.

Lung Cancer

19

Janakiraman Subramanian and Vamsidhar Velcheti

INTRODUCTION

This chapter reviews the physiology of lung cancer, as well as staging and a brief overview of treatment. Lung cancer is first divided into two broad groups: small-cell lung cancer (SCLC) and non-small-cell lung cancer (NSCLC), based on histology. Their clinical behavior and management are different and, therefore, discussed separately. Also reviewed in this chapter is the general workup of a solitary lung nodule.

EPIDEMIOLOGY

Lung cancer is the leading cause of cancer mortality in men and women in the United States. The incidence of lung cancer is continuing to decline in men. However, in women the rates appear to be plateauing after several years of rising incidence. This difference in the gender distribution of lung cancer is due to the rising incidence of tobacco smoking in women. The age-standardized incidence rates of lung cancer are 81.2 cases/100,000 men and 52.3 cases/100,000 women. In the United States, the expected lung cancer mortality for the year 2007 is 160,390 deaths.

RISK FACTORS

Tobacco smoke is the major risk factor for lung cancer and it accounts for 90% to 95% of all lung cancer in men and 85% of women in North America. There is a clear, dose-dependent relationship between **tobacco** use and lung cancer. A major public health goal in reducing total mortality from lung cancer remains reducing the prevalence of smoking. Squamous cell and SCLCs, in particular, are associated with tobacco smoking.

Other exposures have also been associated with lung cancer, including asbestos, radon, bis(chloromethyl)ether, polycyclic aromatic hydrocarbons, chromium, nickel, and arsenic compounds. Genetic predisposition is an important risk factor and there are well-identified familial clusters of lung cancers. A major inheritable lung cancer susceptibility locus has been reported in 6q23-25. Genetic polymorphisms of enzymes regulating tobacco carcinogen metabolism such as exon 7 CYP1A1 polymorphism, GSTM1 null genotype, and GSTP1GG polymorphism are associated with increased lung cancer risk. In addition, polymorphisms of genes regulating DNA repair (ERCC2 and XRCC1) and inflammation (COX-2, IL-6, and IL-8) have also been reported to be associated with increased risk of lung cancer.

NON-SMALL-CELL LUNG CANCER

Classification

NSCLC encompasses four pathologic subtypes.

- **Squamous cell lung cancer** usually arises in proximal bronchi and can cause obstruction of the larger airways.
- **Adenocarcinoma** is the most common subtype, representing 40% of lung cancers in North America. It usually arises in the lung periphery.
- **Bronchoalveolar carcinoma** is a subtype of adenocarcinoma that grows along alveolar septa. It can present as a single nodule or multiple nodules or as a rapidly progressive multilobar disease that radiographically resembles pneumonia. It is not associated with tobacco smoking.
- **Large-cell carcinoma** is the least common subtype.

Clinical Presentation

Symptoms

Presenting signs and symptoms of lung cancer depend on the size, location, and degree of spread of the tumor. Lung cancer can present as an asymptomatic lung nodule found incidentally on chest x-ray (CXR). **Local symptoms** can include cough, wheeze, hemoptysis, dyspnea, postobstructive pneumonia (due to tumors that occlude major bronchi), pain (particularly with pleural or chest wall involvement), dysphagia (due to esophageal compression by tumor or lymphadenopathy), and hoarseness (caused by laryngeal nerve involvement). Apical tumors that invade the lower brachial plexus can present with *Pancoast syndrome*, which is a brachial plexopathy, Horner syndrome, and shoulder pain. Mediastinal lymphadenopathy that compresses the superior vena cava (SVC) can cause *SVC syndrome*, which most commonly presents with dyspnea and facial swelling. **Systemic symptoms** usually accompany disease that is more advanced and can include weight loss, fatigue, and loss of appetite. Metastatic disease also may cause symptoms specific to the involved organs. For example, patients may have pain from bony metastases, dyspnea from pericardial or pleural effusions, or headache and neurologic deficits from brain metastases. Although adrenal and liver metastases are common, they are usually asymptomatic.

Paraneoplastic Syndromes

NSCLC has been associated with numerous **paraneoplastic syndromes.** *Clubbing* results from proliferation of connective tissue at the ends of the digits and usually improves with treatment of the tumor. *Hypercalcemia* may be due to ectopic parathyroid hormone production by the tumor. *Pulmonary hypertrophic osteoarthropathy* is a syndrome consisting of bone and joint pain, clubbing, and increased alkaline phosphatase. It can be diagnosed by plain films (which show periosteal inflammation) or bone scan (which shows increased uptake symmetrically in long bones).

Management

Diagnosis

The goal of the initial workup is to establish the diagnosis of malignancy and to determine accurately the clinical stage of the cancer, so that candidates for potentially curable surgical resection are identified. Strategies for obtaining a pathologic diagnosis of a lung mass include **sputum cytology** (optimally from three early morning sputum collections), biopsy by **percutaneous fine-needle aspiration**, and **bronchoscopy with biopsy.**

Workup

Once the diagnosis of NSCLC has been confirmed, recommended imaging studies include a **CXR and a chest CT scan,** which can reveal the size of the tumor, extent of invasion of local structures, and presence of regional lymph node metastases. **PET scan** is also useful, as it has high accuracy in detecting disease metastatic to lymph nodes and distant sites, and it can aid in the differentiation of benign and malignant lung nodules. *Potential lymph node metastases* identified on imaging studies should be confirmed with direct biopsy. Mediastinoscopy is the most accurate means of staging mediastinal lymph nodes and should be performed when nodal involvement cannot be defined with chest CT. *Pleural effusions* should always be examined by thoracentesis, as a tumor associated with a malignant effusion is inoperable. The best way to identify the presence of distant metastases is with a thorough history and physical exam. Further imaging exams (i.e., head CT, abdominal CT, bone scan) should be directed by the patient's symptoms and are not required in asymptomatic patients who have early-stage tumors. The current staging system for NSCLC is described in Table 19-1.

Treatment Modalities
- **Surgery**, either pneumonectomy or lobectomy, is the best chance for cure for patients with stages I and II disease. **Preoperative workup** includes spirometry, arterial blood gases, and V/Q scan to establish both that the FEV_1 will be >1.2 liters postresection and that the patient does not have hypercapnia or cor pulmonale.
- **Radiation therapy** (RT) is used for cure in unresectable disease, for adjuvant therapy after surgery, or for palliation of locally advanced or metastatic disease. *Toxicities of RT* include pneumonitis (shortness of breath, tachypnea, tachycardia, fever, nonproductive cough, and infiltrate on CXR 1 to 3 months after RT), pulmonary fibrosis, acute esophagitis, pericarditis, and Lhermitte syndrome.
- In locally advanced disease, **chemotherapy** can be combined with surgery and/or RT with curative intent. In stage IIIB with pleural effusion and stage IV disease, chemotherapy is usually the single-treatment modality with the goal of prolongation of survival and palliation of symptoms.

Prognosis
Prognosis correlates with stage (Tables 19-1 and 19-2). Early-stage disease, good performance status, female gender, and absence of weight loss confer a better disease prognosis. Histologic type does not affect prognosis. Overexpression of COX-2, EGFR (epidermal growth factor receptor), MAPK (mitogen-associated protein kinase), p53, and K-ras and loss of FHIT (fragile histidine triad) have been reported to be associated with poor prognosis.

Treatment by Stage

Stages I and II
Stage I and II tumors are considered resectable, as they have extended no further than adjacent resectable structures or first-level lymph nodes. The optimal treatment is surgical resection with lobectomy or pneumonectomy. Patients who are not candidates for surgery because of poor lung function or comorbid conditions should be considered for RT administered with curative intent. RT is administered to resected patients if the resected margins are positive for tumor. Several prospective studies have reported that the addition of adjuvant chemotherapy to resected stage II patients with good performance status significantly improves survival. In stage I patients, there is currently not enough evidence to recommend adjuvant chemotherapy.

Stage III
- For unresectable stage IIIA and stage IIIB disease without malignant pleural effusion, combined modality therapy is the basic approach to care. Several large prospective studies have shown that treatment with concurrent radiation and chemotherapy

TABLE 19-1   TNM STAGING SYSTEM FOR NON-SMALL-CELL LUNG CANCER

Primary tumor (T)

- TX: Primary tumor cannot be assessed, or tumor proven by the presence of malignant cells in sputum or bronchial washes but not visualized with imaging or bronchoscopy
- TO: No evidence of primary tumor
- Tis   Carcinoma in situ
- T1:   Tumor <3 cm in greatest dimension, surrounded by lung or visceral pleura, without bronchoscopic evidence of invasion more proximal than the lobar bronchus a (i.e., not in the main bronchus)
- T2:   Tumor with any of the following features of size or extent: >3 cm in greatest dimension; involves main bronchus, >2 cm distal to the carina; invades the visceral pleura; associated with atelectasis or obstructive pneumonitis that extends to the hilar region but does not involve the entire lung
- T3:   Tumor of any size that directly invades any of the following: chest wall (including superior sulcus tumors), diaphragm, mediastinal pleura, or parietal pericardium; or tumor in the main bronchus <2 cm distal to the carina, but without involvement of the carina; or associated atelectasis or obstructive pneumonitis of the entire lung
- T4:   Tumor of any size that invades any of the following: mediastinum, heart, great vessels, trachea, esophagus, vertebral body, or carina; or tumor with a malignant pleural or pericardial effusion or with a satellite tumor nodule(s) within the ipsilateral primary-tumor lobe of the lung

Regional lymph nodes (N)

- NX: Regional lymph nodes cannot be assessed
- NO: No regional lymph node metastasis
- N1:   Metastasis to ipsilateral peribronchial and/or ipsilateral hilar lymph nodes, and intrapulmonary nodes involved by direct extension of the primary tumor
- N2:   Metastasis to ipsilateral mediastinal and/or subcarinal lymph node(s)
- N3:   Metastasis to contralateral mediastinal, contralateral hilar, ipsilateral or contralateral scalene, or supra clavicular lymph node(s)

Distant metastasis (M)

- MX: Presence of distant metastasis cannot be assessed
- MO: No distant metastasis
- M1:   Distant metastasis present including a separate metastatic tumor nodule(s) in the ipsilateral nonprimary tumor lobe(s) of the lung

Stage grouping: TNM subsets

Stage 0:	Tis: carcinoma in situ
Stage IA:	T1 NO MO
Stage IB:	T2 NO MO
Stage IIA:	T1 N1 MO
Stage IIB:	T2 N1 MO
	T3 NO MO
Stage IIIA:	T3 N1 MO
	T1 N2 MO, T2 N2 MO, T3 N2 MO

(continued)

TABLE 19-1	TNM STAGING SYSTEM FOR NON-SMALL-CELL LUNG CANCER (*Continued*)
Stage IIIB:	T4 N0 M0, T4 N1 M0, T4 N2 M0
	T4 N3 M0
	T1 N3 M0, T2 N3 M0, T3 N3 M0
Stage IV:	Any T, any N, M1

improves long-term survival over radiation alone or sequential radiation and chemotherapy in patients with unresectable stage IIIA without malignant pleural effusion. However, survival benefit was seen only in patients with good performance status. In patients with poor performance status, a palliative treatment approach is preferred.

- In patients with surgically resectable stage IIIA disease, the addition of adjuvant chemotherapy following surgical resection significantly improves survival. In patients with bulky stage IIIA (N2) disease that can be resected only by pneumonectomy, definitive chemoradiation treatment is preferred over resection. The addition of surgery after receiving chemoradiation in patients with stage IIIA disease (N2) has not shown a significant survival advantage; however, it may be considered in patients who have good performance status and are fit to undergo surgery. Patients with stage IIIB disease (invasion of mediastinal organs or contralateral lymph node involvement) are not candidates for surgery and are treated with chemotherapy and radiation. Patients who are classified as having stage IIIB disease because of malignant pleural effusion are treated with chemotherapy only.

Stage IV
- Chemotherapy provides modest improvement in survival. There has been a three- to fourfold improvement in 1-year survival with combination chemotherapy over that with best supportive care. Several new agents have now become available for the management of metastatic NSCLC. They include vinorelbine, gemcitabine, paclitaxel, docetaxel, and irinotecan. The addition of bevacizumab to a carboplatin-paclitaxel

TABLE 19-2	LONG-TERM SURVIVAL IN NON-SMALL-CELL LUNG CANCER
Stage	**5-year Survival (%)**
IA	67
IB	57
IIA	55
IIB	38–39
IIIA	23–25
IIIB	3–7
IV	1

combination has been shown to significantly improve 2-year survival. However, there is an increased risk of hemoptysis/bleeding complications with bevacizumab, and patients with squamous cell cancer were excluded from the study.

- In those patients who fail first-line chemotherapy with a platinum-based regimen, treatment with single-agent docetaxel as second-line chemotherapy has been shown to improve survival. In addition, pemetrexed and erlotinib have also been approved for second-line treatment of NSCLC.

Palliative Care

For patients who have poor performance status and do not benefit from chemotherapy, treatment may focus on palliation of symptoms. A brief palliative course of RT may reduce disease bulk, relieving dyspnea, pain, or other symptoms. Targeted RT may also treat pain and complications from bony or brain metastases.

Follow-up

There is no consensus on the appropriate follow-up for a patient who has had complete resection of NSCLC. Recurrences may be local or distant and will occur in up to 30% of patients with stage I disease and 50% of patients with stage II disease over the subsequent 5 years. After resection, a careful history and physical exam and a CXR should be obtained at intervals of 3 to 4 months, with the frequency of follow-up visits decreasing over time. Regular CXR can be replaced with once-yearly chest CT examinations. In patients with unresectable stage III disease treated with a curative intent, the guidelines for follow-up are similar except that regular CXR is not recommended. Further studies (abdomen or head CT scan, bone scan, PET scan) should be obtained if signs or symptoms suggest recurrent disease. Blood tests and sputum cytology do not have a role in routine follow-up. Unfortunately, even with close follow-up, it is unlikely that recurrent disease will be resectable and curable.

SMALL-CELL LUNG CANCER

SCLC accounts for ~15% of lung cancers in the United States. As opposed to NSCLC, SCLC grows more rapidly, is more often associated with diverse paraneoplastic syndromes, and is (initially) more chemosensitive.

Presentation

Symptoms
The presenting signs and symptoms of SCLC are similar to those of NSCLC. Although SCLCs can present as asymptomatic lung nodules found on imaging studies, most patients with this type of lung cancer present with symptoms, especially cough, dyspnea, and chest pain. Because SCLCs are often centrally located, they can cause hemoptysis, postobstructive pneumonia, and wheezing. Ten percent of patients have SVC syndrome at presentation.

Paraneoplastic Syndromes
Paraneoplastic syndromes associated with SCLC include the following.

- In **syndrome of inappropriate secretion of antidiuretic hormone** (SIADH), antidiuretic hormone production by the tumor leads to hyponatremia.
- In **Cushing syndrome** ectopic ACTH production leads to symptoms of adrenal excess.

- **Neurologic paraneoplastic syndromes,** including peripheral neuropathy and encephalomyelitis, are thought to be due to the production of autoantibodies.
- **Lambert-Eaton syndrome** is caused by an autoantibody that impairs acetylcholine release at the neuromuscular junction, leading to proximal muscle weakness and hyporeflexia. It is diagnosed with electromyography.

Management

The TNM (tumor, node, metastases) staging system is not used to classify SCLC. Instead, SCLC is described either as **limited stage,** with disease confined to one hemithorax that is encompassed in a radiation field, or as **extensive stage,** which describes all other patterns of disease.

Workup

Initial workup should include a comprehensive history and physical exam; screening lab work, including CBC, liver function tests, alkaline phosphatase, and lactate dehydrogenase; and CXR. A **CT scan** is useful for defining the extent of intrathoracic disease and for detecting abdominal metastases. Further workup can include a head CT and bone scan. Once disease has been found outside of the thorax, workup for additional sites of metastasis is not necessary unless a metastasis requiring immediate intervention (e.g., to weight-bearing bone or CNS) is suspected.

Treatment

Chemotherapy is the primary modality used in the treatment of SCLC, and inferior results are obtained when RT is used alone.

- **Limited stage. The role of surgery is controversial** in the management of patients with SCLC. For patients with limited-stage disease, combined modality treatment with chemotherapy and RT to the chest is standard.
- **Extensive stage.** Extensive stage disease is treated with chemotherapy alone. The commonly used standard chemotherapy regimens for SCLC include combinations of carboplatin or cisplatin with etoposide. Irinotecan, topotecan, and epirubicin are acceptable alternatives to etoposide and they have a lower incidence of myelosuppression. Overall, response rate to chemotherapy is ~60%, but nearly all patients eventually relapse.
- **Prophylactic cranial radiation** (PCI) is recommended in patients with limited-stage SCLC who achieve complete response after initial chemoradiation to prevent intracranial metastases. It can also be considered in patients with extensive-stage SCLC with a complete response to treatment. However, it should not be administered to patients with poor performance status or impaired mental function.

Palliative Care

Patients with poor performance status or significant comorbidities may not be able to tolerate aggressive chemotherapy. These patients may receive only RT or attenuated schedules of chemotherapy, with the goal of relieving symptoms.

Prognosis

Stage (limited vs. extensive), performance status, and markers of disease burden such as serum lactate dehydrogenase are the factors that most reliably correlate with outcome. The median survival of limited-stage disease treated with chemotherapy and RT is 15 to 26 months. However, **long-term survival can be achieved in 20% to 40% of patients with limited-stage SCLC with chemoradiation.** The median survival of extensive-stage disease treated with chemotherapy is 7 to 12 months. Only 5% of patients with extensive disease survive to 2 years.

Follow-up

Most patients treated for SCLC will relapse, usually in the first 2 years after diagnosis. Therefore, they should have close follow-up with a medical oncologist for the identification of symptoms, physical exam findings, or lab and CXR abnormalities that suggest recurrent disease.

OTHER TUMORS OF THE LUNG

A small percentage of lung malignancies is **carcinoid tumors,** which are derived from neuroendocrine cells and arise in the bronchi. Carcinoids can produce a variety of systemically active substances that cause the carcinoid syndrome: flushing, diarrhea, and wheezing. They can also cause bronchial obstruction. In the lung, carcinoids tend to grow slowly and are associated with a 5-year survival of 77% to 87%. Please see Chapter 25 for further information. Other malignant tumors of the lung are very uncommon, including adenoid cystic carcinoma and mucoepidermoid tumors, arising from bronchial salivary glands, and sarcomas and other soft tissue tumors.

SOLITARY LUNG NODULE

A solitary lung nodule is a single lesion completely surrounded by lung parenchyma that is <3 cm in diameter. Lung nodules may be malignant or benign. Benign etiologies include infectious granulomas (most common benign lesions), hamartomas, noninfectious granulomas, and adenomas. Lesions >3 cm, termed **masses,** are almost always malignant and should be managed as lung cancer.

Workup

The first goal of the workup of a solitary lung nodule is to assess the probability that the nodule is malignant. It is determined by the nodule size, smoking history, age, and characteristics of nodule margin on CT imaging. **Chest CT** should be performed to provide information on the nodule's size and appearance. Nodules with a spiculated appearance are more likely to be malignant; calcified nodules and nodules that have not increased in size over time are more likely to be benign. Previous x-rays or scans, if available, can provide critical information regarding the evolution of the nodule. **PET scanning** is sensitive and specific for the differentiation of benign and malignant lesion, and it has the advantage of providing staging information if occult nodal or distant metastases are identified. If PET scan is negative, then the nodule is followed with serial chest CT scans.

Follow-up

After the initial assessment, the nodule can be classified as benign, malignant, or indeterminate. *Benign nodules* and *intermediate nodules* <1 cm in diameter should be followed with serial chest CT every 3 to 6 months for 2 years. PET scan is recommended for nodules that have an intermediate probability and are ≥1 cm in diameter.

Diagnosis

Nodules that have a high probability of *malignancy* may be pursued with open biopsy and subsequent possible resection for cure. **Percutaneous fine-needle aspiration** is useful for biopsy of peripheral nodules; larger, central lesions can be biopsied with **bronchoscopy.** **Video-assisted thoracoscopic surgery** with resection of the nodule is the definitive diagnostic procedure; it can be considered in patients with a low surgical risk.

KEY POINTS TO REMEMBER

- Adenocarcinoma is the most common type of lung cancer.
- Paraneoplastic syndromes associated with NSCLC include clubbing, hypercalcemia, and pulmonary hypertrophic osteoarthropathy. Paraneoplastic syndromes associated with SCLC include SIADH, Cushing syndrome, and various neurologic syndromes.
- The staging workup of NSCLC focuses on identifying tumors that can be resected and thereby potentially cured.
- NSCLCs that cannot be resected or that recur after resection have a poor prognosis.
- The staging workup of SCLC focuses on identifying local versus advanced disease.
- Most SCLCs are symptomatic and metastatic at the time of presentation. Chemotherapy with or without radiation is the primary treatment modality.
- Limited-stage SCLC has a 2-year survival rate of 20% to 40% in appropriately treated patients.
- Combined-modality treatment with chemotherapy and RT is the treatment of choice in limited-stage SCLC.

REFERENCES AND SUGGESTED READINGS

Deslauriers J, Gregoire J. Clinical and surgical staging of non-small cell lung cancer. *Chest.* 2000;117 (Suppl 4):96S–103S.

Mountain CF. Revisions in the international system for staging lung cancer. *Chest.* 1997;17(Suppl):S3–S10.

Murren J, et al. Small cell lung cancer. In: DeVita VT Jr, Hellman S, Rosenberg SA, eds. *Cancer: Principles and Practice of Oncology.* 7th ed. Philadelphia: Lippincott Williams & Wilkins; 2005:810–844.

Ost D, et al. The solitary pulmonary nodule. *N Engl J Med.* 2003;348:2535–2542.

Schrump DS, et al. Non-small cell lung cancer. In: DeVita VT Jr, Hellman S, Rosenberg SA, eds. *Cancer: Principles and Practice of Oncology.* 7th ed. Philadelphia: Lippincott Williams & Wilkins; 2005:753–809.

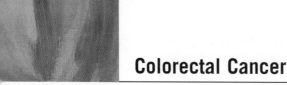

Colorectal Cancer

20

Coy Heldermon

INTRODUCTION

Lower gastrointestinal tract tumors are the third most commonly diagnosed cancers in the United States, and a leading cause of cancer death, but they can be surgically cured in a high percentage of cases. This chapter gives an overview of colon cancer presentation, pathophysiology, and staging and general principles of treatment.

EPIDEMIOLOGY

Colorectal cancer (CRC) is the third most common cancer after prostate and lung in men and breast and lung in women and accounts for ~15% of all cancers diagnosed in the United States. In the United States, there were ~105,000 new cases and 56,000 deaths from colorectal cancer CRC in 2005. The overall incidence of CRC in the United States has been declining since 1985 for unclear reasons. The current incidence of CRC is ~60.4 per 100,000. Incidence increases with age, with ~90% of cases diagnosed in those >50 years old. The median age of newly diagnosed patients is 70 for men and 73 for women. Peak incidence occurs in the eighth decade of life. The lifetime risk for CRC is 6% in average-age-risk persons living in the United States.

PATHOPHYSIOLOGY

Most CRCs are thought to develop from adenomatous polyps that arise from the colonic mucosa. Studies have shown that adenomatous polyps can become malignant over a period of 5 to 20 years. The common histologies of a polyp are tubular, tubulovillous, and villous. Villous adenomas are most likely to become malignant. Other characteristics of a higher propensity for malignancy are a size >1 cm in diameter and a high grade of dysplasia. Adenomatous polyps are found in ~35% of persons in autopsy studies. Up to 5% of polyps are believed to become malignant over time. More than 95% of CRCs are adenocarcinomas. Of these, >80% are moderately differentiated. Other histologic types seen are undifferentiated, squamous, carcinoid, leiomyosarcomas, and hematopoietic and lymphoid neoplasias. *Poor prognosis* is associated with colloid and signet ring subtypes of adenocarcinoma, which together represent ~20% of tumors.

Risk Factors
Risk factors for CRC are listed below.

- First-degree relative with CRC
- Personal history of CRC

- History of other malignancies
- History of radiation therapy to the abdomen or pelvis
- Increasing age
- Ureterosigmoidostomies
- **Inflammatory bowel disease,** especially ulcerative colitis but also Crohn disease
- Family history of a CRC syndrome
- **Familial adenomatous polyposis** (FAP) is an autosomal dominant disease caused by a defect in the APC gene that leads to colon cancer in 100% of patients by the age of 40 if they are left untreated. Affected persons will have up to thousands of adenomatous polyps with malignant potential in their bowel. Persons with FAP should have a prophylactic subtotal colectomy by age 30. Aggressive precolectomy screening for the development of cancer is also indicated. Other cancers such as medulloblastoma, papillary thyroid carcinoma, hepatoblastoma, pancreatic cancer, and gastric cancer are also associated with this syndrome.
- **Hereditary nonpolyposis colorectal cancer** (HNPCC) is inherited in an autosomal dominant manner and often leads to malignancies with mucinous histology in the right side of the colon. Often these tumors may arise without going through a polyp phase and, therefore, are seen as flat adenomas. HNPCC is also associated with cancers of the endometrium, ovary, stomach, and hepatobiliary system. Prophylactic subtotal colectomy is also recommended for persons with HNPCC.
- **Other inherited syndromes** associated with an increased risk of CRC include MYH-associated polyposis, Gardner syndrome, Turcot syndrome, Muir-Torre syndrome, and Peutz-Jeghers syndrome.

Screening

Screening methods used to detect CRC include fecal occult blood testing (FOBT), endoscopy, and barium enema. Early detection improves survival through detection of more curable lesions, and CRC incidence is high enough that screening can be cost-effective with acceptable positive predictive values. Patients with warning signs of CRC require more aggressive investigations, typically colonoscopy.

For the *asymptomatic* patient:

- **FOBT** is the least expensive and most widely used screening test for the detection of CRC. There are problems with its sensitivity, which has been reported to be 18% to 93%, with a specificity of >90%. Sensitivity will be affected by polyp size and frequency of bleeding. Specificity is affected by NSAID use, other sources of gastrointestinal bleeding, consumption of red meat, and consumption of certain vegetables in the diet. Hydration of samples before testing them is not recommended, as this worsens the specificity of the test.
- **Flexible sigmoidoscopy** examines up to 60 cm of the rectum and distal colon and can detect ~50% of CRC cases. Its advantages are that it can be performed in the primary care physician's office and that it has a specificity of nearly 100%. However, it has the disadvantage of not assessing the entire colon, and biopsies cannot be obtained during the procedures. Abnormalities necessitate a follow-up colonoscopy for biopsy.
- **Double-contrast barium enema** is a radiologic method for detection of CRC and is the safest of the visualization methods. It also requires a bowel preparation and, like FOBT, has the disadvantage of requiring subsequent endoscopy for biopsy of identified lesions.
- **Colonoscopy** is considered the gold standard for detection of CRC but is associated with a higher complication rate and a higher cost than the other methods. It also involves more extensive preparation before the procedure and sedation during it. For

the general population after age 50 years, National Comprehensive Cancer Network (NCCN) guidelines recommend colonoscopy every 10 years or annual FOBT combined with flexible sigmoidoscopy every 5 years. If risk factors such as a history of inflammatory bowel disease, family members with CRC, or a known defect such as HNPCC or FAP are present, then more frequent and earlier testing is recommended. For patients with a familial history of colorectal cancer, screening begins 10 years before the age of cancer diagnosis of the affected family member.

CLINICAL PRESENTATION

CRC may present with symptoms such as fatigue, anorexia, failure to thrive, lower gastrointestinal bleeding, and right upper quadrant pain associated with liver metastasis, although it is often asymptomatic until the tumor is large in size. Patients may also present due to a positive screen test. Symptoms associated with CRC are often related to the **location of the tumor** within the bowel. Therefore, *right-sided lesions* often present with symptoms of anemia and, occasionally, of melena. *Left-sided lesions* commonly cause obstruction, tenesmus, constipation, bright-red blood per rectum, and other changes in bowel habits. Patients often have an iron-deficiency anemia and may have symptoms of pica. Because CRC is a cause of anemia, it is important to evaluate any person who presents with unexplained anemia for CRC, especially men and postmenopausal women. CRC most often metastasizes to the liver, lung, adrenals, ovaries, and bone, so symptoms of organ compromise such as abdominal discomfort, shortness of breath, and bone pain may be present in metastatic disease.

Signs of CRC on **physical exam** include gross blood or melanotic stool in the rectal vault, pallor in the conjunctivae and the nail beds, or a palpable mass in the abdomen or the rectum. If liver metastases are present, patients may have hepatomegaly and be tender to palpation in the right upper quadrant. On barium enema, an "apple core" lesion may be seen, which suggests colon cancer. Bacteremia or endocarditis with *Streptococcus bovis* is also a sign of CRC, and these findings should trigger an evaluation for colon cancer.

MANAGEMENT

Diagnosis
Colonoscopy with biopsy is the diagnostic procedure of choice and is potentially curative for benign polyps and carcinoma in situ. Diagnosis depends on tissue pathology consistent with invasive colon cancer.

Workup
Workup for CRC should include the following

- **History and physical**
- **CBC** to evaluate for associated iron-deficiency anemia
- **Chemistry and liver function tests** to evaluate for liver involvement
- **Carcinoembryonic antigen** (CEA): if initially elevated, then a rise in CEA after treatment may indicate a recurrence
- **Chest/abdomen/pelvis CT scan** to rule out metastasis
- **All patients should have the entire colon evaluated by colonoscopy** or barium enema to rule out synchronous lesions. Up to 5% of patients have another focus of CRC in their bowels. Patients should have a tissue biopsy before therapy to confirm the diagnosis.

TABLE 20-1	AMERICAN JOINT COMMITTEE ON CANCER TNM SYSTEM FOR COLORECTAL CANCER STAGING

Tumor
  Tis: Carcinoma in situ: intraepithelial or invasion of the lamina propria
  T1:   Invasion of the submucosa
  T2:   Invasion into the muscularis propria
  T3:   Invasion through the muscularis propria into the subserosa
  T4:   Invasion through visceral peritoneum or invasion into adjacent organs

Node
  N0:   No lymph node metastases
  N1:   Metastases in one to three lymph nodes
  N2:   Metastases in four or more lymph nodes

Metastases
  M0:   No distant metastases
  M1:   Distant metastases present

Adapted from American Joint Committee on Cancer. *AJCC Cancer Staging Manual.* 6th ed. Philadelphia: Lippincott-Raven; 2002.

- **Surgical staging.** Surgery is important for accurate staging of CRC. The preferred staging system for CRC is the American Joint Committee on Cancer (AJCC) TNM (tumor, node, metastases) system (Table 20-1). TNM uses the degree of tumor invasion, the presence of positive lymph nodes, and the presence of distant metastasis to classify the disease in one of four stages. Although the AJCC TNM staging system is the preferred staging system today, the Duke staging system with the Astler-Coller modification is often referred to in older literature (Table 20-2).

Treatment of Colon Cancer

The goals of therapy need to be clearly delineated from the beginning and re-evaluated throughout the patient's course. Colon cancer that has not metastasized is a curable disease

TABLE 20-2	STAGING OF COLORECTAL CANCER BY AMERICAN JOINT COMMITTEE ON CANCER TNM SYSTEM (AND DUKE STAGE EQUIVALENTS)

Stage	Tumor	Node	Metastases	Duke Stage
0	Tis	N0	M0	N/A
I	T1 or T2	N0	M0	A, B1
II	T3 or T4	N0	M0	B2, B3
III	Any T	N1 or N2	M0	C
IV	Any T	Any N	M1	D

N/A, not applicable.

TABLE 20-3	TREATMENT FOR VARIOUS STAGES OF COLON CANCER
Stage	**Treatment**
0	Polypectomy/surgical resection
I	Surgery alone
II	Surgery ± chemotherapy
III	Surgery + chemotherapy
IV	Palliative chemotherapy, metastasis resection (limited cases)

with surgery. Chemotherapy can be added to improve cure rates for stage II or III tumors or as palliation for incurable tumors (Table 20-3).

- **Surgery** is undertaken with intent to cure in 75% of those with colon cancer. Many of the remainder will require surgery to prevent obstruction, perforation, or bleeding. Wide excision of the tumor with a distal margin of ~5 cm is recommended for curative surgery. The length of colon and mesentery resected is determined by vascular anatomy. If the tumor is adherent to or invades another organ, an en bloc excision must be done to prevent seeding and allow the possibility of cure. If the surgical intent is palliation instead of cure, a simple resection or diversion is used to lessen morbidity from the procedure. In stage IV cancer, some patients may benefit from resection of metastases. Five-year survival rates of up to 38% have been obtained with resection of limited liver metastases.
- **Adjuvant chemotherapy** is administered to prevent relapse of CRC, which occurs mainly at distant sites. Overall, 50% of those with macroscopic clearance of their disease through surgery will recur. Either 5-fluorouracil (5-FU), leucovorin, and oxaliplatin (FOLFOX) or 5-FU with leucovorin or capecitabine is the standard of care for stage III colon cancer. Capecitabine is an oral prodrug that is converted to 5-FU in tumor tissues. Adjuvant chemotherapy improves outcome for stage III disease by ~9%. However, controversy remains over adjuvant chemotherapy for stage II disease. Because the 5-year survival rate is 75% to 80% in stage II colon cancer, the reduction in deaths is predicted to be small. Because there seems to be only a small benefit from treating stage II disease, the current focus is on finding subgroups within the stage II colon cancer population that will be more likely to benefit from treatment. For stage II colon cancer, chemotherapy is an option for high-risk disease, including those patients who present with a total obstruction, a perforation, a high grade, lymphovascular invasion, or positive surgical margins.
- **Therapy of metastatic disease** depends on the functional status of the patient but typically involves 5-FU with leucovorin, capecitabine alone, or 5-FU and leucovorin in combination with either the topoisomerase I inhibitor irinotecan (the FOLFIRI regimen) or oxaliplatin (the FOLFOX regimen). Both of the combination regimens are further enhanced by the addition of the vascular endothelial growth factor antibody, bevacizumab (Avastin). After disease progression, patients are usually switched to another one of the primary regimens and may also receive either of the endothelial growth factor receptor inhibitory antibodies, cetuximab (Erbitux) or panitumumab (Vectibix). These agents have a clearly established benefit in the treatment of metastatic colon cancer. Patients with stage IV disease should be referred for clinical trials when possible.

Prognosis

Stage has great significance in the prognosis and treatment of the disease. In the United States between 1996 and 2002, the overall 5-year survival rate for patients with CRC was 65.1%. Five-year survival for stages I/II, III, and IV was 90.4%, 68.1%, and 9.8%, respectively. Five-year survival correlates well with cure of the disease. Other prognostic factors include the number of positive lymph nodes and tumor invasion through the bowel wall into adjacent organs or into veins.

Treatment of Rectal Cancer

Surgery is used in rectal cancer to cure the disease and also plays a role in palliative therapy. The rectum is the distal 15 cm of the large bowel and resides within the bony pelvis. The most important feature of the rectum is the lack of a serosa for these tumors. Because of this anatomy, local recurrence for rectal cancer is high, and adjuvant therapy may be needed to make a tumor resectable. Even with these difficulties, 50% of those who have surgery will be cured. Surgery in the pelvis can be technically demanding because there is a decreased area in which to work. Accordingly, surgery is used in conjunction with radiation or chemoradiation, and this multimodality approach has been associated with decreased recurrence. Approaches aimed at sphincter preservation, obviating the need for colostomy, can often be performed if a 2-cm margin can be obtained.

Compared to colon cancer, rectal cancer is **much more likely to recur locally** than distally. Only about 25% of rectal cancer patients have distant metastases. Therapy is therefore tailored to prevent local recurrence in stage II and III cancers. Currently, stage II rectal cancer is treated with surgery along with FOLFOX, 5-FU, or capecitabine and radiation, leading to significant improvements in overall survival compared to treatment with surgery alone. For stage III tumors, part of the systemic and radiation therapies may be given before surgery to increase resectability.

Complications

Tumor Related

Complications that can result from CRC include **bowel obstruction, anemia,** and **abdominal pain.** More serious complications can include peritonitis after perforation, fistula formation, and malnutrition. Complications can also result from sites of metastatic disease. Liver metastases can lead to hyperbilirubinemia and coagulopathies. Pulmonary metastases, when advanced, may result in cough or shortness of breath. Patients may also develop pain at sites of metastases.

Treatment Related

Complications of treatment are commonly related to surgery and chemotherapy but can also occur with radiation therapy. Postop mortality rates are 1% to 5%. Major morbidity includes bowel and bladder dysfunction, sexual dysfunction, anastomotic leaks, and bowel obstruction. The need for a permanent colostomy can be psychologically upsetting. Chemotherapy complications may include neuropathy (possibly long term), nausea, diarrhea, and hand-foot syndrome. Radiation may cause local radiation dermatitis with pain, desquamation, and color changes.

Follow-up

Current recommendations are for a history, a physical, and CEA every 3 months for 2 years, then every 6 months for another 3 years. At 1 year, a colonoscopy should be performed to look for local recurrence and synchronous disease. If the colonoscopy is negative, then it should be repeated in 3 years and then every 5 years. If the patient had a high-grade tumor or lymphovascular invasion, then a CT of the chest, abdomen, and pelvis should be repeated annually for the first 3 years to monitor for metastatic spread.

ANAL CANCER

Epidemiology

Anal cancer accounts for ~1.6% of all alimentary malignancies in the United States. Its incidence generally increases with age, with the peak incidence in the sixth and seventh decades of life. The incidence is increasing in men <40 years old due to increased risk in the HIV+ population. Histologically, 63% of anal cancers are squamous cell carcinomas. Basaloid transitional cell carcinomas (cloacogenic) make up 23% of cases. More rare types are adenocarcinoma, basal cell, and melanoma.

Risk Factors

The risk factor most commonly associated with anal cancer is **human papilloma virus** (HPV) infection. HPV 16 and HPV 18 have been linked to the disease. This is seen in both men and women. In women, increased anal cancers are seen with HPV-associated cervical cancer. In men, anal cancer is more frequently associated with receptive anal intercourse and HPV. As many as 70% of anal cancers are positive for HPV.

Other risk factors include immunosuppression such as that seen after renal transplant or HIV infection. Current cigarette smoking is also a risk factor for anal cancer, with a relative risk of seven- to ninefold for smokers.

Clinical Presentation and Diagnosis

Anal cancers present with bleeding 50% of the time. Other symptoms include pain, mass, constipation, diarrhea, and pruritus. Often the symptoms are ascribed to hemorrhoids, which may delay diagnosis. Approximately 25% of people are asymptomatic when the cancer is discovered. Physical exam findings include an anal mass and lymphadenopathy. On palpation, an anal mass will often be firm and indurated. Anoscopy, proctoscopy, and transrectal ultrasonography are used to visualize the mass. Diagnosis is made by incisional biopsy of the mass and any inguinal lymphadenopathy.

Workup

Digital rectal exam and inguinal lymph node exam should be accompanied by anoscopy. Notes should be made of the location of the mass, including its position relative to the dentate line. Anal cancers are divided into those of the anal margin and those of the anal canal. The line of demarcation is a zone approximately halfway between the dentate line and the anal verge. Women should have a pelvic exam for cervical cancer screening due to the association with HPV. Men and women should be tested for HIV, especially if any risk factors are present. Chest x-ray or CT, abdominal and pelvic CT, and PET scan should be performed to rule out metastatic disease.

Staging

Staging is based on the TNM system (Table 20-4).

Treatment

Very small tumors at the anal margin may be treated with wide local excision, but combined chemotherapy and radiation therapy has been the preferred treatment for locoregional disease. Treatment is with mitomycin-C and 5-FU, with concurrent radiation. In several trials, 5-year survival varied between 64% and 83% with combined-modality therapy. After treatment, close medical follow-up is needed to screen for recurrence. Recurrences may be treated surgically if resectable or with 5-FU and cisplatin followed by resection. If patients remain unresectable, then consideration should be given to a clinical trial.

TABLE 20-4 STAGING OF ANAL CANCER

Tumor
Tis:	Carcinoma in situ
T1:	Tumor ≤2 cm in diameter
T2:	Tumor between 2 and 5 cm in diameter
T3:	Tumor ≥5 cm in diameter
T4:	Tumor of any size that invades adjacent organs such as the vagina, urethra, or bladder

Node
N0:	No regional lymph nodes involved
N1:	Metastases in perirectal lymph nodes
N2:	Metastases in unilateral internal iliac or inguinal lymph node
N3:	Metastases in perirectal and one inguinal lymph node and/or bilateral internal iliac or inguinal lymph nodes

Metastases
M0:	No distant metastases present
M1:	Distant metastases present

Stage
I:	T1, N0, M0
II:	T2 or T3, N0, M0
IIIA:	T1–T3, N1, M0 or T4, N0, M0
IIIB:	T4, N1, M0 or any T, N2–N3, M0
IV:	Any T, any N, M1

Prognosis

Prognosis is based on staging. T1 and T2 tumors have >80% 5-year survival, whereas T3 and T4 tumors have 5-year survivals of <50%. Inguinal lymphadenopathy and male gender are also related to a poorer prognosis. Tumors in the anal margin have a more favorable prognosis than those in the canal.

KEY POINTS TO REMEMBER

- CRC must be suspected in unexplained anemia in men and postmenopausal women.
- The main risk factors for colon cancer include a personal and family history of colon cancer and age.
- The preferred approach for screening *asymptomatic patients* for CRC is annual FOBT after age 50 combined with flexible sigmoidoscopy every 5 years or colonoscopy every 10 years.
- CRC is a surgically curable disease, with later stages yielding poorer long-term survival rates.
- Chemotherapy for CRC is useful in higher-stage disease.
- Rectal cancer typically has a more difficult operative approach.
- Rectal cancers have a high rate of local recurrence and are, therefore, treated with combined modality treatment in stages II and III disease.
- Anal cancer is associated with HPV infection.

REFERENCES AND SUGGESTED READINGS

Andre T, Boni C, Mounedji-Boudiaf L, et al. Oxaliplatin, fluorouracil, and leucovorin as adjuvant treatment for colon cancer. *N Engl J Med.* 2004;350(23):2343–2351.

Cunningham D, Humblet Y, Siena S, et al. Cetuximab monotherapy and cetuximab plus irinotecan in irinotecan-refractory metastatic colorectal cancer. *N Engl J Med.* 2004;351:337–345.

Flam M, John M, Pajak TF, et al. Role of mitomycin in combination with fluorouracil and radiotherapy, and of salvage chemoradiation in the definitive nonsurgical treatment of epidermoid carcinoma of the anal canal: results of a phase III randomized intergroup study. *J Clin Oncol.* 1996;14:2527–2539.

Fong J, Cohen AM, Fortner JG, et al. Liver resection for colorectal metastases. *J Clin Oncol.* 1997;15:938–946.

Greene FL, Page DL, Fleming I, et al. *AJCC Cancer Staging Manual.* 6th ed. New York: Springer-Verlag; 2002.

Janne PA, Mayer RJ. Chemoprevention of colorectal cancer. *N Engl J Med.* 2000;342:1960–1966.

Jernal A, Murray T, Ward E, et al. Cancer statistics, 2005. *CA Cancer J Clin.* 2005;55:10–30.

Kelly H, Goldberg RM. Systemic therapy for metastatic colorectal cancer: current opinions, current evidence. *J Clin Oncol.* 2005;23(20):4553–4560.

Midgley R, Kerr D. Colorectal cancer. *Lancet.* 1999;353:391–399.

Peeters M, Haller DG. Therapy for early stage colorectal cancer [review]. *Oncology (Huntington)* 1999;13:307–315, discussion 315–317, 320–321.

Petrelli N, Herrera L, Rustum Y, et al. A prospective randomized trial of 5-fluorouracil versus 5-fluorouracil and high dose leucovorin versus 5-fluorouracil and methotrexate in previously untreated patients with advanced colorectal carcinoma. *J Clin Oncol.* 1987;5:1559–1565.

Poon MA, O'Connell MJ, Moertel CG, et al. Biochemical modulation of fluorouracil: evidence of significant improvement of survival and quality of life in patients with advanced colorectal carcinoma. *J Clin Oncol.* 1989;7:1407–1417.

Ryan DP, Compton CC, Mayer RJ. Medical progress: carcinoma of the anal canal. *N Engl J Med.* 2000;342:792–800.

Saltz LB, Cox JV, Blanke C, et al. Irinotecan plus fluorouracil and leucovorin for metastatic colorectal cancer. *N Engl J Med.* 2000;343:905–914.

Schatzkin A, Lanza E, Corle D, et al. Lack of effect of a low-fat, high fiber diet on the recurrence of colorectal adenomas. *N Engl J Med.* 2000;342:1149–1155.

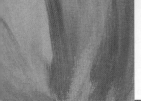

Other Gastrointestinal Malignancies

21

David Kuperman

ESOPHAGEAL CANCER

Introduction

Esophageal cancer is a common neoplasm and is the seventh most common cause of cancer death in the world. There is vast geographic variation in the incidence of this cancer. The incidence in the United States is about 5 per 100,000, although in African American men it may be as high as 18 per 100,000. China and Iran have an incidence of 20 per 100,000. In parts of Africa, Central America, and western Asia, the incidence is only 1.5 per 100,000. In recent years, there has been a shift in the location and histology of esophageal cancers. Adenocarcinoma of the distal esophagus is the most common type diagnosed in the United States, surpassing squamous cell cancer of the midesophagus.

Presentation

The initial symptoms of esophageal cancer may include dysphagia and weight loss. The dysphagia often begins with solid foods, then progresses to liquids. Extraesophageal spread can cause pain, hoarseness (secondary to recurrent laryngeal nerve involvement), aspiration, tracheal narrowing, or tracheoesophageal fistula.

Management

Diagnosis

Upper endoscopy with biopsy is the gold standard for diagnosis of upper gastrointestinal tract tumors. Barium studies may also be used for diagnosis but are less sensitive and do not allow for biopsy of suspicious lesions. Given that ~3% of gastric ulcers are found to be malignant, many gastric ulcers found on upper endoscopy should be considered for biopsy. Repeat endoscopy is frequently done to document resolution of ulcer disease.

Workup
- If an esophageal cancer is found, computed tomography (CT) of the chest and abdomen must be performed. CT is an excellent initial staging tool, but further specialized testing may be necessary. If the patient does not have evidence of metastasis, an endoscopic ultrasound should be performed. This procedure, involving insertion of an ultrasound probe into the esophagus and stomach, allows the most precise assessment of tumor depth, length of esophagus affected, and magnitude of lymph node metastases, particularly paraesophageal and celiac nodes. A biopsy of suspicious lymph nodes can be done during the study.
- Positron emission tomography (PET) scans are an important part of the staging evaluation for patients who do not have clear evidence of metastasis on CT. Fluorodeoxyglucose-avid lymph nodes should be biopsied to confirm metastasis.

The American Joint Committee on Cancer (AJCC) has a TNM (tumor, node, metastases) staging system for esophageal cancer, which is summarized in Table 21-1.

TABLE 21-1	STAGING CLASSIFICATION OF ESOPHAGEAL CANCER		
Primary Tumor (T)	**Regional lymph Nodes (N)**	**Distant Metastasis (M)**	**Stage**
TX: primary tumor cannot be assessed	NX: regional lymph node involvement cannot be assessed	MX: presence of metastasis cannot be assessed	Stage 0: Tis N0 M0
T0: no evidence of primary tumor	N0: no regional lymph node metastasis	M0: no distant metastasis	Stage 1: T1a/b N0 M0
Tis: carcinoma in situ	N1: regional lymph node metastasis	M1: distant metastasis	Stage IIA: T2 N0 M0, T3 N0 M0
T1: tumor invades lamina propria or submucosa	N1a: 1–3 nodes involved	Tumors of the lower thoracic esophagus: M1a, metastasis to celiac lymph nodes; M1b, other distant metastasis	Stage IIB: T1a/b N1 M0, T2 N1 M0
T1a: tumor invades mucosa or lamina propria	N1b: 4–7 nodes involved	Tumors of the midthoracic esophagus: M1a, n/a; M1b, nonregional lymph nodes and/or other distant metastasis	Stage III: T3 N1 M0, T4 any N M0
T1b: tumor invades submucosa	N1c: >7 nodes involved	Tumors of the upper thoracic esophagus: M1a, metastasis to cervical lymph nodes; M1b, other distant metastasis	Stage IVA: any T any N M1a
T2: tumor invades muscularis propria			Stage IVB: any T any N M1b
T3: tumor invades adventitia			
T4: tumor invades adjacent structures			

Treatment

- Surgery is considered the standard therapy for stage I, II, and III esophageal cancers located outside the cervical esophagus. The best chance for surgical cure involves removing the entire tumor and draining lymph nodes with adequate proximal and distal margins. If an early-stage cancer is located in the cervical esophagus, the preferred treatment is a combination of chemotherapy and radiation.
- In order to improve outcomes with surgery, neoadjuvant therapy with chemoradiotherapy, radiation, and combined chemotherapy has been attempted. Neoadjuvant therapy for esophageal cancer is one of the most controversial areas in oncology. Randomized phase III trials have been performed, often with mixed results. Neoadjuvant chemoradiation with cisplatin and 5-fluorouracil (5-FU) remains investigational, but it is a reasonable option for patients with a good performance status and locally advanced disease.
- Postoperative chemoradiotherapy clearly has a role in the treatment of esophageal cancer. Patients with gross or microscopic residual disease following surgery are felt to benefit from combined modality chemotherapy/radiotherapy. Adjuvant chemoradiotherapy in patients without residual disease is less defined. In the current National Comprehensive Cancer Network (NCCN) guidelines, observation is recommended for those with squamous cell carcinoma. Patients with adenocarcinoma who have lymph node-positive disease and large tumors ($\geq$T3) should receive chemoradiotherapy. Chemoradiotherapy is a consideration in patients with T2 N0 adenocarcinoma. Adjuvant chemoradiation in esophageal cancer is most commonly cisplatin and 5-FU along with daily radiation.
- In cases of a locally advanced unresectable esophageal cancer, chemoradiation is the standard therapy. The typical regimen is cisplatin and 5-FU given concurrently with radiation.
- Metastatic esophageal cancer is incurable. Several chemotherapy agents do have activity against esophageal cancer. These include cisplatin, carboplatin, 5-FU, paclitaxel, docetaxel, vinorelbine, oxaliplatin, and irinotecan. In general, platinum-based doublets have the highest response rate and are typically used as first-line therapy. One can also consider treating adenocarcinoma of the lower esophagus like a gastric carcinoma (see below).
- Palliative therapy for swallowing and nutritional support are especially important. There are a number of options for palliation of swallowing. These include esophageal dilation, stent placement, brachytherapy, external-beam radiation, and laser therapy. With regard to nutritional support, patients with metastatic esophageal cancer frequently require a gastrostomy tube.

GASTRIC CANCER

Introduction

Gastric cancer is a relatively less common cancer in the United States, with ~23,000 new cases diagnosed per year. It is much more common in eastern Asia. Risk factors for the development of gastric cancer include a history of atrophic gastritis, cigarette smoking, *Helicobacter pylori* infection, and Barrett esophagitis.

Presentation

Gastric cancer usually presents with nonspecific constitutional symptoms. The most common symptom is weight loss, which occurs in ~80% of patients. Other common symptoms include anorexia, fatigue, vague stomach pain, dysphagia (from gastroesophageal junction tumors), and vomiting (from gastric outlet obstruction). The physical findings in gastric cancer are typically manifestations of metastatic disease. Several eponymic terms have been created to describe specific sites of metastatic gastric cancer. *Virchow node* describes metastasis to the left supraclavicular node. *Sister Mary Joseph node* is a periumbilical lymph node metastasis. A *Krukenberg tumor* is a gastric cancer metastatic to the ovaries. *Blumer shelf* describes a "drop metastasis" into the perirectal pouch. Other common physical findings in patients with metastatic gastric cancer include cachexia, palpable abdominal masses, and malignant ascites.

Management

Workup

Once a diagnosis of gastic carcinoma is made, further staging is necessary. As in esophageal cancer, endoscopic ultrasound may be used to gauge tumor depth and involvement of local lymph nodes. CT scans and PET/CT are used to evaluate for metastatic disease. Unfortunately, metastatic peritoneal deposits may not be seen on routine imaging and a diagnostic laporatomy is necessary to rule this out prior to definitive resection. The AJCC has a TNM staging system for gastric cancer, which is summarized in Table 21-2.

Treatment

- Surgery is the most effective curative therapy for localized gastric cancer. It is, however, usually necessary to give adjuvant or neoadjuvant therapy. In patients with at least stage IB gastric cancer or positive margins at resection, adjuvant concurrent chemoradiation with 5-FU and leucovorin has been shown to have a significant survival benefit.
- Neoadjuvant/perioperative chemotherapy has been tested in order to make unresectable cancers operable and to improve overall survival. The regimen most commonly used is epirubicin, cisplatin, and 5-FU (ECF), with three cycles given before surgery and three cycles afterward. In the MAGIC trial, this regimen showed the ability to downsize tumors and to improve survival versus no adjuvant therapy.
- Combination chemoradiation is considered the standard of care for medically unresectable localized gastic adenocarcinoma. It typically combines 5-FU with 45 to 50 Gy of radiation. Of note, only a very small percentage of patients can be cured with chemoradiotherapy alone.
- Metastatic gastric cancer is incurable. Chemotherapy, however, has been shown to improve survival and quality of life in patients with metastatic gastric carcinoma. Several chemotherapeutic agents have activity in gastric cancer. These include 5-FU, cisplatin, oxaliplatin, irinotecan, capecitabine, anthracyclines, and taxanes.

Screening

Given the rarity of these tumors in the United States, there is no justification for routine screening for esophageal or stomach cancer at this time. However, in countries of high incidence (e.g., Japan), screening for stomach cancer via endoscopy or upper gastrointestinal imaging is standard for those >50 years old.

PANCREATIC CANCER

Introduction

Pancreatic cancer is the fifth leading cause of cancer death in the United States. It has an annual incidence of ~12.3/100,000. Pancreatic cancer can be cured when it is discovered at an early stage, but unfortunately it typically presents at an advanced stage.

Presentation

Many pancreatic tumors are asymptomatic until they are well advanced, especially those located in the tail of the pancreas. Presenting symptoms may include abdominal or back

TABLE 21-2 STAGING CLASSIFICATION OF GASTRIC CANCER

Primary Tumor (T)	Regional lymph Nodes (N)	Distant Metastasis (M)	Stage
TX: primary tumor cannot be assessed	NX: regional lymph node involvement cannot be assessed	MX: presence of metastasis cannot be assessed	Stage 0: Tis N0 M0
T0: no evidence of primary tumor	N0: no regional lymph node metastasis	M0: no distant metastasis	Stage IA: T1 N0 M0
Tis: intraepithelial tumors without invasion of lamina propria	N1: regional lymph node metastasis in 1–6 nodes	M1: distant metastasis	Stage IB: T1 N1 M0, T2a/b N0 M0
T1: tumor invades lamina propria or submucosa	N2: regional lymph node metastasis in 7–15 nodes		Stage II: T1 N2 M0, T2a/b N1 M0, N3 N0 M0
T2: tumor invades lamina propria/ submucosa	N3: regional lymph node metastasis in >15 nodes		Stage IIIA: T2a/b N2 M0, T3 N1 M0, T4 N0 M0
T2a: tumor invades muscularis propria			Stage IIIB: T3 N2 M0
T2b: tumor invades submucosa			Stage IV: T4 any N M0, any T N3 M0, any T any N M1
T3: tumor penetrates serosa (visceral peritoneum)			
T4: tumor invades adjacent structures			

pain, weight loss, nausea, vomiting, painless jaundice, fatigue, and depression. Physical findings such as palpable abdominal mass, jaundice, ascites, Courvoisier sign (painless palpable gallbladder), Virchow node, and Sister Mary Joseph node may occasionally be found. Paraneoplastic syndromes, such as Trousseau syndrome (migratory superficial phlebitis), idiopathic deep venous thrombosis, myositis syndromes, and Cushing syndrome, are rarely seen.

Management

Diagnosis and Workup

When pancreatic cancer is suspected, the initial imaging modality used for staging should be a dynamic-phase spiral CT of the abdomen. This is an excellent modality for evaluating the pancreas as well as common sites of metastasis such as peripancreatic lymph nodes and the liver. Further staging with an endoscopic ultrasound or endoscopic retrograde cholangiopancreatography (ERCP) may also be necessary. Tissue diagnosis can be obtained by percutaneous needle biopsy, laparoscopy, ERCP, or ascitic fluid cytology. CA 19-9 levels may be obtained as a baseline and followed for response/recurrence. Staging is by the TNM system and is reviewed in Table 21-3.

Treatment

Localized Pancreatic Cancer

- **Surgery** is the cornerstone of management for nonmetastatic pancreatic cancer. An experienced surgeon is needed to determine resectability, but patients with positive liver, peritoneal, or distant metastases, or Virchow or Sister Mary Joseph nodes, are typically unresectable. The standard procedure is a pancreaticoduodenectomy with choledochojejunostomy, cholecystectomy, and gastrojejunostomy (Whipple procedure). This is a major surgery with considerable morbidity.
- **Adjuvant therapy** is necessary after resection of the primary. There is considerable controversy as to what is the best adjuvant therapy. Concurrent chemoradiation with 5-FU has traditionally been used in North America. In the Gastrointestinal Tumor Study Group (GITSG) trial published in the mid-1980s, concurrent chemoradiation with 5-FU was found to double the median survival of patients with resected pancreatic tumors compared to radiation therapy alone. Recently, several European trials have cast doubt on the benefit of adjuvant chemoradiation. Other clinical trials have seen a survival benefit with adjuvant chemotherapy with gemcitabine. Currently, the NCCN recommends enrollment in a clinical trial if possible. If a clinical trial is unavailable, the use of either of these approaches or 5-FU-based chemoradiation followed by chemotherapy with gemcitabine can be considered.
- If the cancer is localized but unresectable, 5-FU-based concurrent chemoradiation is the standard therapy. A minority of patients will become resectable using this approach. Even if the patient's tumor cannot be resected, concurrent chemoradiation does provide a survival advantage.

Metastatic Pancreatic Cancer. Metastatic pancreatic cancer is incurable. Chemotherapy has a low objective response rate (6% to 12%) but has been shown to improve quality of life and overall survival. Gemcitabine is the first-line therapy for metastatic pancreatic cancer. A number of agents have been used in combination with gemcitabine in trials, including erlotinib, capecitabine, and cisplatin. These combinations have shown a small improvement in overall survival over gemcitabine alone, but at the price of greater toxicity. The NCCN considers either gemcitabine alone or gemcitabine combinations as acceptable first-line therapy. The data for second-line chemotherapy are less clear. Options include capecitabine and 5-FU/oxaliplatin.

Prognosis

T1 and T2 lesions without distant spread are potentially resectable and are associated with 5% to 35% 5-year survival rates. Median survival for unresectable disease has been as short as 6 months, but many trials are now reporting median survivals of treated patients closer to 12 months.

TABLE 21-3   STAGING CLASSIFICATION OF PANCREATIC CANCER

Primary Tumor (T)	Regional lymph Nodes (N)	Distant Metastasis (M)	Stage
TX: primary tumor cannot be assessed	NX: regional lymph node involvement cannot be assessed	MX: presence of metastasis cannot be assessed	Stage 0: Tis N0 M0
T0: no evidence of primary tumor	N0: no regional lymph node	M0: no distant metastasis	Stage IA: T1 N0 M0
Tis: Carcinoma in situ	N1: regional lymph node metastasis	M1: distant metastasis	Stage IB: T2 N0 M0
T1: tumor limited to the pancreas, ≤2 cm in greatest dimension			Stage IIA: T3 N0 M0
T2: tumor limited to the pancreas, >2 cm in greatest dimension			Stage IIB: T1 N1 M0, T2 N1 M0, T3 N1 M0
T3: tumor extends beyond the pancreas but without involvement of the celiac axis or the superior mesenteric artery			Stage III: T4 any N M0
T4: tumor involves the celiac axis or the superior mesenteric artery			Stage IV: any T any N M1

Complications

Pain management is paramount in pancreatic cancer patients. In addition to standard analgesics, celiac plexus block may be an option in selected patients. Biliary obstruction and subsequent cholangitis should be relieved by stenting or draining procedures.

HEPATOCELLULAR CANCER

Introduction

Hepatocellular cancer is a rare cancer in the United States, but it is a very common tumor in Southeast Asia and Africa. The incidence in the United States, however, has been rising over the last few decades, due to the increase in hepatitis B and C infections. Risk factors for hepatic cancer include hepatitis B, hepatitis C, and cirrhosis of any cause. Cirrhotic patients have a roughly 3% per year risk of developing hepatocellular carcinoma.

Presentation

Patients on presentation may have nonspecific complaints of abdominal pain, malaise, weight loss, or fever. Patients may occasionally have a palpable liver mass.

Management

Diagnosis

Imaging via ultrasound or CT scan is typically the first step to diagnosis, and biopsy is usually performed via percutaneous needle biopsy. Alpha-fetoprotein is elevated in 85% of cases but can be nonspecific.

Workup

- Stage depends on the number and size of tumors, as well as the presence of vascular invasion. Staging workup includes CT scan or MRI to define anatomic relationships and vascular anatomy, but angiography may be needed to completely reveal the anatomy. Multifocal disease is common, especially in patients with a history of cirrhosis.
- Stages can be roughly split into localized resectable, localized unresectable, and advanced cancers. Localized resectable lesions are single masses that may be completely resected with a margin of normal liver for an attempt at cure. Localized unresectable lesions are those that are confined to a localized area of the liver but are not amenable to resection with a tissue margin owing to proximity of vascular structures, amount of tissue resection required, or poor health of the patient. Given that many patients with these tumors are cirrhotic, many cannot tolerate more than a small wedge resection. Advanced liver cancers are metastatic lesions to nodes or other tissues or those that affect both lobes of the liver.

Prognosis

The most important prognostic indicators are size of the tumor mass and degree of hepatic impairment, with cirrhosis conferring a poor outcome.

Treatment

- Surgery is the primary curative modality of treatment for localized resectable lesions. Unfortunately, only 10% of patients are resectable because of advanced disease at presentation. Recurrent local disease may also be treated surgically, with potential for cure.
- Given the frequent association with cirrhosis, liver transplant has been investigated as treatment of both the primary tumor and concomitant cirrhosis. Liver transplant has been used successfully in trials for the treatment of hepatocellular carcinoma, despite the use of immunosuppression after surgery. In one trial, patients with fewer than three lesions smaller than 3 cm or a single lesion smaller than 5 cm had a 4-year survival rate of ~85%.
- For patients with unresectable disease, chemoembolization is a reasonable option. This therapy involves the infusion of lipiodol, Gelfoam, or other materials in the hepatic artery. It may provide a survival benefit. Infusion of lipiodol after resection for cure may also increase survival. Radiation therapy may also be used in unresectable

disease. Radiofrequency ablation and cryosurgery are other potentially promising modalities for unresectable disease.
- Chemotherapy has been used in unresectable localized disease with varying success. Recently, sorafenib was found to provide a survival benefit versus supportive care for unresectable hepatocellular carcinoma. The median overall survival was extended from 7.9 to 10.7 months.

Prevention

Prevention of these tumors may be achieved by decreasing the burden of cirrhosis or chronic liver inflammation. Hepatitis B vaccination is very effective at protecting against the virus, and vaccination in a high-incidence country has been shown to decrease the subsequent incidence of hepatocellular carcinoma. Treatment of hepatitis C with interferon may decrease the subsequent risk of hepatocellular carcinoma. Patients with hepatitis C should be screened with annual alpha-fetoprotein levels and liver ultrasound.

GALLBLADDER CANCER

Introduction

Gallbladder cancer is a rare cancer of the biliary system, with ~5000 cases diagnosed per year in North America. Patients are typically in their 70s and this tumor has a three-to-one female predominance. Gallstones and chronic cholecystitis are the greatest risk factors for gallbladder cancer. Other risk factors include gallbladder polyps, calcification of the gallbladder, and typhoid carriers.

Presentation

These tumors may present with symptoms of acute or chronic cholecystitis, although jaundice and weight loss are more common.

Management

Diagnosis
Liver MRI or abdominal CT can be used for imaging, although ERCP is often needed for tissue diagnosis and demonstration of extent of tumor.

Treatment
- The only curative treatment for gallbladder cancer is surgery, but few patients have resectable disease at the time of presentation. Adjuvant therapy with 5-FU-based concurrent chemoradiation is recommended for most patients with resected gallbladder cancer except for those with very small tumors (T1 N0).
- For patients with unresectable but nonmetastatic gallbladder cancer, therapy with 5-FU-based concurrent chemoradiation is recommended, provided that the patient has an adequate performance status and is not jaundiced. If the patient is jaundiced, biliary decompression is necessary and may be followed by chemotherapy. Chemotherapy with 5-FU or gemcitabine can also be used to treat patients with metastatic disease.

CHOLANGIOCARCINOMA

Introduction

- Cholangiocarcinoma is a rare cancer of the biliary tree, accounting for ~5000 new cases each year in the United States. Patients typically present in their sixties. Men and women are equally affected. Most cases are idiopathic but there are a number of known risk factors including primary sclerosing cholangitis, hepatolithiasis, choledochal cysts, and liver fluke infection.

- Cholangiocarcinoma can be divided into those of intrahepatic and extrahepatic origin. Intrahepatic cholangiocarcinomas arise in the small intrahepatic ductules or the large intrahepatic ducts proximal to the bifurcation of the right and left hepatic ducts. Extrahepatic cholangiocarcinomas originate in any of the major hepatic or biliary ducts. Extrahepatic cholangiocarcinomas are more common.

Presentation

Cholangiocarcinomas typically present with symptoms of biliary obstruction such as jaundice, right upper quadrant pain, and fever. Weight loss is also common. On exam, patients may have jaundice, hepatomegaly, or right upper quadrant mass.

Management

Diagnosis

Imaging with liver MRI, magnetic resonance cholangiopancreatography, or abdominal CT can be used, although ERCP is often needed for tissue diagnosis. Carcinoembryonic antigen (CEA) and CA19/9 are often elevated.

Treatment

- The treatment of intrahepatic and extrahepatic cholangiocarcinoma is slightly different. Surgery is the only cure for either type of cholangiocarcinoma. For intrahepatic cholangiocarcinomas that have positive margins following resection, 5-FU- or gemcitabine-based chemoradiation, radiofrequency ablation, or re-resection can be used. For intrahepatic cholangiocarcinomas that have been completely resected, there is no indication for adjuvant therapy. For extrahepatic cholangiocarcinomas, adjuvant 5-FU-based chemoradiation is typically given.
- Unresectable cholangiocarcinomas can be treated with radiation, chemoradiation, or chemotherapy with 5-FU or gemcitabine. The prognosis is poor, with a median survival of 7 to 12 months. Metastatic disease is typically treated with chemotherapy.

KEY POINTS TO REMEMBER

- Progressive dysphagia is a classic presentation of esophageal cancer.
- The incidence of esophageal cancer has been increasing in the United States, with a predominance of adenocarcinoma as the histologic type. More intensive screening is appropriate for first-generation patients from high-risk countries (Japan, China, Singapore, Costa Rica, and Brazil).
- Upper endoscopy is the diagnostic test of choice in the evaluation of esophageal or stomach cancer.
- Patients with upper digestive tract tumors are at high risk for subsequent aerodigestive tract tumors owing to shared risk factors.
- Pancreatic cancer is typically advanced at time of presentation.
- Hepatocellular cancer is increasing in incidence, likely owing to the burden of hepatitis B and C and alcoholic cirrhosis in this country.
- Patients with hepatitis C should be screened with annual alpha-fetoprotein levels and liver ultrasound.

REFERENCES AND SUGGESTED READINGS

Bosset J, et al. Chemoradiotherapy followed by surgery compared with surgery alone in squamous-cell cancer of the esophagus. *N Engl J Med.* 1997;337:161.

Burris HA, et al. Improvements in survival and clinical benefit with gemcitabine as first-line therapy for patients with advanced pancreas cancer: a randomized trial. *J Clin Oncol.* 1997;15:2403.

Cunningham D, et al. Perioperative chemotherapy versus surgery alone for gastric cancer. *N Engl J Med.* 2006;355:11.

Herskovic A, et al. Combined chemotherapy and radiotherapy compared with radiotherapy alone in patients with cancer of the esophagus. *N Engl J Med.* 1992;326:1593.

Kalser MH, et al. Pancreatic cancer: adjuvant combined radiation and chemotherapy following curative resection. *Arch Surg.* 1985;120:899.

Kelson D, et al. Chemotherapy followed by surgery compared with surgery alone for localized esophageal cancer. *N Engl J Med.* 1998;339:1979.

Llovet J, et al. Sorafenib improves survival in advanced hepatocellular carcinoma (HCC): results of a Phase III randomized placebo-controlled trial (SHARP trial). 2007 ASCO Annual Meeting Proceedings Part 1. *J Clin Oncol.* 2007;25(18S; June 20 Suppl):LBA1 (abstract).

Macdonald J, et al. Chemoradiotherapy after surgery compared with surgery alone for adenocarcinoma of the stomach or gastroesophageal junction. *N Engl J Med.* 2001;345:725.

Malignant Melanoma

22

Mike G. Martin

INTRODUCTION

Background

The incidence of malignant melanoma is increasing more rapidly than that of any other cancer in men, and its increase is second only to lung cancer in women. Melanoma is the fifth most common cancer in American men and the sixth most common in American women. It is principally a cutaneous malignancy and is, hence, often discovered early. With complete excision when it is still localized, 5-year survival is 99%. Unfortunately, metastatic melanoma is rarely curable. Though sun exposure may play a role in the development of melanoma in Caucasians, melanoma may occur in any ethnic group and without a history of significant sun exposure. Public education about sun avoidance, sunscreen use, identification of suspicious lesions, and careful self-screening exams are the patient's best tools for reducing the incidence and mortality of melanoma.

Epidemiology

The American Cancer Society predicted that 62,190 persons would be diagnosed with melanoma in 2006 and 7910 people would die from it. The median age at diagnosis is 58 and the vast majority (~80%) of cases are localized at presentation. Melanoma ranks second to adult leukemia in terms of loss of years of potential life per death. The prevalence is highest in white individuals of European descent, and a white American's lifetime risk of developing melanoma is 1 in 59.

PRESENTATION

Risk Factors

Known risk factors for melanoma include sun exposure; presence of large congenital nevi, dysplastic nevi, or multiple nevi; family or personal history of melanoma; sunburns during childhood; fair complexion; and blue eye color. Ten percent of melanomas are familial.

Clinical Presentation

- The *ABCDE* mnemonic describes common characteristics of melanomas: *asymmetry, border* irregularity, *color* variegation, *diameter* >5 mm, *enlargement,* or *elevation.* Bleeding and ulceration can occur and are associated with worse prognosis. Melanomas have historically been categorized by morphologic appearance. Superficial spreading melanomas are the most common morphologic type. They may have years of radial growth before vertical growth and metastasis occur. Other morphologic types include nodular melanoma, which has early vertical growth; lentigo maligna melanoma, which typically presents on the face of older persons; and acral

233

lentiginous melanoma, which occurs on the palms, on the soles, and under the nails and is the most common presentation of melanoma in individuals of African and Asian descent. Melanoma may also occur in the eye or on mucosal surfaces.

• Screening for potentially malignant skin lesions should be part of a comprehensive physical exam. In addition, patients at risk for melanoma should be encouraged to examine themselves regularly for new or changing skin lesions.

MANAGEMENT

Diagnosis
Suspicious lesions should be examined by excisional biopsy with 1- to 3-mm margins, as other biopsy techniques (such as punch biopsy) may not provide crucial information about lesion thickness.

Workup and Staging
Staging is based on the thickness of tumor and the presence of nodal or distant metastases. Classically, the absolute depth of invasion (millimeters) is referred to as the Breslow thickness and the histological depth is referred to as the Clark level. Staging also incorporates the presence or absence of ulceration, number of nodes involved, and site(s) of distant metastasis. With clinically negative nodes, sentinel lymph node mapping may be employed. Workup should include a detailed history and physical, including a complete skin exam with attention to regional lymph nodes and sign and symptom guided imaging (CT scan, MRI, or PET). A general simplification of the staging system is as follows.

• **Stage 0** is melanoma in situ.
• **Stage I** is a localized lesion <1 mm thick or a 1- to 2-mm-thick melanoma without ulceration.
• **Stage II** is localized and >2 mm thick or >1 mm thick with ulceration.
• **Stage III** has spread to regional lymph nodes or is in-transit disease.
  • Patients with stage III disease should also have a chest x-ray and a lactate dehydrogenase (LDH) level.
• **Stage IV** has distant metastases.
  • Patients with stage IV disease should have an LDH level and a chest CT scan and should be considered for CT of the abdomen and pelvis or PET scan and/or brain MRI.

Treatment
Localized Disease (Stages I and II)
Wide local excision is the standard treatment for stage I and II melanomas. Excision recommendations are 1-cm margins for lesions <1 mm in depth and 2-cm margins for lesions >1 mm in depth. Sentinel lymph node biopsy frequently is performed before wide local excision of ~ 1-mm lesions to rule out subclinical lymph node metastases. After excision of stage I lesions, no further treatment is recommended. Patients with stage II lesions, especially those with lesions >4 mm, can be treated with adjuvant interferon-alpha similar to that used for stage III disease.

Regional Disease (Stage III)
Patients with stage III melanoma can present with a positive sentinel lymph node biopsy, clinically palpable lymph nodes, or in-transit metastasis (i.e., melanoma in the skin or subcutaneous tissue sharing lymphatic drainage with the primary tumor). Preoperative workup for patients with regional disease includes chest x-ray or chest CT, LDH, and other CT scans as clinically indicated. Treatment usually involves lymph node dissection, both

for regional control of disease and for prognostic information, as the number of positive lymph nodes is predictive of survival. In-transit disease can be treated with isolated limb hyperthermic perfusion with melphalan. **Interferon-alpha** is the best-studied adjuvant therapy for stage III melanoma. Most studies have found improved relapse-free and/or overall survival in high-risk patients treated with adjuvant high-dose interferon-alpha for 1 year after resection of the primary tumor and regional lymph nodes. This therapy is relatively toxic, with 50% of patients requiring dose reductions or delays. Common side effects are myelosuppression, hepatotoxicity, neurologic dysfunction, and constitutional symptoms. Radiation therapy to the nodal basin may be considered if macroscopic lymph node metastasis or extranodal extension is present. Adjuvant biochemotherapy (cisplatin, vinblastine, dacarbazine, interleukin-2, and interferon-alpha) offers no benefit over high-dose interferon-alpha. Adjuvant therapy with vaccines derived from melanoma cells shows promise and is currently under study.

Distant Metastatic Disease (Stage IV)

- The most common sites of metastatic melanoma are (in descending order of frequency) skin and lymph nodes, lung, liver, brain, bone, and intestine. Brain lesions are at high risk for hemorrhage due to the vascular nature of melanoma. Presence of visceral metastases (except those to lung) and presence of high LDH are associated with a worse prognosis than metastases limited to skin, lymph nodes, or lung. Workup of patients with metastatic disease includes brain MRI, chest/abdomen/pelvis CT or PET scan, CBC, liver function tests, and LDH. Survival in patients with distant metastases is poor, with 15% alive at 5 years. Resection of solitary skin, lung, or brain metastases can be considered and is usually followed by adjuvant therapy.
- Patients with metastatic melanoma should be enrolled in clinical trials. No chemotherapy regimen has consistently proved superior to single-agent dacarbazine, which has a response rate of 14% to 20%. Temozolomide offers the theoretical advantage of improved CNS penetration but does not improve overall survival compared to dacarbazine. Combination regimens including immunotherapy with interleukin-2 and interferon, and chemotherapy showed promise in phase II trials, though a large phase III trial failed to show a benefit over chemotherapy alone. Of note, a small percentage of patients with metastatic melanoma have a dramatic response to high-dose interleukin-2 (which is an extremely toxic regimen, with patients often requiring vasopressor support), with durable complete remission of disease.

Follow-up

Patients with tumors <1 mm in depth should have follow-up with a dermatologist to screen for new or recurrent melanoma. Patients with tumors 1 to 4 mm in depth should have annual chest x-ray and LDH and dermatology follow-up. Patients with stage III melanoma should follow up with a medical oncologist and dermatologist and have semiannual chest x-ray, LDH, liver function tests, and CBC. Patients with metastatic disease will need close follow-up with a medical oncologist.

Prognosis

Overall 5-year survival for patients with melanoma is 90%, but survival falls off dramatically with increasing stage. Tumor thickness and the presence of ulceration are the most important prognostic factors in localized cutaneous melanoma. Lesions <1 mm in thickness without ulceration are associated with a 10-year survival of almost 90%, whereas lesions >4 mm are associated with a 5-year survival of <60%. The prognosis of regional disease correlates with the number of positive lymph nodes, with a median survival of 90 months for one positive node and 15 months for more than four positive nodes. The overall 5-year survival rate for stage III disease is ~40%. Stage IV melanoma is associated with a median survival of 6 to 9 months. Elevated LDH correlates with the presence of metastatic disease and confers a worse prognosis.

KEY POINTS TO REMEMBER

- The incidence of melanoma has been increasing worldwide over the last 50 years.
- Skin lesions suspicious for melanoma should be removed by excisional biopsy to allow for measurement of lesion depth.
- Prognosis of localized disease depends on the depth of the lesion. Most patients with stage I disease are cured with excision of the melanoma.
- Metastatic melanoma is poorly responsive to chemotherapy and rarely curable, although a few patients have a dramatic response to immunotherapy.

REFERENCES AND SUGGESTED READINGS

Arndt KA, et al. Melanoma. In: Koh HK, Barnhill RL, Rogers GS, eds. *Cutaneous Medicine and Surgery.* Philadelphia: W. B. Saunders; 1996;1576.

Atkins MB, et al. A prospective randomized phase III trial of concurrent biochemotherapy (BCT) with cisplatin, vinblastine, dacarbazine (CVD), IL-2, and interferon alpha-2b (IFN) versus CVD alone in patients with metastatic melanoma: an ECOG-coordinated intergroup trial [abstract]. *Proc Am Soc Clin Oncol.* 2003;22:2847.

Kirkwood JM, Strawderman MH, Ernstoff MS, et al. Interferon alfa-2b adjuvant therapy of high-risk resected cutaneous melanoma: the Eastern Cooperative Oncology Group Trial EST 1684. *J Clin Oncol.* 1996;14:7.

Lotze MT, et al. Melanoma. In: DeVita VT Jr, Hellman S, Rosenberg SA, eds. *Cancer: Principles and Practice of Oncology.* 6th ed. Philadelphia: Lippincott Williams & Wilkins; 2001:2012–2069.

National Comprehensive Cancer Network. NCCN Guidelines: Melanoma. Version 2, 2007. Available at: www.nccn.org. Accessed March 26, 2007.

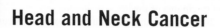

Head and Neck Cancer

23

Yee Hong Chia and David Kuperman

INTRODUCTION

Background

Head and neck cancers are a diverse group of malignancies accounting for ~5% of newly diagnosed invasive malignancies per year. While there are many similarities between head and neck cancers arising from different sites, there are particular differences in anatomy, natural history, and functional consequence that present unique treatment challenges for each site.

Classification

Malignancies of the head and neck are classified by their anatomic location, which is divided into (a) lip and oral cavity, (b) oropharynx, (c) larynx and hypopharynx, (d) nasopharynx, (e) nasal cavity and sinuses, and (f) salivary glands. With the exception of salivary gland tumors, squamous cell carcinoma accounts for >90% of head and neck tumors. As nasopharyngeal cancer and neck masses with unknown primary have different epidemiology and/or management, they are discussed separately.

SQUAMOUS CELL CARCINOMA OF THE HEAD AND NECK (SCCHN)

Epidemiology

Head and neck cancers have a significant male predominance, with a male-to-female ratio of 3:1. These tumors are estimated to account for ~40,000 new cases per year, with an estimated 11,000 deaths per year.

Pathophysiology

SCCHN is an example of the multistep process of carcinogenesis with accumulated genetic mutations that result in changes ranging from hyperplasia to dysplasia to carcinoma in situ to invasive cancer.

Risk Factors

- The main risk factors for development of these malignancies are **tobacco in any form** and **alcohol use**. Tobacco and alcohol are sources of carcinogens that increase the risk of cancer in a dose-dependent fashion and are synergistic in their effects. Field cancerization is a key concept in the natural history of head and neck cancer. Exposure of the mucosa to carcinogens in tobacco is diffuse across the aerodigestive tract. Consequently, tumors may be surrounded by areas of dysplasia or carcinoma in situ. Patients diagnosed with a head and neck cancer are at an increased risk of developing new primary tumors in the head and neck, lung, and esophagus. The risk is estimated to be 3% to 4 % per year. Sun exposure has been associated with an increased risk of carcinoma of the lip.

• Approximately 20% of head and neck cancers, however, occur in people without these established risk factors. A subset of these cancers includes **human papilloma virus** (HPV)-associated tumors of the oropharynx, which portend a better prognosis. Risk factors for HPV-associated tumors of the oropharynx include an increasing number of sexual partners, the practice of oral sex, a history of genital warts, and a younger age at first sexual intercourse. As in cervical cancer, HPV-16 and -18 are thought to play an important role.

PRESENTATION

• The clinical presentation of these malignancies varies depending on the anatomic location of the tumor. **Cancers of the lip and oral cavity** often present with nonhealing lesions in the mouth, pain in the mouth or ear, trismus, weight loss, and "hot potato speech." Leukoplakia and erythroplakia are premalignant lesions of the mucosa and are frequently seen in conjunction with dysplastic changes or invasive carcinoma.

• **Cancers of the nasal cavity** can present with epistaxis, nonhealing ulcer, or obstruction.

• **Cancers of the oropharynx** present with many of the features associated with cancers of the lip and oral cavity. Bleeding from the mouth, alterations in speech, dysphagia, odynophagia, otalgia, and weight loss can be symptoms of oropharyngeal cancers.

• **Cancers of the larynx and hypopharynx** can present challenges in management, as these anatomic structures are intricately associated with the key functions of speech and swallowing. Symptoms include dysphagia, odynophagia, weight loss, dyspnea (including dyspnea with speech), and hoarseness. Symptoms of aspiration should also be elucidated in the history. However, the time of presentation of these cancers varies greatly with their primary site. Supraglottic tumors or tumors in the pyriform sinus may be diagnosed only after cervical metastases occur because symptoms of dysphagia may not become significant until the tumors are quite advanced. On the other hand, glottic carcinomas are associated with symptoms of hoarseness even when they are small, which may lead to earlier detection.

Management

Workup

• The initial workup of suspected head and neck cancers includes a detailed physical examination. Assessment should include a cranial nerve exam, assessment of status of dentition, and examination of tongue movement and atrophy. Lymph nodes in the neck should be palpated, and measurements taken of palpable nodes. Suspicious lesions should be biopsied for histologic confirmation and grading.

• **Imaging studies** should include a chest radiograph, Panorex x-ray for mandibular bony involvement for cancers that abut the mandible, and computed tomography (CT) or magnetic resonance imaging (MRI) of the head and neck to help further delineate disease extent at presentation. **Panendoscopy,** including esophagoscopy with direct laryngoscopy, helps characterize the primary lesion and evaluates for possible second tumors, as there is a 10% to 15% incidence of synchronous primary tumors. A CT scan of the chest should also be performed to rule out pulmonary metastases. Positron emission tomography (PET)/CT may also be helpful in the staging of head and neck cancers and are used at some centers. The staging for head and neck cancer is according to the American Joint Committee on Cancer TNM system, with different staging for SCCHN (Tables 23-1 through 23-6).

TABLE 23-1	AJCC STAGING OF LIP AND ORAL CAVITY CANCER: PRIMARY TUMOR (T)
TX	Primary tumor cannot be assessed
T0	No evidence of primary tumor
Tis	Carcinoma in situ
T1	Tumor ≤2 cm in greatest dimension
T2	Tumor >2 cm but ≤4 cm in greatest dimension
T3	Tumor >4 cm in greatest dimension
T4 (lip)	Tumor invades adjacent structures (e.g., through cortical bone, inferior alveolar nerve, floor of mouth, skin of face)
T4a (oral cavity)	Tumor invades adjacent structures (e.g., through cortical bone, into deep [extrinsic] muscle of tongue, maxillary sinus, skin). (Superficial erosion of bone/tooth socket by gingival primary alone is not sufficient to classify as T4.)
T4b (oral cavity)	Tumor invades masticator space, pterygoid plates, or skull base and/or encases internal carotid artery

From American Joint Committee on Cancer. *AJCC Cancer Staging Manual.* 6th ed. New York: Springer-Verlag; 2002, with permission.

Treatment

- Management of patients requires a multidisciplinary approach, including head and neck surgeons and radiation and medical oncologists, along with allied health professionals including speech language pathologists and nutritionists. Radiation and surgery are the mainstays of treatment with head and neck cancers. Chemotherapy is reserved for patients with regionally advanced disease or metastatic disease.
- **Single-modality treatment** with either surgery or definitive radiation treatment results in similar rates of disease control and survival in 40% of patients who present with **stage I** or **stage II** (node negative with tumor size <4 cm) disease. The choice of treatment modality depends on the accessibility of the tumor and potential side effects of treatment, as well as the patient's general medical condition. Advantages of surgery include avoidance of side effects of radiation and a shorter treatment course. However, in some circumstances, patients may not be able to tolerate surgery secondary to comorbid conditions, or complete surgical resection may have unacceptable morbidities. In these cases, radiation, which is usually administered over a period of 7 weeks, may be used.
- Many patients with head and neck cancers present with **locally advanced disease** (stages III to IVB). Patients with tumors amenable to surgical resection undergo surgery followed by adjuvant therapy with postoperative radiation or concurrent chemoradiation. For patients with locally advanced, unresectable disease, the standard of care is definitive concurrent chemoradiation for patients who can tolerate such therapy. Usually this entails the use of cisplatin, 100 mg/m^2, on days 1, 22, and 43 of a 7-week course of 70 Gy of radiation. More recently, an epidermal growth factor receptor (EGFR) inhibitor, cetuximab (Erbitux), has demonstrated benefits when used concurrently with radiation. In patients who do not achieve a complete tumor response after definitive chemoradiation, surgical resection of residual tumor may improve survival.

TABLE 23-2	AJCC STAGING OF LIP AND ORAL CAVITY CANCER, OROPHARYNX, HYPOPHARYNX, AND LARYNX: REGIONAL LYMPH NODES (N), DISTANT METASTASIS (M)
NX	Regional lymph nodes cannot be assessed
N0	No regional lymph node metastasis
N1	Metastasis in a single ipsilateral lymph node, ≤3 cm in greatest dimension
N2	Metastasis in a single ipsilateral lymph node, >3 cm but not ≤6 cm in greatest dimension; or in multiple ipsilateral lymph nodes, none >6 cm in greatest dimension; or in bilateral or contralateral lymph nodes, none >6 cm in greatest dimension
N2a	Metastasis in a single ipsilateral lymph node >3 cm but not ≤6 cm in greatest dimension
N2b	Metastasis in multiple ipsilateral lymph nodes, none >6 cm in greatest dimension
N2c	Metastasis in bilateral or contralateral lymph nodes, none >6 cm in greatest dimension
N3	Metastasis in a lymph node >6 cm in greatest dimension
MX	Distant metastasis cannot be assessed
M0	No distant metastasis
M1	Distant metastasis

From American Joint Committee on Cancer. *AJCC Cancer Staging Manual*. 6th ed. New York: Springer-Verlag; 2002, with permission.

TABLE 23-3	AJCC STAGE GROUPING: ORAL CAVITY AND LIP, OROPHARYNX, LARYNX, AND HYPOPHARYNX		
Stage 0	Tis	N0	M0
Stage I	T1	N0	M0
Stage II	T2	N0	M0
Stage III	T3	N0	M0
	T1–T3	N1	M0
Stage IVA	T4a	N0–N1	M0
	Any T	N2	M0
Stage IVB	Any T	N3	M0
	T4b	Any N	M0
Stage IVC	Any T	Any N	M1

From American Joint Committee on Cancer. *AJCC Cancer Staging Manual*. 6th ed. New York: Springer-Verlag; 2002, with permission.

TABLE 23-4	AJCC STAGING OF OROPHARYNX CANCER: PRIMARY TUMOR (T)
TX	Primary tumor cannot be assessed
T0	No evidence of primary tumor
Tis	Carcinoma in situ
T1	Tumor ≤2 cm in greatest dimension
T2	Tumor >2 cm but ≤4 cm in greatest dimension
T3	Tumor >4 cm in greatest dimension
T4a	Tumor invades the larynx, deep/extrinsic muscle of tongue, medial pterygoid, hard palate, or mandible
T4b	Tumor invades lateral pterygoid muscle, pterygoid plates, lateral nasopharynx, or skull base or encases carotid artery.

From American Joint Committee on Cancer. *AJCC Cancer Staging Manual.* 6th ed. New York: Springer-Verlag; 2002, with permission.

- In patients with distant metastases, several standard chemotherapeutic agents have significant activity against SCCHN and can provide palliation of symptoms. These include cisplatin, carboplatin, 5-fluorouracil (5-FU), paclitaxel, docetaxel, methotrexate, ifosfamide, gemcitabine, and bleomycin. The most commonly used first-line therapy is a platinum compound combined with a second agent, usually a taxane or 5-FU. First-line therapy typically has a tumor response rate of ~20% to 30%.

TABLE 23-5	AJCC STAGING HYPOPHARYNX CANCER: PRIMARY TUMOR (T)
TX	Primary tumor cannot be assessed
T0	No evidence of primary tumor
Tis	Carcinoma in situ
T1	Tumor limited to one subsite of hypopharynx and ≤2 cm in greatest dimension
T2	Tumor involves more than one subsite of hypopharynx or an adjacent site, or measures >2 cm but ≤4 cm in greatest dimension without fixation of hemilarynx
T3	Tumor measures >4 cm in greatest dimension or with fixation of hemilarynx
T4a	Tumor invades thyroid/cricoid cartilage, hyoid bone, thyroid gland, esophagus, prelaryngeal strap muscles, or subcutaneous fat
T4b	Tumor invades prevertebral fascia, encases carotid artery, or involves mediastinal structures

From American Joint Committee on Cancer. *AJCC Cancer Staging Manual.* 6th ed. New York: Springer-Verlag; 2002, with permission.

TABLE 23-6	AJCC STAGING LARYNX CANCER: PRIMARY TUMOR (T)
TX	Primary tumor cannot be assessed
T0	No evidence of primary tumor
Tis	Carcinoma in situ
T1 supraglottis	Tumor limited to one subsite of supraglottis with normal vocal cord mobility
T1 glottis	Tumor limited to vocal cord(s) (may involve anterior or posterior commissure) with normal mobility
T1a	Tumor limited to one vocal cord
T1b	Tumor involves both vocal cords
T1 subglottis	Tumor limited to the subglottis
T2 supraglottis	Tumor invades mucosa of more than one adjacent subsite of supraglottis or glottis or region outside the supraglottis (e.g., mucosa of base of tongue, vallecula, medial wall of pyriform sinus) without fixation of the larynx
T2 glottis	Tumor extends to supraglottis and/or subglottis, and/or with impaired vocal cord mobility
T2 subglottis	Tumor extends to vocal cord(s), with normal or impaired mobility
T3 supraglottis	Tumor limited to larynx with vocal cord fixation and/or invades either of the following: postcricoid area, pre-epiglottic tissues
T3 glottis	Tumor limited to the larynx with vocal cord fixation
T3 Subglottis	Tumor limited to the larynx with vocal cord fixation
T4a supraglottis	Tumor invades through the thyroid cartilage and/or extends into soft tissues of the neck, thyroid, and/or esophagus
T4a glottis	Tumor invades through the thyroid cartilage and/or to other tissues beyond the larynx (e.g., trachea, soft tissues of neck, including thyroid, pharynx)
T4a subglottis	Tumor invades through cricoid or thyroid cartilage, and/or extends to other tissues beyond the larynx (e.g., trachea, soft tissues of neck, including thyroid, esophagus)
T4b supraglottis	Tumor invades prevertebral space, encases carotid artery, or invades mediastinal structures
T4b glottis	Tumor invades prevertebral space, encases carotid artery, or invades mediastinal structures
T4b subglottis	Tumor invades prevertebral space, encases carotid artery, or invades mediastinal structures

From American Joint Committee on Cancer. *AJCC Cancer Staging Manual.* 6th ed. New York: Springer-Verlag; 2002, with permission.

Targeted therapy also has a significant role in the management of SCCHN. Cetuximab has recently been found to extend survival in recurrent and/or metastatic SCCHN when added to chemotherapy. Cetuximab is also a reasonable option for platinum-resistant disease.

Follow-up

Patients should have close follow-up for evaluation of local recurrence and distant metastases, as well as physical therapy and speech pathology follow-up if needed. In addition, patients should be advised on tobacco and alcohol cessation.

Prognosis

In patients with **distant metastases**, survival is 6 to 8 months in most series. Common sites of distant metastases include the bone, lung, and liver.

Complications

- A multidisciplinary approach is essential to minimize the complications of the malignancy and treatment. **Complications of disease** include weight loss, aspiration, and airway compromise. Nutritional support in the form of oral supplements or enteral feedings may be needed when caloric intake is inadequate. Tracheostomy may be needed in cases of airway compromise. Head and neck tumors may also invade into key structures, such as the carotid artery, leading to major bleeding, which may be a terminal event. Invasion into neural structures may lead to neuropathic pain syndromes. Amitriptyline or gabapentin may be helpful in such cases. The limitation to swallowing imposed by some head and neck cancers can make pain management difficult. In such cases, transdermal fentanyl patches or methadone elixir can be used in conjunction with concentrated opiate elixirs (breakthrough) for pain relief.
- **Complications of treatment** include complications of surgery, acute radiation toxicity, late radiation effects, and complications of chemotherapy. **Acute radiation toxicity** may include severe mucositis, with resulting pain and difficulties with swallowing. Concurrent chemoradiation increases the risk of severe mucositis beyond radiation alone. Oral candidiasis complicating mucositis may be treated with topical or systemic antifungal agents. Many patients find a cocktail of equal volume of diphenhydramine suspension, nystatin, viscous lidocaine, and aluminum hydroxide/magnesium hydroxide ("magic mouthwash") as a topical oral swish-and-swallow solution to be helpful. Opiates can also help in pain management, especially in severe cases. Skin toxicity should be treated with emollients. **Late radiation effects** include xerostomia, dental caries, osteoradionecrosis, and fibrosis of neck tissues resulting in trismus, lymphedema, and loss of range of motion. Xerostomia can be treated with cholinergic stimulants such as pilocarpine to improve salivary flow. Other measures, including topical lubricants, lozenges, coating agents, and artificial saliva, may provide some transient relief. The risk of dental caries should be minimized with good dental care. Osteoradionecrosis may be treated conservatively with antibiotics, hyperbaric oxygen therapy, or surgical débridement. Exercises may help in prevention of trismus associated with radiation therapy. With neck irradiation, hypothyroidism may occur, which can be treated with thyroid replacement therapy.
- The **complications of chemotherapy** are dependent on the agents used. Platinum compounds, a mainstay of chemotherapy in head and neck cancer, are known to cause significant nausea, nephrotoxicity, ototoxicity, myelosuppression, and peripheral neuropathy. 5-FU, another commonly used agent, is associated with mucositis

and myelosuppression. Cetuximab, a newer agent, is associated with rash, diarrhea, and hypersensitivity infusion reactions.

NASOPHARYNGEAL CARCINOMA

Epidemiology and Risk Factors

Nasopharyngeal carcinoma has a different epidemiology and a separate set of risk factors from the other head and neck cancers. Although rare in the United States, it is endemic in the Far and Middle East and in Africa, especially in southern China and Southeast Asia. It accounts for 18% of newly diagnosed malignancies in Southeast China. In these areas, nasopharyngeal cancer is associated with Epstein-Barr virus infection in genetically predisposed individuals. Other risk factors have been implicated, including diet (consumption of salted fish and low intake of fresh fruits and vegetables) and smoking.

Clinical Presentation

Nasopharyngeal cancer can present with a painless neck mass, but other symptoms include nasal obstruction, epistaxis, dysphagia, odynophagia, and Eustachian tube obstruction with otitis media. Tumors may extend through the foramen ovale to access the middle cranial fossa and the cavernous sinus to involve the oculomotor, trochlear, trigeminal, and abducens nerves leading to cranial neuropathy. In advanced cases, the optic nerve and orbital invasion can occur. Headaches, weight loss, trismus, and referred pain to the ear and neck can also be symptoms. Physical examination should include a thorough examination of the nares and oral cavity and the cranial nerves. Proptosis suggests orbital invasion by the tumor.

Management

Workup

Workup of patients with nasopharyngeal cancer should include a thorough physical evaluation and diagnostic imaging with CT or MRI from the skull down to the clavicles. Endoscopy should also be performed. A chest x-ray or CT scan should be done to assess for pulmonary metastases. The staging for nasopharynx is according to the American Joint Committee on Cancer TNM system (Tables 23-7 and 23-8).

Treatment

Nasopharyngeal carcinoma is very sensitive to chemoradiation. Early-stage disease (stages I and II) is typically treated with radiation therapy alone. For local recurrences, surgical resection or repeat irradiation are options for treatment. For advanced disease (stages III and IV), concurrent chemoradiation followed by adjuvant cisplatin and 5-FU has demonstrated benefit in terms of overall survival, progression-free survival, and control of local disease and distant metastases. Metastatic disease is managed with chemotherapeutic agents such as cisplatin, carboplatin, and 5-FU.

SALIVARY GLAND TUMORS

Introduction

Salivary gland tumors may arise either in the major glands, namely, the parotid, submandibular, and sublingual glands, or in the minor glands located in the oral mucosa, palate, uvula, floor of the mouth, posterior tongue, retromolar area and peritonsillar area, pharynx, larynx, and paranasal sinuses. Salivary gland tumors account for ~5% of all head and neck cancers and are varied in their histologic patterns as low- or high-grade

TABLE 23-7	STAGING OF NASOPHARYNX CANCER
Primary tumor (T)	
TX	Primary tumor cannot be assessed
T0	No evidence of primary tumor
Tis	Carcinoma in situ
T1	Tumor confined to the nasopharynx
T2	Tumor extends to soft tissues of oropharynx and/or nasal fossa
T2a	Without parapharyngeal extension
T2b	With parapharyngeal extension
T3	Tumor invades bony structures and/or paranasal sinuses
T4	Tumor with intracranial extension and/or involvement of cranial nerves, infratemporal fossa, hypopharynx, or orbit
Regional lymph nodes (N)	
NX	Regional lymph nodes cannot be assessed
N0	No regional lymph node metastasis
N1	Unilateral metastasis in lymph node(s), ≤6 cm in greatest dimension, above the supraclavicular fossa
N2	Bilateral metastasis in lymph node(s), ≤6 cm in greatest dimension, above the supraclavicular fossa
N3	Metastasis in a lymph node(s)
N3a	>6 cm in dimension
N3b	Extension to the supraclavicular fossa
Distant metastasis (M)	
MX	Distant metastasis cannot be assessed
M0	No distant metastasis
M1	Distant metastasis

From American Joint Committee on Cancer. *AJCC Cancer Staging Manual*. 6th ed. New York: Springer-Verlag; 2002, with permission.

malignancies. Approximately 80% arise from the parotid gland, but of those, 80% are benign. In contrast, 95% to 100% of tumors arising from the sublingual gland are malignant.

Management

Treatment usually involves surgical resection of the gland. Prognosis is more favorable for low-grade tumors and those located in major glands, especially in the parotid. For aggressive or bulky tumors, resection is often combined with postoperative radiation.

NECK MASS WITH AN UNKNOWN PRIMARY

Differential Diagnosis

The differential diagnosis for a malignant neck mass includes squamous cell carcinoma, adenocarcinoma, lymphoma, thyroid neoplasms, and melanoma.

TABLE 23-8	AJCC STAGE GROUPING: NASOPHARYNX		
Stage 0	Tis	N0	M0
Stage I	T1	N0	M0
Stage IIA	T2a	N0	M0
Stage IIB	T1	N1	M0
	T2	N1	M0
	T2a	N1	M0
	T2b	N0	M0
	T2b	N1	M0
Stage III	T1	N2	M0
	T2a	N2	M0
	T2b	N2	M0
	T3	N0	M0
	T3	N1	M0
	T3	N2	M0
Stage IVA	T4	N0	M0
	T4	N1	M0
	T4	N2	M0
Stage IVB	Any T	N3	M0
Stage IVC	Any T	Any N	M1

From American Joint Committee on Cancer. *AJCC Cancer Staging Manual.* 6th ed. New York: Springer-Verlag; 2002, with permission.

Management

Workup

As cancers that originate elsewhere in the body can also present with a neck mass, a thorough history and physical should be performed, along with evaluation for potential primary sites.

Diagnosis

A fine-needle biopsy for cytology may be pursued as the initial step for evaluation of a neck mass without a clear primary. Open biopsy may be helpful if the suspicion for lymphoma is high. If the cytology shows squamous cell carcinoma, then endoscopy with blind biopsy of potential sites in the nasopharynx, tonsils, base of tongue, and pyriform sinus should be performed.

Treatment

If no primary site is found and the tumor is amenable to resection, surgical resection may be the primary therapy. If the surgical pathology shows extracapsular extension or involvement of multiple nodes, postoperative radiation may be given. If the tumor is not amenable to surgical resection, radiation therapy is the primary treatment modality.

- Alcohol and tobacco use in any form are the major risk factors for head and neck cancers. Smoking cessation is a key part of managing patients with head and neck cancers.
- HPV is associated with some cancers of the oropharynx and portends a better prognosis.
- A multidisciplinary team of physicians and allied health professionals is needed to take care of the complex needs of patients with head and neck cancers.
- Single-modality treatment with either surgery or radiation therapy provides equivalent survival rates in early-stage (I or II) head and neck cancers.
- For locally advanced head and neck cancers that are unresectable, concurrent chemoradiation is the definitive treatment. For those with tumors amenable to resection, surgical resection followed by adjuvant radiation is the usual course of treatment.
- Metastatic head and neck cancers are treated primarily with chemotherapy. Survival is typically <1 year.
- Nasopharyngeal cancer is more radiosensitive than other head and neck cancers. Early-stage disease can be managed with radiation alone but more advanced disease is treated with chemoradiation followed by adjuvant chemotherapy.
- Salivary gland tumors most commonly arise from the parotid, of which 75% to 80% are benign.
- Neck mass with an unknown primary may be treated with surgery and/or radiation if no primary site is found on a thorough evaluation of the patient.

REFERENCES AND SUGGESTED READINGS

Bensadoun RJ, Blanc-Vincent MP, Chauvel P, et al. Malignant tumours of the salivary glands. *Br J Cancer.* 2001;84(Suppl 2):42–48.

Bonner JA, Harari PM, Giralt, J, et al. Radiotherapy plus cetuximab for squamous-cell carcinoma of the head and neck. *N Engl J Med.* 2006;354:567–578.

D'Souza G, Kreimer AR, Viscidi, R, et al. Case-control study of human papilloavirus and oropharyngeal cancer. *N Engl J Med.* 2007;356:1944–1956.

Lewin F, Norell SE, Johansson H, et al. Smoking tobacco, oral snuff, and alcohol in the etiology of squamous cell carcinoma of the head and neck. *Cancer.* 1998;82:1367–1375.

Seiwert TY, Salamo JK, Vokes EE. The chemoradiation paradigm in head and neck cancer. *Nat Clin Pract Oncol.* 2007;4(3):156–171.

Spiro RH. Salivary neoplasms: overview of a 35-year experience with 2,807 patients. *Head Neck Surg.* 1986;8:177–184.

Vermoken JB, et al. Results of the Extreme trial. Presented at American Society for Clinical Oncology meeting, Chicago, IL; 2007.

Vermoken JB, Trigo J, Hitt R, et al. Open-label, uncontrolled multicenter phase II study to evaluate the efficacy and toxicity of cetuximab as a single agent in patients with recurrent and/or metastatic squamous cell carcinoma of the head and neck who failed to respond o platinum-based therapy. *J Clin Oncol.* 2007;25(16):2171–2177.

Vokes EE. Head and neck cancer. *Semin Oncol.* 1994;21:279.

Winquist E, Oliver T, Gilbert R. Post-operative chemoradiotherapy for advanced squamous cell carcinoma of the head and neck: a systematic review with meta-analysis. *Head Neck.* 2007;29:38–46.

Sarcoma

Saiama Waqar and David Kuperman

24

BACKGROUND

Sarcomas (from the Greek *sarx* for flesh) are malignancies of the connective tissue. They are a heterogeneous group of tumors comprised of cells of mesenchymal origin. The presenting signs and symptoms depend on the anatomic site of origin and can vary markedly. In general, sarcomas can be divided into two large groups: soft tissue tumors and bone tumors.

EPIDEMIOLOGY

Sarcomas are rare tumors, comprising 1% of adult malignancies and 7% of pediatric malignancies. In the United States, the incidence of soft tissue sarcomas (STSs) and bone sarcomas is 6000 and 2100 cases per year, respectively. Sarcomas occur with equal frequency in both genders.

RISK FACTORS

Most cases of sarcoma are sporadic; however, a number of etiologic factors have been identified, as detailed below.

Radiation
Sarcomas have been found to originate in or near tissues that have received prior external-beam radiation therapy and tend to develop at least 3 years after radiation therapy. The majority of these lesions are high grade, and they are typically osteosarcomas, malignant fibrous histiocytomas, and angiosarcomas.

Chemical Exposure
Thorotrast has been found to cause hepatic angiosarcomas. Other agents such as dioxin and arsenic have also been linked to sarcomas. Alkylating chemotherapy, particularly when used to treat childhood malignancies, has also been associated with the development of sarcomas in adulthood.

Genetic Conditions
Patients with neurofibromatosis type I have a 10% risk of developing a neurofibrosarcoma. Sarcomas also occur in patients with Li-Fraumeni syndrome. Familial retinoblastoma is linked to the development of osteosarcoma, and Gardner syndrome is a risk for fibrosarcoma.

Other Risks Associated with Sarcomas

Lymphangiosarcomas have been known to develop in a lymphedematous arm after mastectomy (Stewart-Treves syndrome). Kaposi sarcoma is associated with HIV disease. Paget disease of bone is a risk factor for the development of osteosarcoma or fibrosarcoma.

SOFT TISSUE SARCOMA

Presentation

Patients typically present with an **asymptomatic mass.** Pain may be present if there is entrapment of neurovascular structures or involvement of bone. Sarcomas may grow quite large before they are obvious on exam.

Extremity Sarcoma

Approximately half of all soft tissue sarcomas arise in the extremities. The majority are first seen as a painless soft tissue mass.

Retroperitoneal Sarcomas

Most patients have an abdominal mass and approximately half have abdominal pain that is vague and nonspecific. Weight loss is seen less frequently, with early satiety, nausea, and emesis occurring in <40% of patients. Neurologic symptoms, particularly paresthesia, occur in up to 30% of patients.

Physical Exam

Physical examination of a patient presenting with a soft tissue mass should include an assessment of the size of the mass and its mobility with respect to the underlying tissue. If a mass is >5 cm and deep, it should be presumed to be sarcoma until proven otherwise. High-grade sarcomas may have significant necrosis and can be confused with hematoma or abscess. A site-specific neurovascular examination should also be performed.

Differential Diagnosis

The differential diagnosis includes benign soft tissue tumors as well as carcinoma, lymphoma, and melanoma. The most common benign tumors include lipoma, desmoid tumor, neurofibroma, hemangioma, and schwannoma.

Workup

Patients with masses suspicious for sarcoma should undergo **radiologic evaluation and biopsy.** The studies needed for adequate staging vary depending on the site of disease. Sarcoma of the head and neck or extremities should be evaluated with **plain films** and **MRI.** Plain films may reveal soft tissue mineralization (which is typical for synovial sarcoma) or may reveal skeletal reaction to the tumor. MRI is valuable for assessing fat and distinguishing it from surrounding tissues. This may assist in the diagnosis of the lesion and allows for planning of the biopsy and subsequent surgery. For retroperitoneal and abdominal sarcomas, CT is the imaging modality of choice, as this provides the best anatomic definition of the tumor.

In addition to evaluating the primary lesion with imaging, **distant metastatic disease** may also be assessed. STS spreads *hematogenously*, and the lung is the most common site of metastasis. Chest x-ray may be sufficient for small, low-grade lesions, but in patients with high-grade tumors or tumors larger than 5 cm, a staging CT of the chest should be performed.

Diagnosis

An accurate biopsy diagnosis is essential for STS. Any lesion >5 cm or any rapidly growing lesion should be biopsied. The placement of the biopsy tract is also critical, as it will be seeded with tumor and must be excised at the time of resection. Generally, the preferred technique is open incisional biopsy performed by a surgeon with experience in resection of STS. Hemostasis is also very important, as a hematoma may require enlarging radiation fields or may interfere with planned resection.

Pathology

Histologic evaluation should be performed at an experienced center, as **grade is critically important to determining prognosis.** STSs are named for their tissue of origin based on light microscopy examination, and there are many possible histological types (Table 24-1). Tumors are also carefully evaluated for grade, which takes into account cellularity, mitotic activity, nuclear atypia, and necrosis. In general, the *grade, size,* and *depth* are more important factors than the histologic type. Immunohistochemistry studies are sometimes used to subclassify STS. The three most common types of STS are malignant fibrous histiocytoma, liposarcoma, and leiomyosarcoma.

Prognosis

- The most important prognostic factors for STS are **size, grade, depth,** and **relationship to fascial planes.** The American Joint Committee on Cancer (AJCC) staging system for STSs incorporates histologic grade (G), size of the primary (T), nodal involvement (N), and distant metastasis (M) (Table 24-2).
- Grade of the tumor is the predominant feature predicting early metastatic recurrence and death. Beyond 2 years of follow-up, the size of the lesion becomes as important as the histologic grade.
- Stage I carries a survival of 99%. Stage II has a survival of 82%. Stage III has a survival of 52%, and metastatic disease carries a survival of 20%.

Treatment

Early-Stage Disease (Stages I to III)
Extremity Soft Tissue Sarcomas
- **Surgery.** Surgery is the mainstay of therapy for early-stage STSs of the extremities. Sarcomas grow along planes and grossly appear to be well encapsulated. However, they usually extend into the pseudocapsule (an area around the tumor that is composed of tumor fimbriae and normal tissue), and "shelling-out" of lesions is associated with high local recurrence rates, 37% to 63%. In the past, radical excision and amputation were utilized to avoid this problem. Over the past 20 years, there has been a gradual shift in the surgical management of extremity soft tissue sarcomas

TABLE 24-1	GUIDELINES TO THE HISTOLOGIC GRADING OF SARCOMAS
Low-Grade Sarcomas	**High-Grade Sarcomas**
Good differentiation	Poor differentiation
Hypocellularity	Hypercellularity
Increased stroma	Minimal stroma
Hypovascularity	Hypervascularity
Minimal necrosis	Much necrosis
<5 mitoses per high-power field	>5 mitoses per high-power field

Adapted from Hajdu SI, Shiu MH, Brennan MF. The role of the pathologist in the management of soft tissue sarcomas. *World J Surg.* 1988;12:326–331, with permission.

TABLE 24-2 AJCC STAGING SYSTEM FOR SOFT TISSUE SARCOMA

Primary Tumor (T)	Regional Lymph Nodes (N)	Distant Metastasis (M)	Grade (G)	Stage
TX: primary tumor cannot be assessed	NX: Regional lymph node involvement cannot be assessed	MX: presence of metastasis cannot be assessed	G1: Low, well differentiated	Stage I: T1a,b N0 M0 G1; T2a,b N0 M0, G1
T0: no evidence of primary tumor	N0: no regional lymph node metastasis	M0: no distant metastasis	G2: Intermediate, moderately well differentiated	Stage II: T1a,b N0 M0, G2–3; T2a N0 M0, G2–3
T1: tumor is <5 cm in greatest dimension	N1: regional lymph node metastasis	M1: distant metastasis	G3: High; poorly differentiated	Stage III: T2b N0 M0, G2–3
T1a: tumor is located above and without invasion of the superficial fascia				Stage IV: any T N1 M0, any G; Any T N0 M1, any G
T1b: tumor is located below and/or with invasion of the superficial fascia				
T2: tumor is >5 cm in greatest dimension				
T2a: tumor is located above and without invasion of the superficial fascia				
T2b: tumor is located below and/or with invasion of the superficial fascia				

From American Joint Committee on Cancer. *AJCC Cancer Staging Manual*. 6th ed. New York: Springer-Verlag, 2002, with permission.

away from radical ablative surgery toward limb-sparing surgery. Amputation is only required in ~5% of patients today.

- **Radiation therapy.** Wide local excision alone is all that is necessary for small (T1), low-grade, STSs of the extremities, with a local recurrence rate of <10%. **Adjuvant radiation therapy**, however, is required in a number of situations: (a) virtually all high-grade extremity sarcomas, (b) lesions larger than 5 cm (T2), and (c) positive or equivocal surgical margins in patients for whom re-excision is impractical. When adjuvant radiation is planned, metal clips should be placed at margins of resection to facilitate radiation field planning. **Neoadjuvant radiation** may be needed prior to definitive resection. This is most commonly performed for tumors that are borderline resectable or for tumors located adjacent to the joint capsule. A phase III National Cancer Institute of Canada trial comparing adjuvant (postoperative) and neoadjuvant (preoperative) radiation demonstrated similar local control rates, metastatic outcome, and overall survival rates between the two arms. However, patients receiving preoperative radiation had a significantly higher incidence of wound complications (35% vs. 17%) (O'Sullivan et al. 2002).
  - **Radiation as definitive therapy** alone in the treatment of unresectable or medically inoperable soft tissue sarcoma patients yields a 5-year survival rate of 25% to 40% and a local control rate of 30%. Radiation doses should be at least 65 Gy, if feasible, given the site of the lesion. **Brachytherapy** also has been used in treatment for sarcomas. Iridium-192 is the most commonly used agent. It has similar local control rates to adjuvant external beam radiation and has the advantage of a decrease in the patient's entire treatment from 10–12 weeks to 10–12 days. In addition, smaller volumes of tissues are irradiated, which may be useful if important structures, such as joints, are nearby.
- **Adjuvant chemotherapy.** The benefit of adjuvant chemotherapy for extremity STSs is controversial. The only exception to this is rhabdomyosarcomas, in which adjuvant chemotherapy is accepted as standard of care.
  - A formal meta-analysis of individual data from 1568 patients who participated in 13 trials was performed by the Sarcoma Meta-Analysis Collaboration. The analysis demonstrated a significant reduction in the risk of local or distant recurrence in patients who received adjuvant chemotherapy. There also was a decrease in the risk of distant relapse (metastasis) by 30% in treated patients. Overall survival, however, did not meet criteria for statistical significance between the control group and adjuvant chemotherapy arm, with a hazard ratio of 0.89 (Sarcoma Meta-Analysis Collaboration 1997). Most of the randomized trials examined in this meta-analysis were limited by patient numbers, inclusion of all subtypes of STS and of low-grade tumors, heterogeneous patient and disease characteristics, and varied chemotherapy regimens.
  - Certain subgroups of patients, such as those with high-grade lesions, may benefit from adjuvant chemotherapy, but further studies are needed.

Retroperitoneal Sarcomas

- **Surgery.** As with other soft tissue sarcomas, surgery is the primary treatment of retroperitoneal sarcomas. Tumors that are <5 cm and not located close to adjacent viscera or critical neurovascular structures are considered resectable. If a tumor is thought to be a sarcoma and is resectable, a preoperative biopsy is not necessary. One should consider a preoperative CT-guided core biopsy if an incomplete resection is a reasonable possibility to allow neoadjuvant therapy.

Unfortunately, only 50% of patients with early-stage retroperitoneal sarcomas are able to undergo complete surgical resection. Of the tumors removed, approximately half will develop a local recurrence. Adjuvant therapy, therefore, plays an important role in the management of retroperitoneal sarcomas.

- **Radiation therapy. Adjuvant radiation** therapy is most frequently recommended for patients with high-grade tumors or positive margins. The radiation is typically started 3 to 8 weeks following surgery to allow wound healing. Two-year local control rates of 70% have been reported with the addition of postoperative radiation therapy. **Neoadjuvant radiation therapy** can be given to patients with marginally resectable tumors and to those in whom one would expect postoperative radiotherapy to be required. It has a number of advantages over postoperative radiotherapy including smaller radiation portals and reduction of the extent of the surgical procedure.
- **Management of unresectable, locally advanced retroperitoneal sarcomas.** Unresectable retroperitoneal sarcomas can be managed in a number of ways. Radiation therapy can be given for palliation and with the hope that the tumor could be made resectable. Palliative surgery to reduce local symptoms can be performed. Chemotherapy can also be administered (see management of metastatic patients for specific regimens). An asymptomatic patient can be observed.

Metastatic Soft Tissue Sarcomas. Metastatic STSs can be divided into limited metastasis and extensive metastasis. **Limited metastatic disease** is defined as resectable metastasis involving one organ system. The prognosis of these two subsets of patients is very different. **It is possible to cure limited metastatic disease,** whereas patients with extensive metastatic disease can only be palliated.

- **Management of limited metastatic disease.** For patients with a limited number of pulmonary metastases, metastasectomy has been performed with some improvement in survival compared with no surgery. Three-year survival rates range from 23% to 42% if a complete resection is performed. In patients with visceral sarcomas and limited liver metastasis, it is sometimes possible to perform a metastasectomy by surgery, chemoembolization, or radiofrequency ablation.
- **Management of extensive metastatic disease.** The goal of therapy for patients with metastatic sarcoma is palliation and prolongation of survival. Cure is no longer a viable goal. Systemic chemotherapy is the primary modality of treatment. Radiation and surgery may be used with a goal of palliation.

Numerous chemotherapy agents have been used as single agents or in combination for the treatment of soft tissue sarcomas. These include doxorubicin, ifosfamide, cyclophosphamide, gemcitabine, and taxanes.

BONE SARCOMA

Introduction

Bone sarcoma may arise from any tissue within the bones. The most common bone sarcomas are osteosarcoma, chondrosarcoma, and Ewing sarcoma.

Classification

Osteosarcoma

Osteosarcoma is the most common primary bone tumor, accounting for 40% to 50% of bone sarcomas. They present with pain and swelling. Approximately 60% occur in adolescents and children. Ten percent may occur in the third decade. There is a second peak in the fifth and sixth decades, which is frequently due to radiation-associated osteosarcoma or transformation of existing lesions. They are spindle cell neoplasms that produce bone and are more common in long bones. Most osteosarcomas occur in the metaphyseal region, near the growth plate, of skeletally immature long bones. The distal femur, proximal tibia, and proximal humerus are common sites. The majority is classified as "classic," and this type is more common at between 10 and 20 years of age. Most of these lesions are high grade and highly vascular.

Chondrosarcoma

Chondrosarcoma is the second most frequent malignant primary bone tumor, representing approximately 20% of bone sarcomas. They generally occur between the fourth and the sixth decades. They tend to develop in flat bones, including the shoulder and pelvic girdles. They may arise de novo or from pre-existing lesions. They are indolent and are generally low grade. Chondrosarcoma may arise peripherally or centrally. Imaging studies may be bland, particularly in central lesions, which may make it difficult to distinguish between benign and malignant lesions. New pain, increasing size, and signs of inflammation point toward malignant lesions. In general, these malignancies are resistant to chemotherapy and radiation.

Ewing Sarcoma

Ewing sarcoma accounts for 10% to 15% of bone sarcomas, and incidence peaks in the second decade. It is the second most common malignant tumor of the bone in childhood and adolescence. It tends to occur in the diaphysis of long bones. The femoral diaphysis is the most common location. These are highly aggressive tumors and are best considered a systemic disease. A characteristic chromosomal translocation, t(11:22), is associated with this sarcoma and with peripheral primitive neuroectodermal tumor (PPNET). Ewing sarcoma is one of the small, round, blue cell tumors.

Presentation

History

Localized pain and swelling are the hallmark clinical features of bone sarcomas. The pain is initially insidious but can become unremitting. Occasionally, a pathologic fracture will bring the patient to medical attention. If the tumor arises in the lower extremities, the patient may have a limp. Constitutional symptoms are rare but can be observed in patients with Ewing sarcoma or patients with metastatic disease. A pertinent history should note how long a lesion has been present and any change in it. Rapid growth or change in a lesion favors a malignant etiology.

Physical Exam

Physical exam may reveal a palpable mass. A joint effusion may be observed, and range of motion of the joint may be limited, with stiffness or pain. Neurovascular and lymph node examinations are usually normal.

Management

Workup
- Patients who are suspected to have bone sarcoma should undergo imaging studies, including plain films, MRI, and biopsy.
- **Plain films** may demonstrate characteristic lesions for bone sarcoma. Osteosarcoma is associated with destructive lesions showing a moth-eaten appearance. In addition, a spiculated periosteal reaction and cuff of periosteal new bone may be seen. Plain films in chondrosarcoma show lesions with a lobulated appearance with punctate or annular calcification of cartilage. Ewing sarcoma is associated with an "onion peel" periosteal reaction and soft tissue mass. Metastatic disease may be associated with either osteolytic or osteoblastic lesions, depending on the type of primary malignancy.
- **MRI** is the imaging modality of choice to evaluate the relationship of the tumor to surrounding structures and determine resectability. CT scan of the primary site may

be considered in place of MRI to demonstrate cortical destruction more accurately and for evaluation of pelvic tumors. CT scan of the chest is used to evaluate for pulmonary metastases. **Bone scan** helps to evaluate for the local extent of the tumor as well as to evaluate for other lesions.

Diagnosis

An accurate tissue biopsy is needed for diagnosis. Imaging studies may be suggestive of tumor type; however, it can be difficult to distinguish benign and malignant bone tumors. Biopsy specimens are used to determine the histologic type of tumor as well as the grade. As with STSs, **open incisional biopsy is preferred for bone sarcomas.** The biopsy should be performed by a surgeon experienced in sarcoma so that it does not compromise the definitive surgical procedure.

Staging

Bone sarcomas are staged using the American Joint Committee on Cancer staging system based on grade, tumor size, and metastatic disease as reported in Table 24-3. Adverse prognostic indicators include elevated lactate dehydrogenase (LDH), elevated alkaline phosphatase, and an axial primary. Patients with Ewing sarcoma should have bilateral bone marrow biopsies as part of staging.

Treatment

The treatment of bone sarcoma, in contrast to STS, is more dependent on histologic subtype.

General Principles of Local Therapy

- Surgical excision is the mainstay of treatment for patients with low-grade bone sarcomas. For high-grade tumors, multimodality therapy is indicated. As an example, for high-grade osteosarcomas, preoperative multiagent chemotherapy is followed by surgical removal of the tumor and then further adjuvant chemotherapy. Physical therapy and prosthetics are of great importance in these patients because of the highly invasive nature of the treatment.
- The Musculoskeletal Tumor Society and the National Comprehensive Cancer Network (NCCN) recognize wide excision, either by amputation or by a limb-salvage procedure, as the recommended surgical approach for all high-grade bone sarcomas. Currently, 75% to 80% of patients may be treated with a limb-sparing surgery. This type of resection is predicated on complete tumor removal, effective skeletal reconstruction, and adequate soft tissue coverage.

Osteosarcoma Therapy. The 5-year survival for osteosarcoma with surgery alone is <20%. This occurs because microscopic dissemination is likely to be present in 80% of patients at the time of diagnosis. The addition of adjuvant chemotherapy has improved survival for high-grade osteosarcoma, permitting long-term survival as high as 80%.

- **Neoadjuvant and adjuvant chemotherapy.** Neoadjuvant chemotherapy began as a strategy to permit limb-sparing surgery, allowing time for creation of custom-made prosthetics. Since its acceptance, other advantages have been recognized with this approach. It permits earlier treatment of occult micrometastatic disease, preventing emergence of resistant clones and potentially debulking the primary to improve chances for limb-sparing surgery.

Chemotherapeutic agents active in osteosarcomas include doxorubicin, cisplatin, ifosfamide, and high-dose methotrexate with leucovorin rescue. These agents are typically used in combination to improve response, although the optimal combination and duration of therapy remain controversial. Currently, the NCCN recommends a combination of at least two of the above agents for six cycles, with two of the cycles given prior to surgery.

TABLE 24-3 AJCC STAGING SYSTEM FOR BONE SARCOMA

Primary Tumor (T)	Regional Lymph Nodes (N)	Distant Metastasis (M)	Grade (G)	Stage
TX: primary tumor cannot be assessed	NX: regional lymph node involvement cannot be assessed	MX: presence of metastasis cannot be assessed	G1: low, well differentiated	Stage IA: T1 N0 M0, G1; T1 N0 M0,G2
T0: no evidence of primary tumor	N0: no regional lymph node metastasis	M0: no distant metastasis	G2: intermediate, moderately well differentiated	Stage IB: T2 N0 M0, G1; T2 N0 M0, G2
T1: tumor ≤8 cm in greatest dimension	N1: regional lymph node metastasis	M1: distant metastasis	G3: High; poorly differentiated	Stage IIA: T1 N0 M0, G3; T1 N0 M0,G4
T2: tumor is >8 cm in greatest dimension		M1a: lung metastasis	G4: undifferentiated (Ewing sarcoma)	Stage IIB: T2 N0 M0, G3; T2 N0 M0, G3; T2 N0
T3: discontinous tumors in the primary bone site		M2b: other sites of metastasis		Stage III: T3 N0 M0, any G
				Stage IVA: any T N0 M1a, any G
				Stage IVB: any T any N M1b, any G; any T N1 any M, any G

From American Joint Committee on Cancer. *AJCC Cancer Staging Manual.* 6th ed. New York: Springer-Verlag, 2002, with permission.

Histologic response to preoperative therapy is recognized as a significant prognostic factor. Various systems have been developed for grading histologic response to chemotherapy, but >90% necrosis of tumor cells is associated with the best prognosis. If the tumor has been resected to negative margins and had a good histologic response to chemotherapy, the patient continues on chemotherapy for an additional 2 to 12 cycles. If the tumor was fully resected but has <90% necrosis, salvage chemotherapy with agents not used in induction is attempted, but the effect of this change in chemotherapy on outcomes is unclear. If the tumor margins are positive, additional local surgery should be attempted.

- **Radiation therapy.** Radiation is not routinely used in the therapy of osteosarcoma but may prove helpful in patients who refuse definitive resection or in palliation of patients with metastatic disease.
- **Management of metastatic disease.** Approximately 10% to 20% of patients with osteosarcoma have evidence of metastatic disease at presentation. Some of these patients may be candidates for surgical resection of pulmonary metastases. For patients with more extensive metastatic disease, chemotherapy is used to provide control of disease and palliation of symptoms.

Therapy for Ewing Sarcoma. Therapy for Ewing sarcoma and the related primitive peripheral neuroectodermal tumors uses a combined-modality approach.

- **Treatment of the primary tumor.** The optimal treatment for local tumor control is not well defined. Historically, radiation therapy has been the mainstay of local therapy, but there has been a recent trend toward surgery. No prospective randomized trials have been performed to compare the two modalities, but retrospective data suggest improvements in local control and survival when surgery is done with a complete resection of the tumor. Patients with unresectable disease or positive margins require radiation therapy to improve local control.
- **Chemotherapy.** Before the availability of effective chemotherapeutic agents, <10% of patients with Ewing sarcoma survived beyond 5 years, despite the fact that only 15% to 35% of patients with Ewing sarcoma/primitive peripheral neuroectodermal tumors have evidence of metastatic disease at presentation. This suggests that many patients with Ewing sarcoma have occult microscopic dissemination of the disease at the time of diagnosis. The current standard regimen is to use vincristine, actinomycin D, and cyclophosphamide (VAC) alternating with ifosfamide and etoposide (IE).
- **Recurrent metastatic Ewing sarcoma.** In this setting, cure is not a realistic goal. Palliation and prolongation of survival are more realistic expectations. Fortunately, aggressive combination chemotherapy (VAC or IE) and radiation therapy can still lead to prolonged progression-free survival.

KEY POINTS TO REMEMBER

- STSs are a rare, heterogeneous group of tumors best treated by experts.
- Treatment of STS consists mainly of limb-sparing surgery and radiation, with chemotherapy having a less defined role.
- Bone sarcoma is rare, and treatment depends on histologic subtype. Conversely, treatment of STS is more dependent on grade, size, and depth than histologic subtype.

REFERENCES AND SUGGESTED READINGS

Beech DJ, Pollock RE. Surgical management of primary soft tissue sarcoma. *Hematol Oncol Clin North Am.* 1995;9(4):707–718.

Bramwell V. Adjuvant chemotherapy for adult soft tissue sarcoma. *J Clin Oncol.* 2001;19(5):1235–1237.

DeVita VT, Hellman S, Rosenberg SA, eds. *Cancer: Principles and Practice of Oncology.* 6th ed. Philadelphia: Lippincott Williams & Wilkins; 2001.

Fauci AS, et al. *Harrison's Principles of Internal Medicine.* 14th ed. New York: McGraw-Hill; 1998:744–747.

Ferguson WS, Goorin AM. Current treatment of osteosarcoma. *Cancer Invest.* 2001;19(3):292–315.

Kattan MW, Leung, DH, Brennan, MF. Postoperative nomogram for 12-year sarcoma-specific death. *J Clin Oncol.* 2002; 20:791–796.

O'Sullivan B, Davis AM, Turcotte R, et al. Preoperative versus postoperative radiotherapy in soft-tissue sarcoma of the limbs: a randomised trial. *Lancet.* 2002;359(9325): 2235–2241.

Pirayesh A, Chee Y, Helliwell TR, et al. The management of retroperitoneal soft tissue sarcomas. *Eur J Surg Oncol.* 2001;27:491–497.

Rougraff B. The diagnosis and management of soft tissue sarcomas of the extremities in the adult. *Curr Probl Cancer.* 1999;23:7–41.

Sarcoma Meta-Analysis Collaboration. Adjuvant chemotherapy for localized resectable STS of adults. *Lancet.* 1997;350:1647–1654.

Wunder JS, et al. A comparison of staging systems for localized extremity soft tissue sarcoma. *Cancer.* 2000;88:2721–2730.

Endocrine Malignancies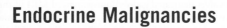

Mark A. Schroeder

INTRODUCTION

Endocrine neoplasms may develop in any of the endocrine organs or in the amine precursor uptake and decarboxylation cells. Overall, this heterogeneous group represents only 1.5% of noncutaneous malignancies. However, certain population subsets, such as those who inherit one of the autosomal dominant multiple endocrine neoplasia (MEN) syndromes, are predisposed to developing these relatively rare cancers. Clinical presentations of endocrine tumors vary, and patients do not always have an associated clinical endocrinopathy. This chapter discusses neoplasms of the endocrine glands—pituitary, thyroid, parathyroid, and adrenal cortex—as well as the diffuse endocrine system—gastroenteropancreatic neuroendocrine tumors, pheochromocytoma, and MEN syndromes.

PITUITARY NEOPLASMS

Introduction

Pituitary neoplasms are rare endocrine malignancies arising from epithelial origin in the adenohypophysis. Pituitary adenomas account for 10% to 15% of intracranial tumors. Their incidence peaks in the third and fourth decades of life. In general, males and females are affected equally, with the exception of some subtypes such as adrenal corticotropin hormone (ACTH) and prolactin secreting adenomas, which are more common in females.

Previously classified by histopathology (acidophilic, basophilic, chromophobic), pituitary adenomas are now classified by the hormones they secrete, that is, prolactin, growth hormone, ACTH, gonadotropins, and thyroid stimulating hormone (TSH). Tumors that do not secrete hormones above physiologic levels are termed nonfunctional adenomas.

Pathophysiology

Like other malignancies, pituitary adenomas are a result of oncogenes and defects in tumor suppressor genes. Examples include the pituitary tumor transforming gene (PTTG) and tumor suppressors such as p53. The exact mechanism of pituitary transformation is unknown.

Presentation

Clinical Presentation
Initial clinical presentation includes symptoms of headache, visual disturbance, and increased intracranial pressure, as well as syndromes related to the type of hormone secreted (Cushing syndrome, acromegaly, hirsutism, hyperprolactinemia, hyperthyroidism).

Evaluation

Initial evaluation involves dedicated gadolinium-enhanced MRI of the pituitary and laboratory evaluation for active adenomas with a panel consisting of growth hormone (GH), insulinlike growth factor 1 (IGF-1), prolactin (PRL), TSH, free T4, T3, ACTH, cortisol, luteinizing hormone (LH), follicle stimulating hormone (FSH), and testosterone. Diagnosis is made on imaging, substantiated by hormone levels in active adenomas, and, when appropriate, confirmed pathologically by transsphenoidal biopsy or resection. No TNM staging classification exists for these rare tumors and prognostic markers include levels of hormone secreted, size of tumor, and extent of suprasellar extension.

Management

Management of pituitary adenomas depends on the type, but in general, transsphenoidal surgical resection is the favored curative approach. The exceptions are prolactin secreting microadenomas, which are managed by dopamine agonists, or inactive adenomas, which remain stable in size on serial imaging. The goals of surgery are to alleviate mass effect while preserving pituitary function and abating endocrine hyperactivity. Postoperative management depends on the type of pituitary adenoma.

Prolactin Secreting Adenomas

- Prolactin secreting adenomas are the most commonly diagnosed pituitary tumor, representing ~30% of cases. Symptoms of hyperprolactinemia include galactorrhea and hypogonadism (oligomenorrhea or amenorrhea, dry vaginal mucosa, sterility, decreased libido, and impotence). Prolactinomas are usually slow-growing microadenomas in premenopausal women but can grow to a larger size (macroadenomas) in men and postmenopausal females. Macroadenomas can cause mass effect, classically manifested by visual disturbances (bitemporal hemianopsia) and headaches.
- The **differential diagnosis** of hyperprolactinemia includes pregnancy, prolactin stimulating drugs, hypothyroidism, and renal failure. The definitive diagnosis requires radiographic evidence of an adenoma and a persistently elevated prolactin level (>200 ng/mL in females and >100 ng/mL in males), with other etiologies of hyperprolactinemia having been ruled out.
- **Treatment** of prolactinomas is dependent on size. Microadenomas are treated medically since 95% of them do not increase in size and surgery is rarely curative. Medical treatment is achieved with dopamine agonists (bromocriptine and cabergoline), where the response rates are 70% to 80% for tumor shrinkage and 80% to 90% for restoration of ovulation. In cases where dopamine agonist therapy is not tolerated (~30% of cases) or fertility is not a concern, oral contraceptives containing estrogen and progesterone can be used to treat symptoms of hypogonadism. In cases of macroadenomas with significant suprasellar involvement or in pregnancy (which stimulates growth of adenomas), surgery or radiation therapy can be used, often in combination with dopamine agonists. Cure by surgery is rare in tumors >2 cm and with prolactin levels >200 ng/mL.
- **Follow-up** should include yearly prolactin levels. If prolactin increases to >250 ng/mL or neurological symptoms develop, repeat MRI is indicated. For patients with macroadenomas, visual field testing and MRI at 6 months after commencement of therapy should be performed. When prolactin levels are normalized for 2 years and at least 50% tumor reduction is observed, a trial of tapering the dopamine agonist may be considered.

Growth Hormone Secreting Adenomas

- These adenomas account for 30% of pituitary adenomas. Growth hormone excess results in acromegaly (coarse facial features, macroglossia, acral growth). Growth hormone leads to an increase in IGF-1, which affects bone and tissue growth and can ultimately lead to organomegaly, hypertension, cardiomyopathy, arthropathies, and restrictive lung diseases. Symptoms include arthralgias, oily skin, hyperhidrosis, headaches, and fatigue.

- The **diagnosis** is suggested by physical exam showing acromegaly, elevated IGF-1 level (preferred over fasting GH because the levels are more stable), oral glucose suppression test failing to suppress IGF-1, elevated GH, and pituitary adenoma on MRI.
- The **treatment** of choice is transsphenoidal resection. In patients not eligible for surgery, external-beam radiation may be used. Medical treatment with dopamine agonists or somatostatin analogues such as octreotide are not curative but may be used for symptomatic control of acromegaly, with response rates of 30% to 50%.
- **Follow-up** should include monitoring GH and IGF-1 levels. Monitoring for hypopituitarism after radiation is also essential.

Adrenal Corticotropin Hormone Secreting Adenomas

- These less common pituitary adenomas result in Cushing disease. Cushing disease is more common in women. The clinical presentation is most often a result of endocrinopathy and less commonly secondary to mass effect. Increased ACTH results in adrenal hyperplasia and hypercortisolism. Hypercortisolism results in centripetal obesity, moon facies, buffalo hump, hirsutism, abdominal striae, and acne (i.e., Cushing syndrome). Clinical signs include hypertension, bone loss, myopathies, diabetes, and psychiatric disorders.
- The **diagnosis** is made by confirming hypercortisolism with measurement of 24-hour urinary cortisol. The pituitary origin of cortisol is demonstrated by failure of the low-dose dexamethasone suppression test to suppress serum cortisol to <10 μg/dL. Finally, serum ACTH should be elevated to rule out an adrenal adenoma. Ectopic ACTH syndrome is excluded if the high-dose dexamethasone suppression test results in reduction of cortisol levels to <50% of baseline. If the above laboratory testing is inconclusive, inferior petrosal sinus sampling for ACTH can be performed to confirm the pituitary etiology. Imaging studies are less reliable, as 50% of ACTH secreting adenomas may not be detectable by MRI; nonetheless, MRI remains essential to guiding therapy and is performed in all cases.
- The **treatment** of choice is transsphenoidal resection, with cure rates ranging from 76% to 94%. External-beam radiation can be used for poor surgical candidates or as adjuvant therapy to surgery. Medical therapy with ketoconazole or mitotane can be used for symptom control in those unable to tolerate surgery or in relapsed cases.
- **Follow-up** requires replacement hormonal therapy for up to 1 year after surgery and monitoring for hypopituitarism after radiation.

Gonadotropin Secreting Adenomas and Nonsecreting Pituitary Adenomas

- These adenomas account for 30% of pituitary tumors. They are associated with an older population. Most are nonsecretory but demonstrate secretory granules containing FSH and LH. **Clinical presentation** typically occurs secondary to mass effect, with symptoms of headaches, visual changes, and hypopituitarism.
- The **diagnosis** is suggested by increased LH and FSH and by MRI findings of a macroadenoma. Postmenopausal women may have naturally elevated FSH and LH and diagnosis relies on final surgical pathology.
- The **treatment** is primarily transsphenoidal resection. Adjuvant external-beam radiation therapy may be considered in patients with residual tumor on imaging postoperatively. **Follow-up** several months postoperatively with repeat MRI is essential since most tumors are nonsecretory.

TSH Secreting Adenomas
- TSH secreting adenomas are the least common pituitary tumor, comprising ~1% of pituitary adenomas. Clinical presentation is typically with symptoms of hyperthyroidism (heat intolerance, diarrhea, weight loss, or exophthalmos) or mass effect.
- The **differential diagnosis** includes primary hyperthyroidism and pituitary resistance to thyroid hormone. The diagnosis is made by demonstrating increased TSH despite elevated T4 and T3. MRI may confirm the presence of an adenoma.
- **Treatment** is primarily transsphenoidal resection. Adjuvant external-beam radiation is used in refractory cases. Palliative medical therapy with octreotide has been used in refractory cases, with response rates of 90%. **Follow-up** requires monitoring of TSH, T4, and T3 levels.

THYROID CARCINOMA

Introduction

Multiple histologic subtypes of thyroid cancer exist (Table 25-1), and together they account for >90% of all endocrine malignancies. Thyroid cancer is nearly twice as

TABLE 25-1	THYROID CANCER HISTOLOGIC SUBTYPES AND KEY FEATURES	
Histologic Subtype	**% of Thyroid Cancers**	**Characteristics**
Well-differentiated		Typically affect younger patients Course is relatively benign and indolent. Metastases occur late and to bone, lungs, cervical lymph nodes, and skin. Surgery and radioactive iodine are treatments of choice.
Papillary	80	Psammoma bodies present on histology in 50%.
Follicular	12–20	Hürthle cell variety (3%) is more aggressive form.
Anaplastic (spindle cell)	2	Typically affect older patients and may arise from differentiated thyroid carcinomas or from a multinodular goiter. Aggressive tumors with local invasion common and always considered stage IV. Metastases to lung common and advanced diseases are uniformly fatal. External-beam radiation is marginally effective.
Medullary thyroid carcinoma	5–9	Neoplasia of the parafollicular/C cells for which sporadic and inherited forms exist. Secrete calcitonin and occasionally ACTH. May cause diarrhea in advanced disease. Metastases to inferior surface of liver capsule typical. Treatment is surgical.

common in women as in men, and it is the eighth most common malignancy diagnosed in women. Peak incidence occurs at about age 50 for females and age 65 for males. Previous radiation exposure is the main risk factor for well-differentiated thyroid malignancy, with an average lag time of 25 years to cancer presentation. The former use of radiation in treatment of benign childhood conditions during the early to mid-20th century partially accounts for the increase in follicular carcinomas seen since 1970. Cancers of the parafollicular cells, termed medullary thyroid carcinomas (MTCs), are not known to be related to radiation exposure and can occur sporadically (two thirds) or in individuals who have either MEN II syndrome or familial MTC (one third). Although the behavior of thyroid cancer can be variable, the course is usually indolent. Thus, if the cancer is discovered early, cure rates are high.

Presentation

- There are three main histologic variants of thyroid cancer: differentiated (papillary, follicular, and Hürthle), medullary, and anaplastic. Initial presentation is typically with a solitary thyroid nodule. Evaluation of the thyroid nodule is a relatively common medical issue (present in 5% of adults >50 years old). The majority of thyroid nodules are benign, and the history and exam assist in directing further investigation. For all cases, the chance of a thyroid nodule being malignant is 5% to 10% and the lifetime risk of thyroid carcinoma in the U.S. population is 1%. The risk of malignancy is increased in men, individuals younger than 15 or older than 60, those with a positive family history, those with other diseases associated with MEN II (hyperparathyroidism, marfanoid habitus, pheochromocytoma, or mucosal neuromas), and those having previous radiation exposure. A solitary, firm, immobile nodule or a rapid change in size is also of greater concern, as are symptoms of hoarseness, dyspnea, dysphagia, or new Horner syndrome.
- **Physical exam** should evaluate for nodule size, firmness, mobility, and local lymphadenopathy. Symptoms of diarrhea and flushing are occasionally seen in advanced MTC due to hormone secretion. Nodules <1 cm in a patient without other risk factors may be followed with a repeat exam in 6 to 12 months. However, nodules >1 cm or a nodule of any size in a patient with one of the previously listed risk factors warrants further evaluation.

Management

Diagnosis

In the clinically euthyroid patient, diagnosis is made by histologic evaluation. Fine-needle aspiration is the initial approach. If malignancy cannot be excluded (in 6% to 30% of fine-needle aspiration samples), a lobectomy is usually performed to obtain adequate tissue and to determine correct diagnosis. Ultrasound of the thyroid is also recommended; central hypervascularity, irregular borders, and/or microcalcifications suggest malignancy. Radioactive isotope scans and serologic testing with TSH and serum thyroglobulin assays are only useful in postoperative follow-up; they are not useful in making the diagnosis of thyroid malignancy. Calcitonin levels, however, should be checked at presentation and at follow-up exams for patients with MTC, as calcitonin serves as a sensitive tumor marker. In addition, those with MTC need to be evaluated for the *RET* proto-oncogene mutation and submit a 24-hour urine for vanillylmandelic acid, catecholamines, and metanephrines to evaluate for possible pheochromocytoma as part of MEN II syndrome.

Workup

- Once the diagnosis of malignancy is made, all individuals should have a chest x-ray to evaluate for metastases to the lung. An extensive staging workup is necessary only in anaplastic thyroid cancers, as they are often metastatic at presentation. Patients with anaplastic tumors should receive complete imaging of the neck with ultrasound or MRI and have a contrast-enhanced CT scan of the chest. Consideration should be given to abdominal imaging with CT or MRI. A thyroid scan is usually performed before thyroidectomy. The malignant nodule will appear cold.

• The **staging** of thyroid cancer (Tables 25-2 and 25-3) depends on tumor histology, size, and patient age at presentation. In MTC staging, information comes from evaluation of the total thyroidectomy and ipsilateral cervical lymph node dissection. For patients <45 years old, well-differentiated papillary or follicular cell carcinomas are never classified higher than stage II, which correlates with metastatic disease. On the other hand, anaplastic tumors are classified as stage IV regardless of anatomic extent due to their aggressive nature and high potential for metastasizing. Staging of MTC is based on tumor size, local or nodal involvement, and presence of metastases.

Prognosis

Overall, the **course** for most of these neoplasms is indolent, but some subsets of follicular and papillary tumors may be more aggressive or undergo transformation to an anaplastic carcinoma. Well-differentiated thyroid carcinomas have an excellent prognosis. Cure rates reach nearly 100% at 10 years, even with capsular invasion, as long as there is no vascular

TABLE 25-2	TNM CLASSIFICATION OF THYROID CANCER
Tumor	
Tx:	Primary tumor cannot be assessed
T0:	No evidence of primary tumor
T1:	Tumor ≤2 cm in maximum dimension, limited to the thyroid
T2:	Tumor >2–4 cm in maximum dimension, limited to the thyroid
T3:	Tumor >4 cm in maximum dimension, limited to the thyroid, or any tumor with limited extrathyroid extension (e.g., perithyroid soft tissue or sternothyroid muscle)
T4a:	Tumor of any size extending beyond the thyroid capsule and invading subcutaneous soft tissues, larynx, trachea, esophagus, or recurrent laryngeal nerve
T4b:	Tumor invades prevertebral fascia or encases carotid artery or mediastinal vessels
Nodes	
Nx:	Regional lymph nodes cannot be assessed
N0:	No regional lymph node metastasis
N1:	Regional lymph node metastasis
N1a:	Metastasis to level VI (pretracheal, paratracheal, and prelaryngeal lymph nodes
N1b:	Metastasis to unilateral, bilateral, or contralateral cervical or superior mediastinal lymph nodes
Metastasis	
Mx:	Distant metastasis cannot be assessed
M0:	No distant metastasis
M1:	Distant metastasis

TABLE 25-3 STAGING THYROID CANCER

	Stage	Tumor	Node(s)	Metastasis
Papillary or follicular				
<45 years old	I	Any T	Any N	M0
	II	Any T	Any N	M1
>45 years old	I	T1	N0	M0
	II	T2	N0	M0
	III	T1	N1a	M0
		T2	N1a	M0
		T3	N0–N1a	M0
	IVA	T1	N1b	M0
		T2	N1b	M0
		T3	N1b	M0
		T4a	N0–N1b	M0
	IVB	T4b	Any N	M0
	IVC	Any T	Any N	M1
Medullary carcinoma				
	I	T1	N0	M0
	II	T2	N0	M0
	III	T1	N1a	M0
		T2	N1a	M0
		T3	N0–N1a	M0
	IVA	T1	N1b	M0
		T2	N1b	M0
		T3	N1b	M0
		T4a	N0–1b	M0
	IVB	T4b	Any N	M0
	IVC	Any T	Any N	M1
Anaplastic carcinoma				
	IVA	T4a	Any N	M0
	IVB	T4b	Any N	M0
	IVC	Any T	Any N	M1

involvement. However, in individuals >45 years with distant metastases, disease is classified as stage IV, and 20-year disease specific mortality is >75%. Anaplastic tumors carry a grim prognosis, often leading rapidly to death within the first few years after diagnosis regardless of treatment. MTCs have 5-year survival rates >80% in stage I and II disease but <40% in stage III or IV disease.

Treatment

- **Treatment** of the three main types of thyroid cancer varies significantly. Radioactive iodine, external-beam radiation, surgery, and systemic chemotherapy each have their role in comprehensive therapeutic regimens.
- **Well-differentiated thyroid carcinoma (i.e., papillary, follicular, and Hürthle)** is mainly treated by surgical resection in all stages. Patients younger than 40 have an excellent prognosis with thyroidectomy alone. Factors increasing the chance of recurrence include advanced age and tumor size >1 cm. For these patients, a total thyroidectomy is recommended. Recurrent laryngeal nerve damage resulting in hoarseness is an uncommon complication of thyroid lobectomy. A total thyroidectomy carries the additional risk of hypocalcemia from hypoparathyroidism.

- In more advanced disease, dissection of the central and lateral cervical lymph nodes should be considered. However, the increased morbidity is often not compensated with a substantial effect on prognosis. Residual disease should be treated with radioactive iodine therapy. Even with spread to bone or lung, a cure may be attained with one or more administrations of iodine-131 (^{131}I), as long as the tumor is of low volume. Chemotherapeutic agents, including platinum, taxane-based regimens, and doxorubicin, have all been attempted but are rarely administered because they are typically less effective and have a worse side-effect profile than radioactive iodine.

- Short-wave beta **radiation** from ^{131}I induces cytotoxicity and is the key adjuvant therapeutic agent. External-beam radiation therapy rarely has a role in differentiated thyroid carcinomas. There are two main indications for use of ^{131}I. The first is to ablate residual normal thyroid tissue post–total thyroidectomy to improve the sensitivity of subsequent diagnostic ^{131}I scans in detecting recurrence. The second is to treat metastatic disease and destroy microscopic malignant foci. Radioactive iodine therapy requires withdrawal of thyroid hormone for ≥2 weeks until TSH levels reach 30 mU/L before administration. Follow-up imaging with ^{131}I determines treatment efficacy by revealing residual normal tissue as well as carcinoma. Treatment ends when there is no further radioactive iodine uptake present. Recent studies show that, for follow-up diagnostic scans, a two-dose regimen of exogenously administered recombinant TSH effectively mimics hormone withdrawal for imaging purposes, but not for treatment.

- **Adjuvant hormonal therapy** with exogenous thyroid hormone is routinely used in well-differentiated thyroid carcinomas to suppress TSH. Both normal and neoplastic thyroid tissue depends on TSH for growth. Thyroid hormone is also necessary to prevent symptoms of hypothyroidism. One should keep in mind, however, the potential side effects of higher rates of bone loss and an increased incidence of atrial fibrillation during this period. **Suppression of TSH** to undetectable levels for the initial 5 to 10 years is reasonable. After this time, if there is no evidence of recurrent disease, exogenous thyroid hormone supplementation may be decreased such that the TSH levels rise to the lower limits of normal.

- **MTC** is sporadic in most cases, but about 20% of cases are part of inherited tumor syndromes (MEN IIA and IIB and familial MTC). This possibility makes ruling out a *RET* proto-oncogene mutation or hyperparathyroidism and pheochromocytoma essential to the initial preoperative management, along with calcitonin measurement. Total thyroidectomy with bilateral central neck dissection is the mainstay of therapy for MTC because of the high frequency of bilateral disease. Although MTC is somewhat indolent in its progression, no effective systemic chemotherapy regimens exist, and MTC cells take up radioactive iodine poorly. For this reason, patients with genetic predisposition to the disease (i.e., *RET* mutations) should be highly encouraged to undergo prophylactic total thyroidectomy with central lymph node dissection. Surgical techniques vary, but many surgeons choose to remotely autograft the parathyroid glands during the operation to avoid hypoparathyroidism. Complications of local MTC invasion mirror those of anaplastic tumors, yet progression is less rapid. Doxorubicin (Adriamycin, Doxil) is the most effective cytotoxic chemotherapeutic agent, but an objective response is seen in <40% of patients, with no patients having a complete response.

- **Anaplastic thyroid carcinoma** is poorly responsive to therapy and is often locally invasive, if not metastatic, at the time of presentation. These poor prognostic features mean that they are always classified as stage IV at diagnosis regardless of size, grade, node involvement, or metastasis. The invasive nature makes tumor resection difficult or even impossible. At initial presentation, the tumor may encompass the carotid arteries, esophagus, and/or trachea. Recurrent or superior laryngeal nerve damage may also occur. The complications of local invasion account for the major morbidity of this cancer, often leading patients to require gastrostomy tubes or a tracheostomy. If the imaging reveals limited disease, resection should be pursued for improved local control and delay of these complications, although survival is not altered. Radioactive iodine is rarely taken up by anaplastic carcinoma cells so external-beam radiation therapy is a necessary component of treatment, and administration should be undertaken concurrently with systemic radiosensitizing chemotherapy. Doxorubicin is the most commonly used agent. End-stage care typically includes managing local complications, with ~50% of patients dying from airway obstruction.

Follow-Up
For routine follow-up of well-differentiated thyroid carcinoma, physical exam, TSH, thyroglobulin level measurement, and chest x-ray are recommended twice yearly for 4 years, then once yearly for 10 years. Thyroglobulin levels are expected to be <5 ng/mL if complete thyroid ablation has been successful. For MTC, serum calcitonin and carcinoembryonic antigen levels should initially be followed at 2 to 3 months postoperatively, then yearly. Abnormal serum markers should trigger diagnostic imaging evaluation.

Prognosis
- Prognosis for differentiated thyroid carcinomas is good. The two most important predictors of mortality are age (>45) and tumor stage at the time of initial therapy. Relative survival at 10 years for papillary, follicular, and Hürthle cell carcinomas is 93%, 85%, and 76%, respectively. Thirty percent of patients will have a recurrence, the majority locally, with distant recurrence mainly involving the lungs. Fifty percent of patients with recurrent distant metastasis die of cancer. Treatment options for recurrence include metastectomy and external-beam radiation, radio-iodine, or, as a last resort because of poor response rates, doxorubicin-based chemotherapy.
- Prognosis for MTC is adversely affected by increasing patient age (>40), increasing stage, and elevated tumor markers postoperatively. Patients <40 years old have a 5-year disease-specific survival rate of 95%; this declines to 65% for those older than 40. Prognosis is poor for anaplastic carcinoma, with mortality approaching 100%. Median survival from diagnosis is 3 to 7 months and 5-year survival rate is 5%.

PARATHYROID CARCINOMA

Introduction

Although adenomas of the parathyroid glands are a common endocrine abnormality, parathyroid carcinoma is quite rare. Primary hyperparathyroidism is categorized pathologically into three groups: single parathyroid adenoma (83% to 85%), multiglandular hyperplasia (15%), and parathyroid carcinoma (0.5% to 3%). Unlike benign hyperparathyroidism, which is found primarily in the postmenopausal female population, parathyroid carcinoma is found equally in both genders at younger ages. With an incidence of only 0.015 in 100,000, parathyroid cancer is classified as one of the rarest human cancers. Although no etiologic causes are known, parathyroid cancer is seen in the autosomal dominant disease of MEN I.

Presentation

Patients with parathyroid carcinoma often present initially with either hypercalcemia or a neck mass. On physical exam, 30% to 50% of patients with parathyroid carcinoma have palpable masses in the central neck region. A hyperfunctional parathyroid tumor leads to excessive production of parathyroid hormone and, ultimately, the clinical syndrome of primary hyperparathyroidism. Clinical signs and symptoms include fatigue, renal stones, bone disease, and neuromuscular/neuropsychiatric disturbances related to hypercalcemia. Grossly elevated calcium levels lead to nausea, vomiting, polyuria, and dehydration. In addition to hypercalcemia, markedly elevated parathyroid hormone levels are typically found on laboratory evaluation. Cytologic examination of a needle aspirate is considered an unreliable criterion for diagnosis of malignancy. Definitive diagnosis of parathyroid carcinoma is made in the operating room, where local invasion and metastasis can be assessed.

Management

- The mainstay of treatment is surgical exploration of the neck and complete en bloc resection of the tumor along with the ipsilateral thyroid lobe and central cervical lymph nodes. There is no effective adjuvant therapy. Likewise, the only effective therapy for recurrent or metastatic disease is complete resection. The value of radiation therapy is under scrutiny. The management of severe hypercalcemia includes saline hydration, furosemide diuresis, and bisphosphonates. Octreotide as well as calcimimetic agents is occasionally used to lower calcium in patients refractory to other therapeutic interventions.
- The prognosis for parathyroid carcinoma depends on the adequacy of initial en bloc resection. Recurrence rates are reported to range from 22% to 42%. The most common site of recurrence is locally (50% to 75%) followed by lung, liver, and bone, in order of decreasing incidence. Early recurrence correlates with death from the disease. The overall survival is ~85% at 5 years and 50% to 70% at 10 years. The major cause of death is hypercalcemia.

ADRENAL CORTICAL TUMORS

Introduction

Adrenal cortical carcinomas are rare (2/1 million) and aggressive tumors. Only 50% of tumors are endocrinologically active. Incidence is highest in the fourth to sixth decades, with men who smoke heavily and women exposed to oral contraceptives at higher risk.

Presentation

- Adrenal "incidentalomas" can be found on 1% to 3% of CT scans of the abdomen. The differential diagnosis includes benign adenomas and metastases. The chance of malignancy is directly related to the size of the mass (<3 cm, benign; >6 cm, malignant), with most carcinomas presenting as large masses.
- Adrenal carcinomas can secrete cortisol, sex hormones, or aldosterone, or can be inactive. The clinical presentation is dependent on the predominant hormone secreted. The most common clinical presentation is Cushing syndrome, which results from cortisol excess. This clinical syndrome consists of muscle weakness, easy bruising, irritability, and weight gain. Sex hormone excess can lead to acne, oligomenorrhea, and virilization/hirsutism in women and feminization in men. Rarely, these carcinomas may produce aldosterone, resulting in hypertension and hypokalemia.
- The **staging** of adrenal carcinoma depends on tumor size, nodal involvement, and presence of distant metastasis. Tumors <5 cm with no nodal involvement are stage I; those >5 cm without nodal involvement, stage II; those with nodal involvement, stage III; and those with distant metastasis, stage IV.

Management

- The **diagnosis** is suggested by enhancement of the adrenal mass with contrast, as well as elevated hormone levels. The definitive diagnosis is obtained by surgical pathology. High urinary free cortisol and serum cortisol, low ACTH, and lack of suppression in a high-dose dexamethasone suppression test occur in the instance of cortisol secreting carcinoma. Virilizing sex hormone-secreting carcinomas demonstrate high levels of testosterone, androstenedione, and DHEA-S, while feminizing tumors demonstrate high estradiol levels. Some tumors are nonsecretory and definitive diagnosis relies on pathologic diagnosis.

- Initial **evaluation** involves staging with imaging, typically with CT of the abdomen and pelvis, and determination of hormone levels, which are used to monitor for recurrence and progression. Surgical resection is the treatment of choice even in advanced disease. Debulking of the tumor and metastectomy are often considered. Adjuvant chemotherapy can be considered in advanced disease but seems minimally effective (response rates, 10% to 50%), with not enough evidence to support any single regimen. Multiple prospective trials are currently ongoing and should be considered. Typical agents include doxorubicin, vincristine, platinums, taxanes, 5-FU, and etoposide. In patients ineligible for surgery combined modality therapy with etoposide + doxorubicin + cisplatin + mitotane has been used with a response rate of 50% and time to progression of 18 months. Most chemotherapeutic regimens will include mitotane, which selectively targets the adrenal cortex and results in selective chemical ablation. Overall response rate to mitotane is ~33%, but its effect on overall and disease-free survival has not been conclusively determined in prospective trials; nonetheless, a recent retrospective study suggested improved disease-free survival for those patients undergoing surgery followed by adjuvant mitotane (42 vs. 10 months). Other medical therapies aimed at palliating symptoms include ketoconazole and aminoglutethimide. Finally, adjuvant external-beam radiation therapy may also be effective for local control after resection or for symptomatic metastasis.
- The **prognosis** of adrenal carcinoma depends on initial stage and resectability. For surgically resectable tumors, the median overall survival is almost 6 years, but with medical therapy alone <10% of patients live to 6 years. **Follow-up** with repeat CT scans and hormone levels at 6-month intervals is recommended.

DIFFUSE ENDOCRINE SYSTEM TUMORS

Some endocrinologically active tumors are not localized to any one organ but share the common embryonic origin of the neural crest and neuroectoderm. These include gastroenteropancreatic neuroendocrine tumors, pheochromocytoma, and MEN syndromes.

GASTROENTEROPANCREATIC NEUROENDOCRINE TUMORS

Introduction

Tumors of the gastroenteropancreatic axis are classified according to their secretory products: insulinoma, gastrinoma, somatostatinoma, glucagonoma, vasoactive intestinal peptide-oma (VIPoma), and carcinoid. Some are nonsecretory and classified as extrapulmonary small-cell carcinomas. Half of neuroendocrine tumors are of the carcinoid variant, followed by gastrinomas, insulinomas, VIPomas, and glucagonomas, in order of decreasing incidence.

Presentation

Most neuroendocrine tumors are malignant and are commonly identified at the time of metastatic disease, with the exception of insulinomas, which are slow growing. Clinical presentation depends on the hormones secreted and site of disease. The initial laboratory analysis should focus on specific hormones associated with those clinical symptoms as outlined in Table 25-4.

TABLE 25-4	HORMONE STUDIES AND CLINICAL SYMPTOMS IN NEUROENDOCRINE TUMORS	
	Laboratory Test(s)	**Clinical Symptom(s)**
Carcinoid	5-HIAA 24-h urine Chromogranin A	Carcinoid syndrome: flushing/diarrhea/wheezing
Gastrinoma	Gastrin	Ulcer disease
Insulinoma	Proinsulin Insulin/glucose ratio >0.3 C-peptide	Hypoglycemia
VIPoma	VIP	Watery diarrhea and hypokalemia
Glucagonoma	Glucagon Serum glucose CBC	Dermatitis/diabetes/deep vein thrombosis
Other pancreatic islet cell tumors	Chromogranin A Somatostatin Pancreatic polypeptide Calcitonin Parathyroid hormone-related peptide	Diabetes/steatorrhea/ gallbladder disease Hypercalcemia Hypocalcemia
Pheochromocytoma	Metanephrines (plasma and urine) Urine catecholamines	Cyclic hypertension

5-HIAA = 5-hydroxyindolacetic acid.

Adapted from Clark OH, et al. Neuroendocrine tumors. *J Natl Compr Canc Netw.* 2006;4(2):102–138.

Management

Tumor localization is essential for successful management of limited disease. CT and MRI may detect larger tumors, but often scintigraphy or angiography with venous hormone sampling may be required to localize tumors. Therapy varies from surgical resection for localized tumors, to medical therapies and dietary changes to palliate symptoms, to chemotherapy and arterial embolization. Chemotherapy has variable activity depending on the type of gastroenteropancreatic tumor. Typical agents used include 5-FU, streptozotocin, doxorubicin, and dacarbazine. Octreotide is commonly used in the treatment of gastroenteropancreatic malignancies for symptom relief (e.g., flushing, wheezing, and diarrhea); it also has a direct inhibitory effect on tumor growth and is used in the perioperative setting as suppressive therapy.

CARCINOID TUMORS

Introduction

Carcinoid tumors are the most common neuroendocrine tumors, with a yearly incidence of 1.5 in 100,000 in the United States. Benign and malignant tumors occur at approximately equal frequency, and either type may be symptomatic. Although relatively rare, they are important, as some secrete various vasoactive substances, including histamine, serotonin, catecholamines, and prostaglandins. The small bowel is the most common location for these tumors, but they may occur in the appendix, colon, rectum, lung, stomach, or ovary as well. Symptomatic carcinoid tumors usually result from small bowel tumors with metastases to the liver and do not occur with rectal carcinoid. **Carcinoid syndrome** is due to excessive production of serotonin and other bioactive compounds that then have direct access to the systemic circulation.

Presentation

- More than 95% of gastrointestinal carcinoids arise from the rectum, appendix, or small intestine. Appendiceal and small (<1 cm) rectal tumors rarely metastasize, cause symptoms, or affect survival. Small bowel tumors are more likely to be problematic. One third of small intestine tumors are multicentric, and the chance of metastases increases with increased tumor size (tumors >2 cm have a high rate of metastatasis). In general, the progression of small intestinal carcinoid tumors is indolent. However, once metastasis of tumor cells occurs, prognosis is considerably worse. Five-year survival with localized disease, with only nodal involvement, and, finally, with liver metastases is ~95%, 65%, and 20%, respectively. Urinary 5-hydroxyindoleacetic acid levels inversely correlate with survival.
- Approximately 40% of carcinoid tumors found in living patients are hormonally active, leading to **carcinoid syndrome** in 10% of cases. This syndrome rarely occurs without liver metastasis. Symptoms may include facial flushing and edema, abdominal cramping and diarrhea, bronchospasm, hypotension, and cardiac valvular lesions (typically on the tricuspid and/or pulmonic valve if the tumor secretions originate in the bowel). Alcohol, stress, or exercise may precipitate symptoms. Tumors that are not endocrinologically active can also cause devastating effects such as bowel obstruction, appendicitis, or painful liver metastases.

Management

Diagnosis

An elevated 24-hour urinary 5-hydroxyindoleacetic acid level is often used for diagnosis but is not useful for detecting carcinoid at early stages when it is curable. Levels >25 mg/day are the typical finding (normal value of excretion is <9 mg/day). Patients should avoid excessive intake of nuts, bananas, avocados, and pineapples for ~2 days prior to testing, as these may result in erroneously high levels. Plasma **chromogranin A** level may also be a useful test with a high sensitivity and without significant variability or need for a 24-hour urine collection. Other routine tests should be aimed at identifying tumor location. Routine blood tests, with attention to liver function tests, hepatic and upper gastrointestinal system imaging, a chest x-ray, and eventual tissue acquisition should all be part of the workup. If available, somatostatin receptor scintigraphy is a useful imaging test. There is not an accepted staging system for carcinoid. Finally, pathologic diagnosis is confirmed with positive stains for chromogranin, synaptophysin, and neuron-specific enolase.

Treatment

For localized disease, surgical resection is the standard curative modality, with a 5-year overall survival of 70% to 90%. In metastatic disease, overall survival is ~2 years, with the focus of therapy on palliating symptoms both surgically and medically. As survival with untreated carcinoid tumors can exceed 10 years, therapy is usually focused on controlling symptoms. Dietary tryptophan restriction, along with serotonin antagonists and other symptom-controlling drugs, is the initial mainstay of therapy. The somatostatin analogue **octreotide**, used at doses of 100 to 600 mcg SC/day in two to four divided doses, is effective at symptom alleviation in nearly 90% of patients. A depot formulation of octreotide available as monthly dosing has become standard. Histamine (H1 and H+) blockers, prochlorperazine, and cyproheptadine (4 to 6 mg qid) may decrease flushing. Atropine, diphenoxylate, and cyproheptadine can be used for diarrhea. Monoamine oxidase inhibitors (MAOIs) are contraindicated. **Surgery** can be risky, as anesthesia often precipitates attacks. However, resection is indicated and highly successful in localized carcinoid tumors. Preoperative administration of octreotide is necessary to prevent carcinoid crisis. **Radiation** and various **chemotherapy** regimens are typically reserved for symptomatic control of metastases in advanced disease.

PHEOCHROMOCYTOMA

Introduction

Pheochromocytomas arise from chromaffin cells primarily in the adrenal medulla (90%), although they can also arise along the aorta, within the carotid body, intracardiac, and even within the urinary bladder. This widespread distribution reflects the location of chromaffin cells associated with the sympathetic ganglia. Pheochromocytoma is present in only 0.1% of hypertensive patients who undergo urinary catecholamine quantification. The incidence of malignancy in pheochromocytomas ranges from 5% to 45% in several series. Extra-adrenal tumors are more commonly malignant. Pheochromocytomas are associated with several inherited disorders. Bilateral adrenal medullary pheochromocytomas are elements of the inherited MEN IIA and MEN IIB neuroendocrine syndromes. Although ~25% of patients with von Hippel-Lindau disease develop pheochromocytomas, <1% of patients with neurofibromatosis and Von Recklinghausen disease are found to have the tumor.

Presentation

The most common presenting complaint of patients with pheochromocytomas is severe hypertension unrelated to physical or emotional stress. The production of catecholamines results in the clinical symptoms of episodic or sustained hypertension and anxiety attacks. Pheochromocytomas have been known to produce other hormones, including ACTH, somatostatin, calcitonin, oxytocin, and vasopressin. Classically, patients describe spells of hypertension, palpitations, headaches, and diaphoresis. Other presenting findings include lactic acidosis, hypovolemia, and unexplained fever. Clinically, the cluster of symptoms can be recalled by remembering the five "Ps": pain, pressure, palpitation, perspiration, and pallor. However, it should be appreciated that many patients do not exhibit these "classic" episodes and may also have persistent hypertension, rather than episodic. The "rule of 10" is also useful in recognizing general features of pheochromocytomas: 10% are malignant, 10% are extra-adrenal, and 10% are bilateral.

Management

Diagnosis

Diagnosis and localization of pheochromocytomas are critical, as death secondary to hypertensive crisis, cerebrovascular accident, or myocardial infarction is associated with this relatively rare tumor. Pheochromocytomas represent a potentially curable cause of hypertesion with tumor resection. Traditionally, diagnosis has been based on a 24-hour measurement of catecholamines and metabolites, including vanillylmandelic acid and metanephrines, in the urine. New data suggest that a random plasma metanephrine level is extremely sensitive (~99%) in diagnosing pheochromocytoma and, therefore, is an excellent choice for initial screening. Although rarely used in clinical practice today, the clonidine suppression test has been used in the past. Normally, clonidine suppresses plasma levels of epinephrine and norepinephrine. In the presence of pheochromocytomas, no such suppression is observed.

Workup

After diagnosis, tumor localization and operative preparation are indicated, as **surgical resection** represents the mainstay of curative therapy. Localization of a pheochromocytoma is accomplished by chest and abdominal imaging with CT or MRI. Nuclear scanning after the administration of labeled metaiodobenzylguanidine can be done if the tumor is not localized by either of these other methods. Metaiodobenzylguanidine is structurally similar to norepinephrine and is selectively taken up by adrenergic tissue.

Treatment

- **Preoperative alpha-adrenergic blockade** is necessary for patients with pheochromocytomas. Traditionally, phenoxybenzamine has been used to control hypertension. Propranolol may be used to control tachycardia but must always follow alpha-adrenergic blockade to avoid hypertensive exacerbation due to unopposed vasoconstriction. Intraoperative hypertensive episodes are controlled with alpha-adrenergic blockers or sodium nitroprusside.
- **Malignant pheochromocytomas** are difficult to distinguish from benign pheochromocytomas by pathology alone. Natural history, secondary tumor sites, and recurrence help determine the nature of the pheochromocytoma. Aggressive disease may require combination chemotherapy with cyclophosphamide, vincristine, and dacarbazine. Routine **follow-up** consists of blood pressure measurements and urinary catecholamines in addition to regularly scheduled CT, MRI, or metaiodobenzylguanidine scanning to monitor for recurrence.

MULTIPLE ENDOCRINE NEOPLASIA SYNDROMES

MEN syndromes are a group of rare genetic disorders that confer an increased risk of malignancy of endocrine tissues. These disorders are grouped by the major cell type of malignancy that the affected patients are at risk for developing (Table 25-5). They share a common cell of origin (amine precursor uptake and decarboxylation [APUD] neuroendocrine cells) and are inherited in an autosomal dominant pattern.

TABLE 25-5	FEATURES OF MULTIPLE ENDOCRINE NEOPLASIA (MEN) SYNDROMES
Syndrome	**Associated Tumors and Abnormalities**
MEN I	Pituitary adenomas Pancreatic islet cell tumors or duodenal (35%–75%) Parathyroid hyperplasia (90%)
MEN IIA	Medullary carcinoma of thyroid Pheochromocytoma (bilateral) Parathyroid hyperplasia
MEN IIB	Medullary carcinoma of thyroid Pheochromocytoma (bilateral) Multiple mucosal ganglioneuromas Colonic and skeletal abnormalities with marfanoid body habitus
FMTC	Medullary carcinoma of thyroid

FMTC, familial non-MEN medullary thyroid carcinoma.

Multiple Endocrine Neoplasia I (Werner Syndrome)

This syndrome has high penetrance, with **parathyroid glands** most frequently involved. One third of gastrinomas are associated with MEN I, and pituitary adenomas can also be discovered. The MEN I gene locus has been mapped to 11q13 and codes for a tumor suppressor gene. Inheritance of the mutation is autosomal dominant. Morbidity and mortality are predominately related to duodenopancreatic malignancies. Treatment is directed by sites of tumor involvement. Patients require close follow-up for evidence of additional sites of involvement in the pituitary, parathyroid, pancreas, duodenum, adrenals, thymus, and lungs.

Multiple Endocrine Neoplasia IIA (Sipple Syndrome) and IIB

MEN II syndromes demonstrate autosomal dominant inheritance of an activating mutation of the *RET* proto-oncogene, located on chromosome 10. Nearly all patients develop MTC, which is typically multifocal and bilateral and occurs at a young age. Other features of these syndromes are expressed variably and are reported in Table 25-5. Treatment is directed by sites of tumor involvement. All patients presenting with MTC should be considered for genetic screening for *RET* proto-oncogene mutations. Furthermore, all patients with MTC should be evaluated for possible pheochromocytoma before undergoing thyroidectomy to avoid life-threatening hypertensive crisis.

Familial Non-Multiple Endocrine Neoplasia Medullary Thyroid Carcinoma (FMTC)

This disease is also associated with an autosomal dominant inheritance of the *RET* **proto-oncogene;** however, these patients develop MTC without other abnormalities associated with MEN II syndromes. Patients with MEN IIA and FMTC almost invariably develop MTC at an early age, and therefore, prophylactic thyroidectomy should be considered in patients with a known mutation.

KEY POINTS TO REMEMBER

- Endocrine malignancies are uncommon and do not necessarily result in a clinical endocrinopathy.
- The most common pituitary adenoma is the prolactinoma, and treatment is medical via dopamine agonists.
- Thyroid cancer is the most common endocrine cancer and is divided into subtypes based on original cellular histology as well as level of differentiation.
- Papillary and follicular thyroid tumors generally have an excellent prognosis in the young. These individuals can frequently be cured via surgery and radioactive iodine administrations, if necessary. Negative prognostic indicators include age >45 and distant spread.
- Anaplastic thyroid tumors are the undifferentiated versions of papillary and follicular tumors. These very aggressive cancers carry a poor prognosis, as treatment options are almost never curative.
- Medullary thyroid cancers derive from the parafollicular cells and produce calcitonin. Both sporadic and inherited forms exist. Individuals in whom genetic testing indicates MEN II or NMTC should be advised to undergo prophylactic thyroidectomy.
- Adrenal cortical carcinoma is a rare and aggressive tumor, and surgery is the treatment of choice even in advanced disease.

(*continued*)

KEY POINTS TO REMEMBER (continued)

- Carcinoid tumors may secrete vasoactive hormones. The liver can usually process and deactivate these hormones. However, when metastases reach the liver, a collection of symptoms, including flushing, edema, bronchospasm, and diarrhea (carcinoid syndrome), may result.
- Pheochromocytoma is a rare neuroendocrine tumor. It may present with a severe hypertensive episode, palpitations, diaphoresis, headaches, and/or skin pallor. Surgery is the primary therapy, although adjuvant chemotherapy is occasionally used.
- MEN syndromes are inherited in an autosomal dominate nature and MEN II is associated with *RET* proto-oncogene mutation.

REFERENCES AND SUGGESTED READINGS

Berruti A, et al., Etoposide, doxorubicin and cisplatin plus mitotane in the treatment of advanced adrenocortical carcinoma: a large prospective phase II trial. *Endocr Relat Cancer.* 2005;12(3):657–666.

Brandi ML, et al. Guidelines for diagnosis and therapy of MEN type 1 and type 2. *J Clin Endocrinol Metab.* 2001;86(12):5658–5671.

Clark OH, et al. Neuroendocrine tumors. *J Natl Compr Canc Netw.* 2006;4(2):102–138.

Hundahl SA, et al. A National Cancer Data Base report on 53,856 cases of thyroid carcinoma treated in the U.S., 1985–1995 [see comments]. *Cancer.* 1998;83(12):2638–2648.

Hundahl SA, et al. Two hundred eighty-six cases of parathyroid carcinoma treated in the U.S. between 1985-1995: a National Cancer Data Base Report. The American College of Surgeons Commission on Cancer and the American Cancer Society. *Cancer.* 1999;86(3):538–544.

Kearns AE, Thompson GB. Medical and surgical management of hyperparathyroidism. *Mayo Clin Proc.* 2002;77(1):87–91.

Kulke MH. Clinical presentation and management of carcinoid tumors. *Hematol Oncol Clin North Am.* 2007;21(3):433–455.

Mann SJ. Severe paroxysmal hypertension (pseudopheochromocytoma): understanding the cause and treatment. *Arch Intern Med.* 1999;159(7):670–674.

Mazzaferri EL, Jhiang SM. Long-term impact of initial surgical and medical therapy on papillary and follicular thyroid cancer. *Am J Med.* 1994;97(5):418–428.

Pacak K, et al. Recent advances in genetics, diagnosis, localization, and treatment of pheochromocytoma. *Ann Intern Med.* 2001;134(4):315–329.

Pei L, Melmed S. Isolation and characterization of a pituitary tumor-transforming gene (PTTG). *Mol Endocrinol.* 1997;11(4):433–441.

Schlechte JA. Clinical practice. Prolactinoma. *N Engl J Med.* 2003;349(21):2035–2041.

Schlumberger MJ. Papillary and follicular thyroid carcinoma. *N Engl J Med.* 1998;338(5):297–306.

Sherman SI, et al. Thyroid carcinoma. *J Natl Compr Canc Netw.* 2007;5(6):568–621.

Terzolo M, et al. Adjuvant mitotane treatment for adrenocortical carcinoma. *N Engl J Med.* 2007;356(23):2372–2380.

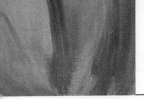

Urological Malignancies 26

Bryan A. Faller and James C. Mosley, III

PROSTATE CANCER

Introduction

Prostate cancer is the most common noncutaneous cancer among men in the United States. It was predicted to account for 29% of male cancers diagnosed in 2007 and is the third leading cause of cancer deaths in men. Although only a fraction of those with the disease will die from it, many more may suffer from its complications. These include, but are not limited to, bleeding, pain, and urinary obstruction. American men have an ~18% lifetime risk of developing cancer of the prostate and a 3.4% risk of dying from this disease. Its course, fortunately, is often indolent, and the average age at presentation is late in life. As a result of widespread screening, most patients today are diagnosed with asymptomatic, prostate-confined disease.

Epidemiology and Risk Factors

Age is the most significant risk factor. Autopsy studies show rates of >10% in men aged 40 to 49 years and up to 80% in men older than 80 years. Increased risk is conferred to patients with a positive family history and those of African American descent. High-fat diets also correlate positively with prostate cancer development. Symptomatic benign prostatic hypertrophy and history of vasectomy are *not* risk factors.

Screening

- Recommendations regarding screening for prostate cancer in asymptomatic patients remain controversial. Although treatment outcomes of patients diagnosed with early disease are substantially better than those diagnosed with late-stage disease, high-quality randomized controlled trials have yet to prove that screening decreases the morbidity or mortality of prostate cancer. Epidemiologic data, however, do suggest a benefit to screening. The mortality rate from prostate cancer has declined steadily since the introduction of the **prostate-specific antigen (PSA)** test in 1989. Several randomized studies from Canada and Italy are suggestive that screening may affect long-term outcome. Additionally, large trials suggest that tumors discovered by use of PSA screening are more likely to be confined to the prostate, a stage in which radical prostatectomy has been shown to be of significant benefit (44% relative risk reduction in cancer-specific mortality compared with expectant management). Finally, a recent analysis estimated that PSA screening has a higher positive predictive value and is more cost-effective than screening mammography for breast cancer. However, physicians should take age and comorbidities into account when deciding with their patients whether to pursue screening.
- Potential drawbacks to PSA screening include morbidity from overdiagnosis and treatment of clinically insignificant tumors. The U.S. Preventive Services Task Force

does not recommend routine screening; however, the American Cancer Society and the American Urological Association both recommend PSA screening beginning at age 50 years in patients with a life expectancy >10 years or at age 40 years if risk factors for early disease are present. In addition, annual digital rectal exams (DREs) are recommended starting at age 40.

Clinical Presentation

- Often, patients with prostate cancer are asymptomatic. However, obstructive symptoms as well as dysuria, back or hip pain, and hematuria can be initial presenting symptoms. In some cases, disease may become evident only after investigation of metastatic symptoms such as spinal cord compression, deep venous thrombosis with pulmonary embolus, and bone pain.
- Clues from **physical exam** are dependent on the DRE. The sensation of a hard and irregular nodule(s) is characteristic for the disease. Carcinoma of the prostate sometimes develops within the posterior surfaces of the lateral lobes, which are palpable during the DRE. However, deeper lesions are not detectable on routine DRE. One should recognize that detection sensitivity varies significantly between examiners owing to differences in experience and technique. Trials for detecting early disease suggest that the physical exam, or even an ultrasonography (U/S) exam, is less sensitive than measurement of PSA. Locally invasive disease may also be detectable on exam. On occasion, disease disseminates to the lymph nodes, causing evidence of scrotal or lower-extremity lymphedema.

Management

Diagnosis

- Because signs and symptoms are often nonspecific or nonexistent, diagnosis is often suggested by use of serum markers. The relatively high sensitivity (70% to 80%) and noninvasive nature of the **total serum PSA assay** have made it the most often used test. Although PSA levels fall on a continuum, a normal level is considered to be <4 ng/mL. Studies have shown that the sensitivity may increase, along with a decrease in specificity, if a cutoff value of 2.5 ng/mL is used, especially in men younger than 60. Of note, levels typically elevate with age and following prostatic massage. The PSA may be elevated, as well, in other conditions, such as benign prostatic hypertrophy and prostatitis. In the general population, a PSA level of 4 to 10 ng/mL has a positive predictive value (PPV) of 20% to 25%, whereas a level >10 ng/mL has a PPV of ~50%. Studies show that with both an abnormal DRE and a PSA >4 ng/mL, the PPV reaches 60%. Perhaps the most important feature of PSA testing is the ability to follow its change over time (PSA velocity). An increase of >0.75 ng/mL/year suggests cancer if the same assay is used.
- Although **transrectal U/S** has been used for screening in some situations, its greatest use is to guide prostatic biopsies. It should then be the next step in diagnosis if screening tests are abnormal or if a nodule is felt on exam.
- **Biopsy** is essential for diagnosis. PPVs of a first biopsy attempt range from 75% to 80% and increase to 95% with a second separate biopsy. The sensitivity can also be increased when more needle cores are obtained. A minimum of six cores is standard, although many patients routinely have 8 to 12 cores/biopsy session.
- Histologic **grade** is an important determinant of disease course and patient survival. Adenocarcinomas represent >95% of prostate cancers and are graded histologically using the **Gleason scoring system**. This system takes the two most predominant histologic patterns in the area of the tumor and assigns each a number from 1 to 5. These numbers are then added together to give the total score. *Higher scores* correlate with more poorly differentiated tumors and worse prognosis. Squamous and transitional

cell tumors make up the majority of the remaining prostate tumors, with another important subset being the high-grade neuroendocrine or small-cell tumors. Imaging studies, although well studied, have unclear utility in the initial staging. CT scans of the abdomen and pelvis and nuclear bone scans, in particular, are likely to be useful in identifying extraprostatic disease when the serum PSA exceeds 10 ng/mL. Table 26-1 reports the current TNM (tumor, node, metastasis) staging system and basic treatment guidelines, although each individual's case must be considered separately.

Treatment
- The key determinants in considering the optimal treatment of prostate cancer are estimates of life expectancy and risk of cancer progression. The risk of cancer progression can be estimated using the **pathologic stage**, which is determined by the clinical stage (based on DRE), preoperative PSA, and biopsy Gleason score. The National Comprehensive Cancer Network publishes a staging monogram based on these three features in their Clinical Practice Guidelines in Oncology. It is freely accessible at http://www.nccn.org/.

TABLE 26-1	STAGING AND TREATMENT FOR CANCER OF THE PROSTATE	
Stage	**Description**	**Initial Therapy Based on Life Expectancy**[a]
T1a	Nonpalpable; ≤5% resected tissue with cancer	<10 years: EM or RT >10 years: RadP ± PLND, RT, EM
T1b	Nonpalpable; >5% resected tissue with cancer	Same as for T1a
T1c	Nonpalpable; elevated PSA	Same as for T1a
T2a	Palpable; ≤50% of one lobe	Same as T1a
T2b	Palpable; >50% of one lobe only	<10 years: EM, RT ± PLND, or RadP ± PLND >10 years: RadP ± PLND, or RT ± PLND
T2c	Palpable; involves both lobes	Same as for T2b
T3a	Palpable; unilateral extracapsular invasion	ADT + RT, or RT, or RadP + PLND
T3b	Palpable; bilateral extracapsular invasion with seminal vesicle involvement	RT + ADT, or ADT
T4	Tumor is fixed or invades adjacent structures other than seminal vesicles	Same as for T3b
M	Distant metastases	Same as for T3b

ADT, androgen deprivation therapy; EM, expectant management; PLND, pelvic lymph node dissection; RadP, radical prostatectomy; RT, radiation therapy.

[a]For localized tumor with Gleason score = 7, or PSA level of 10 to 20 ng/mL, initial therapy is the same as for T2b. If Gleason score is 8 to 10 or PSA level is >20 ng/mL, initial therapy is the same as for T3a.

- **Expectant management.** Prostate cancer is often indolent in nature, allowing expectant management, also referred to as "watchful waiting," to be reasonable in some patients. In general, this option is reserved for patients whose life expectancy is <10 years and/or who have clinically localized disease with a low histological grade and PSA. Mortality rates from prostate cancer in this group range from 9% to 15% in the first 10 years but rise dramatically after 15 to 20 years. Younger, healthier men rarely qualify for expectant management.
  - If expectant management is chosen, regular follow-up is required and frequency varies based on estimated life expectancy. If life expectancy is >10 years, DRE and PSA testing is recommended every 6 months, with repeat needle biopsy as often as annually. If life expectancy is <10 years, PSA, DRE, and prostate biopsy may be performed less frequently. Cancer progression and alternative therapy should be considered if primary Gleason grade 4 or 5 cancer is found on repeat biopsy, a greater percentage of prostate core biopsies is involved by tumor, PSA doubling time is <3 years, or PSA velocity is >0.75 ng/year.
- **Radical prostatectomy.** Surgical therapy is indicated for all men with an estimated life expectancy >10 years and in whom disease is believed to be localized to the prostate. Earlier detection of less advanced disease, partly achieved by screening patients with serum PSA assays, has resulted in a higher number of patients receiving surgery before extracapsular spread of their cancer. In these patients, 15-year survival reaches 90%. **Complications** specific to this procedure include urethral strictures, erectile dysfunction, and urinary incontinence. Many of these men are able to benefit from the less extensive, nerve-sparing radical retropubic prostatectomy, which offers preserved erectile function. Select centers are now performing laparoscopic and robot-assisted radical prostatectomies offering the potential for decreased risk of blood loss and long-term urinary incontinence. Pelvic lymph node dissection is recommended as an adjunctive therapy when the predicted probability of lymph node metastasis is ≥7%.
- **External-beam radiation therapy** (RT). This is another viable option for patients with clinically localized (T1 or T2), low-risk disease. In several case series, the progression-free survival after RT has been found to be similar to that after radical prostatectomy, although the surgical series include longer follow-up times. Improved three-dimensional imaging techniques combined with increasingly focused radiation delivery systems, termed *conformal RT*, are allowing for delivery of higher cumulative doses of radiation, with reduced risks of toxicities. This has led to improved outcomes and tolerability of this treatment modality. The **side effects** of erectile dysfunction (40% to 50%), incontinence (1% to 2%), and urethral stricture (3% to 8%) still remain, and radiation proctitis occurs in 5% to 15% of patients. Up to 50% of patients will experience some temporary bladder or bowel symptoms during the 8 to 9 week course of treatment. External-beam RT is also the treatment of choice in patients with high-risk cancers. These patients benefit from the addition of neoadjuvant androgen deprivation therapy (ADT; see below) and bilateral pelvic lymph node irradiation. Adjuvant ADT is continued following RT for 2 to 3 years but may be abbreviated to 4 to 6 months if no more than one high-risk feature is present.
- **Brachytherapy.** This form of RT, which involves the placement of a radioactive source into the prostatic tissue, is an option for low-risk, clinically organ confined (T1c–T2a, Gleason grade 2 to 6, PSA <10 ng/mL) tumors. The benefits of **brachytherapy** include convenience (treatment is completed in 1 day), cancer-control rates comparable to radical prostatectomy for appropriate patients, and decreased risk of incontinence and early erectile dysfunction. The disadvantages include the need for general anesthesia and the risks of acute urinary retention or

prolonged irritative voiding symptoms. Brachytherapy combined with external-beam RT and neoadjuvant ADT may be effective for patients with intermediate-risk cancers, but this approach is associated with increased rates of complications.

- **Androgen deprivation therapy.** Numerous treatment options are available based on the principle that prostate cancers are testosterone dependent. These hormonal treatment options are typically used for patients who cannot tolerate other interventions but are symptomatic from localized disease, or in advanced prostate cancer. In low-risk, clinically localized disease, ADT has been found to confer no additional survival benefit. An **orchiectomy** is a simple and effective method of decreasing serum testosterone and has the benefit of being free of compliance issues for those who chose this option. **Ketoconazole** at very high doses induces a chemical castration in a short period of time, but hepatotoxicity limits its long-term use. **Estrogen therapy** with diethylstilbestrol is also effective but may increase cardiovascular mortality and cause painful gynecomastia. **Luteinizing hormone-releasing hormone** (LHRH) **agonists,** used initially with an androgen antagonist, are equally effective as bilateral orchiectomy at long-term testosterone suppression. They are the current first-line therapy for ADT. This treatment option is more expensive but has psychological advantages over surgical castration or estrogen use.
  - **Androgen antagonists** are useful for attenuating symptoms related to the initial flare of testosterone that is produced when initiating LHRH agonist therapy. Their use in conjunction with ADT or orchiectomy, however, provides no additional proven benefit. They can therefore be discontinued 7 days after the initiation of an LHRH agonist.
  - The main **adverse effects** of ADT include hot flashes, decreases in libido, and loss of muscle mass. Data also suggest that osteoporosis occurs at a higher rate with long-term androgen deprivation. For this reason, a baseline bone density screen is recommended prior to initiation of ADT. Supplementation with calcium and vitamin D is recommended for all men receiving long-term ADT. **Bisphosphonate therapy** should also be offered to men who are found to be osteopenic or osteoporotic.
  - In general, ADT should be continued in patients whose cancer relapses, as the androgen receptor remains active. For patients on a LHRH agonist alone at the time of cancer relapse, an androgen antagonist, followed by other hormonal therapy, such as estrogen or ketoconazole, may be considered.
- **Chemotherapy.** Many men receiving ADT will eventually develop increasing PSA values despite continued therapy. This progression of disease is termed androgen-independent prostate cancer and is due to adaptations at the cellular level that allow the prostate cancer cell to grow despite a low-androgen environment. It is now common practice to use systemic **chemotherapy** in treating this stage of disease. A **docetaxel**-based regimen with prednisone is the current standard-of-care therapy for patients with androgen-independent prostate cancer, based on a demonstrated survival benefit over mitoxantrone- and corticosteroid-based regimens in two recent phase III trials (Southwest Oncology Group [SWOG] 9916 and TAX 327). **Bisphosphonate therapy** should also be considered in all patients with androgen-independent prostate cancer, as it is postulated to prevent skeletal related events in addition to improving bone mineral density.

RENAL CELL CARCINOMA

Introduction

Less prevalent than prostate cancer, renal cell carcinoma represents ~2% of all cancers. However, it rarely produces symptoms or signs until later stages of the disease, at which time the chances of cure have drastically diminished.

Epidemiology and Risk Factors

The overall incidence of renal cell carcinoma is on the rise, but it remains twice as common in men as women, with equal incidence in blacks and whites. The higher incidence in males may change as smoking rates equalize between men and women. As with most cancers, age is the major risk factor. Accordingly, disease predominantly presents in the seventh and eighth decades of life. Other apparent, but not absolute, risk factors include cigarette smoking, obesity, hypertension, and heavy metal or petroleum product exposure. Although hereditary forms of the disease occur uncommonly, one clear genetic linkage is with von Hippel-Lindau disease. Nearly 40% of these individuals develop multifocal renal cell carcinoma with clear cell histology.

Presentation

Hematuria, abdominal pain, and a palpable flank or abdominal mass is the classic triad for diagnosis of renal cell carcinoma, but this triad occurs in combination only 10% of the time. In general, most small tumors produce very few symptoms. Other nonspecific symptoms include fever, night sweats, feeling of malaise, and weight loss. One interesting potential presenting symptom in men is a left-sided varicocele, secondary to obstruction of the left testicular vein. Diagnosis of earlier stages of renal cell carcinoma has improved, predominantly because of incidental findings during an abdominal CT or U/S performed for other indications. At diagnosis, 20% to 30% of tumors are overtly metastatic, often to the lung, bone, liver, and brain. Paraneoplastic syndromes are rare but include erythrocytosis and hypercalcemia from overproduction of erythropoietin or parathyroid hormone-related protein, respectively.

Management

Diagnosis

Contrast-enhanced CT has a >90% sensitivity in detecting tumors of ≤3 cm. Sensitivity of U/S is ~80% for similar tumors. CT scans are also highly useful in determining cancer staging preoperatively. MRI with gadolinium enhancement is superior to CT imaging and is appropriate in those who have an IV contrast allergy or in whom inferior vena cava involvement is suspected. Despite the high sensitivity of available imaging techniques, diagnosis still relies on histologic exam of tissue. In addition to renal cell carcinoma, differential diagnosis of a renal mass includes squamous and transitional cell carcinoma of the renal pelvis, Wilms' tumor, sarcoma, and metastatic disease.

Staging and Prognosis

The current standard TNM staging system of the American Joint Committee on Cancer is most often employed for assigning renal cell carcinoma a pathologic stage. This stage is the most important factor in determining survival. Other prognostic factors affecting 5-year survival include tumor grade, local extent of the tumor, presence of regional nodal metastases, and evidence of metastatic disease at presentation. Table 26-2 lists 5-year overall survival rates based on pathologic stage.

Treatment

- The mainstay of therapy in stage I to II, localized disease is **surgical resection.** Radical nephrectomy (resection of kidney and perirenal fat) and nephron-sparing surgery (partial nephrectomy) have both been studied. For patients without large superior-pole tumors or abnormal-appearing adrenal glands on CT scan, overall patient survival data are similar between the two procedures. While indications for partial nephrectomy classically include bilateral tumors or a functional/anatomic solitary kidney, this method is also increasingly used in patients with small unilateral lesions (up to 7 cm).

TABLE 26-2	STAGING OF RENAL CELL CARCINOMA AND 5-YEAR SURVIVAL RATES	
Description of Disease Extent	**AJCC Equivalent**	**5-year Survival (%)**
Confined to renal capsule		65–85
≤7 cm	I	
>7 cm	II	
Extends through renal capsule but not through Gerota's fascia	III	45–80
Renal vein, IVC, or regional nodal involvement	III	15–50
Extends through Gerota's fascia, >1 lymph node, or distant metastases	IV	0–10

AJCC, American Joint Committee on Cancer; IVC, inferior vena cava.

Adapted from American Joint Committee on Cancer. *AJCC Cancer Staging Manual.* 6th ed. New York: Springer-Verlag; 2002.

- After surgical resection, patients should be followed with repeat imaging for evidence of recurrence. Approximately 20% to 30% of all patients with localized disease who undergo surgical resection will relapse.
- Patients with metastatic disease at diagnosis should still be considered for nephrectomy if their medical condition allows. Patients with single sites of metastases that are amenable to resection can undergo metastectomy, with increased disease-free survival. Patients with multiple sites of metastatic disease can be considered for cytoreductive surgery.
- Although numerous regimens have been tried, chemotherapeutic and hormonal therapies have been largely ineffective at treating metastatic renal cell carcinoma. Until recently, use of **immunomodulatory therapies,** including those with high-dose interleukin-2 and/or interferon-alpha had been the standard of care. Overall response rates up to 20% had been noted and up to 5% of patients treated with these regimens attained prolonged complete responses. However, these regimens are quite toxic and poorly tolerated.
- Currently, the standard of care for metastatic renal cell carcinoma includes the use of **targeted therapies.** In recent studies, the oral, small-molecule, multi-tyrosine kinase inhibitors sunitinib and sorafenib have been demonstrated to significantly increase progression-free survival, as well as to likely increase overall survival. These medications are generally well tolerated, with common side effects of hand-foot syndrome and worsening hypertension. The MTOR inhibitor temsirolimus also improves progression-free and overall survival.

TESTICULAR CANCER

Introduction

Germ cell tumors, which comprise 95% of malignant testicular tumors, are relatively uncommon, accounting for 2% of all human malignancies. Although testicular cancer is relatively rare, it is an important cancer to recognize, as it typically affects younger patients. It also is amenable to screening by patient self-exam and is a highly curable tumor in most circumstances.

Epidemiology

Testicular cancer is the most common cancer among men aged 15 to 35 years. Incidence is much higher in whites than blacks. Family history of a germ cell tumor, cryptorchidism, and Klinefelter syndrome are additional predisposing factors. Orchiopexy to the undescended testis does not modify the risk of malignancy in cryptorchidism, but it does allow for easier testicular examination.

Causes

The **differential diagnosis** consists of infections as well as benign masses, such as epidermoid cyst, spermatoceles, and varicoceles. Lymphoma is the second most common testicular tumor. Metastases to the testicles are rare.

Pathology

Testicular tumors are divided into **seminomas** and **nonseminoma tumors.** The nonseminoma tumors include embryonal carcinomas, teratomas, choriocarcinomas, and mixed germ cell types. Leydig, granulosa, and Sertoli cell tumors occur rarely. Nonseminomas are clinically more aggressive tumors. If elements of both seminoma and nonseminoma are found on biopsy, management follows that for nonseminomas.

Presentation

A painless testicular mass is the classic presenting symptom and sign, but diffuse testicular pain or swelling is present in many patients. Physical exam should focus on the testicles, lymphadenopathy (particularly supraclavicular), scrotal edema, and evaluation for gynecomastia. Early metastases to bone are rare but possible, and back pain can result from bulky retroperitoneal lymphadenopathy. Patients are often treated initially with a course of antibiotics for possible epididymitis or orchitis.

Management

Diagnosis and Workup

- If symptoms persist after a course of antibiotics or if a mass is palpated, scrotal U/S is the initial test of choice. Unless U/S results indicate otherwise, an orchiectomy by inguinal approach is necessary for diagnosis.
- **Serum tumor markers**—beta human chorionic gonadotropin (β-hCG), lactate dehydrogenase, and alpha-fetoprotein—are important in diagnosis and monitoring therapeutic response. All three markers may be present in nonseminomas, with β-hCG being present in 100% of choriocarcinoma subtype tumors. Seminomas occasionally express β-hCG, but never express alpha-fetoprotein.
- Other preoperative workup should include a chest x-ray in addition to routine chemistry and hematology. Testicular U/S is an optional study, especially when the diagnosis is clinically obvious, but it is useful in helping to define the lesion and in examining the contralateral testicle. Abdominal and pelvic CT exams are useful in assessing nodal enlargement and for staging. In general, stage I disease is localized to the testis, stage II disease has spread to retroperitoneal lymph nodes, and stage III disease is metastatic or has spread to lymph nodes above the diaphragm.
- Finally, the option of sperm banking should be discussed prior to the initiation of any therapy.

Prognosis

The **prognosis** for GCTs is generally very favorable. More than 90% of patients diagnosed with these tumors are cured, including 70% to 80% of patients with advanced tumors treated with chemotherapy.

Treatment

- **Surgery.** Transinguinal orchiectomy is the preferred surgical approach and is necessary for staging and diagnosis. The transscrotal approach has increased risk of tumor seeding. An open inguinal biopsy of the contralateral testis should be performed in cases of cryptorchidism, in cases of marked testicular atrophy, or if abnormalities are seen on U/S.
- **Surveillance.** Some patients with early-stage disease who are anticipated to be highly compliant with follow-up and for whom RT is relatively contraindicated may be observed after orchiectomy without adjuvant therapy. This option is rarely recommended for the treatment of seminomas given the low morbidity of RT for this indication, and the high relapse rate (15% to 20%) seen following orchiectomy without adjuvant RT.
- **Treatment of Seminomas.** Seminomas are highly radiosensitive, and thus infradiaphragmatic RT is the preferred adjuvant therapy for stage I and stage II tumors without bulky lymphadenopathy. For stage I disease, **chemotherapy,** consisting of a single dose of carboplatin, has been shown in one randomized trial not to be inferior to RT for progression-free survival and offers another alternative to adjuvant RT. If nonbulky nodal involvement is present, RT along with orchiectomy is the preferred approach for stage II tumors. Chemotherapy with etoposide and cisplatin remains an alternative option for patients in whom RT would not be tolerated. For bulky stage II or stage III disease, chemotherapy is the preferred management, with etoposide and cisplatin ± bleomycin.
- **Treatment of nonseminomatous tumors.** These tumors are less radiosensitive, and patients often require additional surgical therapies following orchiectomy. In general, most patients with nonseminoma will undergo sympathetic nerve-sparing, retroperitoneal lymph node dissection for either diagnostic or therapeutic purposes. The major morbidity of this surgery is retrograde ejaculation with resulting infertility, which occurs in ~10% of cases using an open nerve dissection technique. Adjuvant chemotherapy is often recommended if the surgical resection reveals lymph node involvement or in stage III disease. Etoposide and cisplatin ± bleomycin is the chemotherapeutic regimen of choice. Residual tumor following chemotherapy often consists of chemoinsensitive teratomas. These should be removed surgically.

Follow-up

Patients with testicular cancer should have close **follow-up** after diagnosis and treatment. This includes serial chest x-rays, CT scanning of the abdomen and pelvis, and blood work for relevant tumor markers, in addition to a detailed clinical exam. PET scanning may have a role in surveillance, but this has yet to be fully determined. Screening for **late effects** of platinum-based chemotherapy, most commonly dyslipidemias, cardiovascular disease, and cerebrovascular diseases, should be included in follow-up as well. High-frequency hearing loss and Raynaud phenomenon are other commonly experienced side effects, as well as a slightly higher than background risk of acute leukemia.

CANCER OF THE URINARY BLADDER

Introduction

Bladder cancer is the fourth most common cancer in men and the eighth most common in women. It represents a significant source of morbidity and mortality in the United

States, accounting for ~13,000 deaths in 2006. Similar to prostate cancer, the median age at presentation is late in life (65 years), and therefore medical comorbidities and life expectancy play key roles in management decisions.

Epidemiology

Bladder cancer is primarily a malignancy of the epithelium, occurring in individuals >60 years old. Urothelial (transitional cell) carcinomas are the most common histological subtype and account for >90% of bladder tumors. There is a male predominance (roughly 2.7:1), and nearly three fourths of all cases can be linked to cigarette smoking or exposure to industrial dyes and solvents. Occupational exposure to aromatic amines in the dye industry is a risk factor. Similarly, occupational exposure can also occur in the rubber, leather, textile, paint, printing, and hairdressing industries. Although uncommon in the United States, squamous cell carcinoma is a prevalent subtype in areas endemic for *Schistosoma haematobium*.

Presentation

Symptoms are not always appreciated by patients, but **hematuria** is present in ~90% of individuals with bladder cancer. This may be intermittent or constant, frank or microscopic, and is occasionally associated with symptoms of urinary frequency or urgency.

Management

Diagnosis and Workup

- Urine cytology may yield the diagnosis, but the gold standard is cystoscopy with biopsy. If bladder cancer is found on cystoscopy, a transurethral resection of the bladder tumor (TURBT) should be arranged, preferably following a CT of the abdomen and pelvis if invasive or high-grade features are present. Intravenous pyelogram and retrograde pyelogram should be performed to evaluate the upper urinary tracts. Other imaging modalities, including MRI, U/S, and bone scintigraphy, may be useful for disease staging and may be performed as clinically indicated.
- Staging of bladder cancer is primarily based on pathologic findings, including depth of invasion, tumor grade, and spread outside of the bladder. Fifty percent to 80% of bladder cancers are superficial at presentation, having not yet reached muscular layers of the bladder, lymph nodes, or other distant sites. Proper treatment by transurethral resection and intravesicular chemotherapy may lead to prolonged disease-free survival in >80% of these patients.

Treatment

Local treatment of the bladder, via urethral catheter with **intravesicular chemotherapy**, is used as adjuvant treatment following TURBT to eradicate remaining disease and reduce the risk of recurrence. Bacillus Calmette-Guérin (BCG) is the most common and effective intravesicular agent used, but others, including mitomycin-C, interferon, and doxorubicin, are also used. If imaging and initial transurethral resection reveal more advanced cancer, a partial or radical cystectomy with lymph node dissection may be necessary. The role of RT has not been well defined. RT has been recommended for treatment of patients who would not tolerate cystectomy or in those who hope to preserve their bladder. For both of these indications, combination treatment with chemotherapy may be warranted based on individual patient characteristics. The role of **chemotherapy** in the treatment of resectable bladder cancers is also controversial. Increasing data support the role of neoadjuvant chemotherapy before cystectomy in patients with tumor invading the muscle or perivesical tissue. Definitive recommendations on adjuvant chemotherapy await well-designed randomized controlled trials, but there is evidence to suggest it is effective at delaying recurrences of high-risk malignancies. In patients found to have unresectable or metastatic disease on presentation (~15%), chemotherapy ± RT is the treatment of choice. In general, cis-platin-based regimens are recommended as first-line therapy. More recently, gemcitabine and taxane regimens have also been shown to provide effective control.

KEY POINTS TO REMEMBER

- Prostate cancer is the most common cancer among men, but many men die *with* the disease rather than *from* it.
- The preferred approach to screening for prostate cancer includes the serum PSA test in combination with the DRE. Because no study has unequivocally proven that screening decreases morbidity or mortality, the decision to screen patients may be individualized.
- Because of prostate cancer's indolent course, treatment options are based on an individual patient's life expectancy, along with risk of tumor progression.
- Renal cell carcinoma's classic triad—hematuria, abdominal pain, and a palpable flank or abdominal mass—is present in only 10% of patients.
- Surgery is currently the mainstay of therapy for renal cell carcinoma.
- The paradigm of treatment for metastatic renal cell carcinoma has changed recently, and first-line therapies include the oral multi-tyrosine kinase inhibitors, sorafenib and sunitinib.
- Testicular cancer is the most common cancer in men aged 15 to 35 years and often presents as a painless testicular mass.
- Treatments for testicular cancer are highly successful, with cure rates of >85% for most cases. Orchiectomy is necessary for diagnosis and treatment.
- Seminomas are exquisitely sensitive to RT if cancer spreads to the retroperitoneal lymph nodes.
- Most bladder cancers are superficial at the time of diagnosis and can be treated by transurethral excision and intravesicular chemotherapy.

REFERENCES AND SUGGESTED READINGS

DeVita VT, Hellman S, Rosenberg SA, eds. *Cancer: Principles and Practice of Oncology*. 7th ed. Philadelphia: Lippincott Williams & Wilkins; 2004.

National Comprehensive Cancer Network: NCCN Practice Guidelines in Oncology: Bladder Cancer. Version 1: 2007. Available at: http://www.nccn.org/. Accessed May 13, 2007.

National Comprehensive Cancer Network. NCCN Practice Guidelines in Oncology: Prostate Cancer. Version 2: 2007. Available at: http://www.nccn.org/. Accessed May 13, 2007.

National Comprehensive Cancer Network: NCCN Practice Guidelines in Oncology: Testicular Cancer. Version 1: 2007. Available at: http://www.nccn.org/. Accessed May 13, 2007.

Stephenson A, Kuritzky L, Campbell S. Screening for urological malignancies in primary care: pros, cons, and recommendations. *Cleve Clin J Med*. 2007;74(Suppl 3):S6–S14.

Wilson SS, Crawford ED. Screening for prostate cancer: current recommendations. *Urol Clin North Am*. 2004;31:219–226.

Gynecologic Oncology

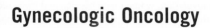

Andrea R. Hagemann and Israel Zighelboim

INTRODUCTION

Tumors of the female reproductive tract are often diagnosed and managed by the combined efforts of the primary care physician, gynecologist, gynecologic oncologist, and radiation oncologist. This chapter describes the approach to common gynecologic oncology evaluations, as well as briefly discussing selected gynecologic tumors.

VAGINAL BLEEDING

Differential Diagnosis

Vaginal bleeding can be caused by exogenous hormones, endocrine imbalances including hyper- or hypothyroidism and diabetes mellitus, anatomic causes such as fibroids, polyps, or cervical lesions, hematologic causes such as coagulopathy, infectious causes such as cervicitis from *C. trachomatis*, and neoplasia. Organic causes are either related to genital tract pathology or secondary to a systemic disease. Cervical and endometrial cancers are the most common malignancies that result in vaginal bleeding. Dysfunctional uterine bleeding (DUB) is considered a diagnosis of exclusion and is the term used to describe abnormal bleeding for which no specific structural cause can be identified.

Presentation
History
A thorough medical and gynecologic history, with careful attention to last menstrual period and amount and duration of bleeding, should be obtained.

Physical Exam
A careful gynecologic exam, including a speculum exam and pelvic exam, should be performed. A Papanicolaou (Pap) smear should be obtained, and any suspicious cervical or vulvar lesions should be biopsied. A rectal exam with stool Guaiac should also be performed.

Management
Lab Analysis
Appropriate laboratory studies include a complete blood count to detect anemia or thrombocytopenia and a pregnancy test in reproductive-aged women. In certain individuals, thyroid stimulating hormone and screening coagulation studies may be appropriate to rule out thyroid dysfunction and a primary coagulation problem, respectively. Von Willebrand disease is a common cause of heavy menses, especially in adolescent women (see Chap. 7).

Diagnosis

Women with chronic anovulation, women with obesity, and those older than 35 years of age require further evaluation. A vaginal ultrasound can be helpful in evaluating for anatomic abnormalities, and assessment of endometrial stripe thickness may prove useful in postmenopausal women. Endometrial sampling, accomplished in the office using disposable plastic cannulae, should be performed in these women, as they are at risk for polyps, hyperplasia, or carcinoma of the endometrium.

Treatment

- In most cases, abnormal bleeding can be managed medically. Hormonal management, including oral contraceptives, can be used to significantly reduce blood flow. When estrogen is contraindicated, progestins can be used, including cyclic oral medroxyprogesterone acetate, depot forms of medroxyprogesterone acetate, and the levonorgestrel-containing intrauterine device, which has been shown to decrease menstrual blood loss by 80% to 90%.
- Surgical management ranges from endometrial ablation, hysteroscopy with resection of uterine polyps or leiomyomas, myomectomy, uterine artery embolization, magnetic resonance-guided focused ultrasonography ablation, and, most definitively, hysterectomy.
- Acute, profound vaginal bleeding should first be managed by assessing for a primary coagulation disorder. If anovulatory bleeding is established as the working diagnosis, hormonal therapy with oral or intravenous estrogen will usually control bleeding. If hormonal management fails, a structural cause of bleeding is more likely.

PELVIC MASS

Differential Diagnosis

A variety of entities may result in the development of a pelvic mass. These may be gynecologic in origin or, alternatively, may arise from the urinary or gastrointestinal (GI) tracts. Gynecologic causes of a pelvic mass may be uterine, adnexal, or, more specifically, ovarian. Age is an important determinant of the likelihood of malignancy.

Ovarian Masses

Ovarian masses can be functional or neoplastic; neoplastic masses can be either benign or malignant.

- **Ovarian cysts.** Functional ovarian cysts include follicular cysts, corpus luteum cysts, and theca lutein cysts. Women with endometriosis can develop ovarian endometriomas. Follicular cysts, defined by a diameter >3 cm, are most common, and are most often <8 cm. They usually resolve spontaneously and only require expectant management. Corpus luteum cysts can rupture, leading to hemoperitoneum, which may occasionally require surgical management. Theca lutein cysts are usually bilateral and occur with pregnancy due to ovarian stimulation by human chorionic gonadotropin (hCG). These cysts may be prominent in certain conditions such as multiple and molar pregnancies. Combination monophasic oral contraceptives can reduce the incidence of these functional cysts.
- **Neoplastic masses.** The most common benign ovarian neoplasm is the mucinous cystadenoma. Eighty percent of cystic teratomas (dermoid cysts) occur during the reproductive years. Epithelial tumors of the ovary increase with age, and benign tumors of this type include serous and mucinous cystadenomas, fibromas, and Brenner tumors. Malignant ovarian neoplasms are discussed in the following section.
- **Other.** Adnexal masses arising from the fallopian tube are primarily related to inflammatory causes in the reproductive age group. Examples of masses in this category include ectopic pregnancy, tubo-ovarian abscesses, and paraovarian or paratubal cysts.

Uterine Masses

Uterine leiomyomas, commonly referred to as fibroids, are the most common benign uterine tumors. Asymptomatic fibroids are present in up to 50% of women older than age 35. Degenerative changes can occur in these tumors. Smooth muscle tumors of the uterus rather represent a continuum that ranges from benign lesions (leiomyoma or fibroid) to malignant neoplasms (leiomyosarcoma). Smooth muscle tumors of uncertain malignant potential have 5 to 9 mitoses per 10 high-power fields (hpf) and do not demonstrate nuclear atypia or giant cells. Leiomyosarcomas typically have ≥10 or more mitoses/hpf and demonstrate nuclear atypia.

Presentation

History

History should include any history of urinary or GI symptoms, pelvic pain, or vaginal bleeding.

Physical exam

A complete pelvic exam, including a rectovaginal exam and Pap test, should be performed. Evidence of ascites or a pleural effusion heightens the suspicion for a malignant ovarian tumor.

Management

Workup

Pelvic ultrasonography, usually done transvaginally, will help to clarify the origin of the mass. Endometrial sampling with an endometrial biopsy or dilatation and curettage is necessary if both a pelvic mass and abnormal bleeding are present. Laboratory studies should include cervical cytology, complete blood count, testing of stool for occult blood, and a pregnancy test in reproductive-age women. CA-125 is a nonspecific tumor marker that may be obtained, but be aware that a number of benign conditions, including leiomyomas, pelvic inflammatory disease, pregnancy, and endometriosis can cause elevations of this marker. A barium enema or other study of the GI tract may be indicated to exclude a GI etiology.

Management and Follow-up

Once a nongynecologic problem is excluded, management depends on the size of the mass and age of the patient. Premenopausal women with an adnexal mass <8 cm, with predominantly cystic features, can be followed with close observation and/or hormonal suppression. Women with a mass >8 cm, those with complex, solid, or suspicious features on ultrasound, and those whose masses persist or progress with close follow-up should be managed surgically by a gynecologist or a gynecologic oncologist. Recently, the American College of Obstetrics and Gynecologists, along with the Society of Gynecologic Oncologists, released guidelines for referral to a gynecologic oncologist for a pelvic mass. In these guidelines, they state that premenopausal women with any of the following should be referred: CA-125 >200 U/mL, ascites, evidence of abdominal or distant metastasis (by imaging or exam), or family history of breast or ovarian cancer in a first-degree relative. The criteria for referral for postmenopausal women are slightly different: CA-125 >35 U/mL, ascites, evidence of abdominal or distant metastasis (by imaging or exam), and family history of breast or ovarian cancer in a first-degree relative. Surgery can be done laparoscopically or by laparotomy depending on the size of the mass and concern for malignancy. Most postmenopausal women with an adnexal mass should undergo surgery to rule out an ovarian malignancy.

CERVICAL CANCER

Epidemiology

It was estimated that in 2007, there would be ~11,150 new cases of invasive cervical cancer in the United States, resulting in more than 3600 deaths. Worldwide, 370,000 cases are identified each year. Despite the fact that screening programs are becoming more established, cervical cancer is still the leading cause of death from cancer among women in developing countries and second only to breast cancer worldwide.

Natural History

Invasive cancer of the cervix is considered a preventable disease. There is a long preinvasive state (cervical dysplasia), and cytologic screening programs as well as effective treatments are readily available. Cervical intraepithelial neoplasia is a precancerous lesion of the cervix.

Risk Factors

Several risk factors for cervical cancer have been identified. These include young age at first intercourse (<16 years), multiple sexual partners, cigarette smoking, immunosuppression, African American or Hispanic ethnicity, high parity, and lower socioeconomic status. Human papilloma virus infection is detected in up to 99% of women with squamous cell cervical cancer.

Screening

The Pap smear is the standard screening test for cervical cancer. Annual cervical cytology screening should begin ~3 years after the initiation of sexual intercourse but no later than age 21. Women younger than 30 years should undergo annual cervical cytology screening. Women aged 30 years and older who have had three consecutive negative cervical cytology screening test results, with no history of high-grade dysplasia, are not immunocompromised and were not exposed to diethylstilbestrol in utero may extend the interval between cytology examinations to 2 to 3 years. The combination of cytology and screening for high-risk subtypes of human papilloma virus can be appropriate for women older than age 30. If such combined screening results are negative, they should be screened no more often than every 3 years. Gardasil, a quadrivalent vaccine against human papilloma virus types 6, 11, 16, and 18, is now approved for girls ages 9 to 26. Cytologic screening is still recommended for those receiving the vaccine.

Classification

The most common histologic types identified in cases of invasive cervical cancer are squamous cell carcinoma (85%) and adenocarcinoma (5%). Less common histologies include neuroendocrine carcinoma, melanoma, and sarcomas (embryonal rhabdomyosarcoma in children and young adults).

Clinical Presentation

The most common symptom in women with cancer of the cervix is vaginal bleeding, which can often be postcoital. Asymptomatic women are usually diagnosed on the basis of abnormal cytology. Advanced disease may present with symptoms of malodorous discharge, weight loss, or obstructive uropathy. Physical exam may reveal a palpable cervical mass, and palpation of the inguinal and supraclavicular nodes may reveal lymphadenopathy.

Diagnosis

If a gross lesion is present, cervical biopsy should be performed. Abnormal cytologic screening should be evaluated as indicated with colposcopy and directed biopsies, along with endocervical curettage. Cervical cancer is a clinically staged disease, often via an exam under anesthesia to yield the most accurate assessment. Cystoscopy, proctoscopy, chest radiographs, and intravenous pyelograms may be used for staging purposes. CT, MRI, and PET scan are commonly used in the evaluation of disease extension and for treatment planning. However, such imaging modalities should not alter the clinical stage.

Treatment

The treatment of cervical cancer is determined by the clinical stage of disease, with the underlying principal that therapy should consist of either radiation or surgery alone in order to prevent increased morbidity that results when the two are combined.

Surgical Management

Surgical management is generally limited to patients with disease limited to the cervix or with limited involvement of the upper vagina. Depending on the clinical stage, fertility goals, and physical condition of the patient, surgical treatment ranges from cone excision of the cervix, to simple hysterectomy, to radical trachelectomy (where the cervix and parametria are removed with preservation of the uterine corpus), to radical hysterectomy.

Radiation Therapy

Radiation therapy can be classified as either primary or adjuvant therapy. Primary therapy combines external radiotherapy to treat parametria and regional lymph nodes and to lessen tumor volume with brachytherapy to target the central tumor. Brachytherapy is delivered by intracavitary or interstitial implants. Intensity modulated radiotherapy utilizes computer algorithms to distinguish between normal and diseased tissues in order to optimize the delivery of radiation to the affected area while minimizing radiation complications. Adjuvant radiotherapy is often used postoperatively for patients with metastases to pelvic lymph nodes or channels, invasion of paracervical tissue, deep cervical invasion, or positive surgical margins. This has been shown to decrease pelvic recurrence but not necessarily to improve 5-year survival rates. Complications of radiation therapy include vasculitis and fibrosis of the bowel and bladder, as well as bowel and bladder fistulas.

Chemotherapy

Randomized trials have shown that the addition of chemotherapy to radiation therapy (known as chemoradiation) improves survival in patients with locally advanced cervical cancer. Chemotherapy allows for systemic treatment as well as sensitization of cancer cells to radiation therapy to improve local and regional control. Cisplatin-based adjuvant chemotherapy is the treatment of choice for patients with locally advanced cervical cancer. Single-agent platinum or multiagent chemotherapy with platinum in combination with topotecan or paclitaxel are usually prescribed in cases of advanced or recurrent cervical cancer. Multiagent chemotherapy may offer improved response rates and modest survival benefits at the expense of increased toxicity.

Recurrence

Patients treated for cervical cancer require careful follow-up with clinical exams, Pap smears, and various imaging modalities, as indicated. Pelvic recurrences in patients initially treated by surgery are usually treated with radiation therapy. Cases of isolated central recurrences after radiation may be salvaged by radical or ultraradical (exenterative) surgical procedures. Systemic recurrences are most often treated with platinum-based chemotherapy.

Prognosis

The 5-year survival rate for early stage cervical cancer is ~85% with either radiation therapy or radical hysterectomy. For patients with locoregional extension, 5-year survival falls to ≤40%.

OVARIAN CANCER

Epidemiology

In the United States, 1 in 70 women will develop ovarian cancer in her lifetime (lifetime risk, ~1.4%). In 2007, it was estimated that 22,430 new cases of ovarian cancer would be diagnosed in the United States, and 15,280 deaths were expected to occur as a result of ovarian cancer. Epithelial ovarian cancer, which accounts for ~90% of all ovarian cancers, is the leading cause of death from gynecologic cancer in the United States. This type of cancer is often diagnosed at an advanced stage, as patients usually remain asymptomatic until metastasis occurs. The peak incidence of invasive epithelial ovarian cancer is 56 to 60 years of age. Germ cell and sex cord stromal tumors are less common and typically occur in adolescents and younger women.

Risk Factors

Ovarian cancer has been associated with low parity and infertility; risk factors include early menarche and late menopause. Oral contraceptive use for ≥5 years has been shown to reduce the likelihood of ovarian cancer by 50%. Mutations in BRCA-1 and BRCA-2, along with Lynch or hereditary nonpolyposis colorectal cancer syndrome (HNPCC), are important risk factors for ovarian cancer. In some patients, prophylactic oophorectomy may be a reasonable approach, but this decision must be highly individualized.

Screening

There is considerable public controversy regarding ovarian cancer screening, but unfortunately, the value of tumor markers and ultrasonography to screen for epithelial ovarian cancer has not been clearly established by prospective studies. Recently, the tumor marker CA-125 has played an important role in the diagnosis, management, and follow-up of patients with ovarian cancer. Particularly in premenopausal women, CA-125 testing and transvaginal ultrasonography have not been shown to be cost effective and should not be used routinely to screen for ovarian cancer in the general population. Different screening strategies are an active area of study in ovarian cancer research.

History

Symptoms from ovarian cancer can be vague and nonspecific, and many women remain asymptomatic for long periods of time. Abdominal distention, nausea, vomiting, early satiety, and increased abdominal girth may be reported. In premenopausal women, irregular or heavy menses may be noted. The Society of Gynecologic Oncologists has recently presented the Ovarian Cancer Symptoms Consensus Statement in an attempt to educate the general public about the signs and symptoms of ovarian cancer. The document states that women who have certain symptoms (bloating, pelvic and abdominal pain, difficulty eating, and early satiety as well as urinary urgency or frequency) on a daily basis for more than a few weeks should be specifically evaluated to rule out the possibility of ovarian cancer by means of a skillful pelvic exam, ultrasound examination, and CA-125 determination, as indicated.

Physical Exam

The most important sign on physical exam is the presence of a pelvic mass or ascites. Pleural effusions are not uncommon.

Diagnosis

The diagnosis of ovarian cancer must be made by surgical exploration and pathologic confirmation. Prior to exploratory laparotomy, a CA-125 level should be drawn, and other primary cancers metastatic to the ovaries should be excluded, specifically colon, gastric, or breast (via barium enema or colonoscopy, upper GI, and mammogram, respectively). Preoperative evaluation may also include a CT of the chest, abdomen, and pelvis to assess for extra-abdominal disease and parenchymal liver lesions.

Treatment

- Treatment of ovarian cancer begins with surgical staging and cytoreduction. Thorough surgical staging is essential, as subsequent treatment will be based directly on the surgical stage. Cytoreduction, or debulking, refers to removing as much gross tumor as technically feasible. Optimal debulking, where the residual macroscopic tumor is <1 to 2 cm, and ideally <0.5 cm, has been shown improve survival as well as responsiveness to subsequent chemotherapy. After cytoreductive surgery, adjuvant chemotherapy with a taxane- and platinum-containing compound is used unless precluded by toxicity. Multiple studies have evaluated the role of intraperitoneal chemotherapy in patients with ovarian cancer. Recently, a randomized prospective Gynecologic Oncology Group study has shown that intraperitoneal cisplatin with intravenous paclitaxel improves disease-free and overall survival compared to intravenous cisplatin and paclitaxel in patients with optimally cytoreduced ovarian cancer. In general, the administration of intraperitoneal chemotherapy involves significant toxicity. However, quality of life 1 year after treatment is comparable in patients treated intravenously versus intraperitoneally.

- Approximately 85% of patients with early-stage and 50% of patients with advanced ovarian cancer experience a complete response after initial treatment with cytoreductive surgery and combination chemotherapy. However, a large number of patients, especially those with advanced disease, will eventually recur and require additional treatment. Treatment in the recurrent setting usually consists of chemotherapy. Selected patients will undergo secondary cytoreductive surgery. In general, patients who present with recurrence or progression more than 6 months after platinum-based chemotherapy are "platinum sensitive" and therefore treated with combination chemotherapy including platinum compounds. Those who have recurrences within 6 months of platinum-based therapy are considered platinum resistant. These patients are treated with second-line chemotherapy agents such as pegylated liposomal doxorubicin, topotecan, and gemcitabine, among others. Biologic and/or hormonal agents are used in selected cases, alone or in combination with cytotoxic chemotherapy.

Prognosis

Surgical staging is the most important prognostic variable for patients with ovarian cancer. Five-year survival rates are estimated to be 75% to 95% for patients with disease limited to the ovaries and 10% to 25% for those with extensive peritoneal disease or extraperitoneal metastases at diagnosis. Other independent prognostic variables include extent of residual disease after primary surgery, histologic grade, volume of ascites, patient age, performance status, and platinum-free interval before recurrence. Following initial treatment, patients are followed with serial CA-125 levels, pelvic exams, and CT scans, as indicated.

ENDOMETRIAL CANCER

Epidemiology

Endometrial cancer is the most common gynecologic malignancy diagnosed in developed countries and accounts for more than 90% of malignancies affecting the uterine corpus. It was estimated that in 2007, ~39,000 new cases of uterine cancer would be diagnosed and 7400 women would die of this disease in the United States. The median age at diagnosis is 63 years.

Classification

Patients with endometrial carcinomas can be generally classified in two groups. The largest group is represented by estrogen-dependent or type I tumors. These patients tend to be younger at diagnosis. Unopposed estrogenic stimulation of the endometrium in these cases is thought to cause endometrial hyperplasia and well- to moderately differentiated endometrioid carcinomas. Tumors of this type usually carry an overall better prognosis. Risk factors for type I endometrial cancer include iatrogenic unopposed stimulation of estrogenic receptors in the uterus (estrogens or selective estrogen receptor modulators such as tamoxifen), chronic anovulation, truncal obesity, diabetes mellitus, hypertension, nulliparity, and late menopause. Type II patients are on average older at diagnosis and lack evidence of sustained unopposed estrogenic endometrial exposure as their main risk factor. Tumors in this group tend to be poorly differentiated and include more uncommon and aggressive histologic subtypes such as clear cell and papillary serous carcinoma.

Presentation

Screening

- Since only about 50% of cases of endometrial cancer will have abnormalities on a Pap smear, evaluation of the endometrial cavity to rule out malignancy requires histologic evaluation. Several biopsy devices are currently available and allow for endometrial sampling to be performed in the office setting with a sensitivity >90%. However, screening for endometrial cancer at the general population level is currently not recommended.
- Biopsy of the endometrium for screening purposes should be reserved for women at high risk. This includes postmenopausal women who have been treated with unopposed estrogen replacement therapy, premenopausal women with prolonged untreated chronic anovulation, and patients with estrogen-producing tumors. Tamoxifen use does not represent an indication for endometrial surveillance with ultrasound or biopsy in asymptomatic patients.
- Endometrial cancer is associated with Lynch syndrome (HNPCC) as well as other familial cancer syndromes. Women diagnosed with Lynch syndrome have a 40% lifetime risk of developing endometrial cancer. Prophylactic hysterectomy with bilateral salpingo-oophorectomy is an effective strategy for preventing endometrial and ovarian cancer in these women.

Clinical Presentation

More than 90% of cases will initially present with abnormal uterine bleeding. Therefore, the presence of abnormal peri- or postmenopausal bleeding should prompt immediate and thorough evaluation to rule out the presence of a gynecologic malignancy. If cervical stenosis is present, pyometra or hematometra may develop. Physical exam is usually unremarkable. Slight uterine enlargement may occasionally be present.

Physical Exam

A detailed history and physical should be performed. Physical examination may offer evidence of chronic anovulation. Pelvic and rectal exams will allow complete evaluation of the genital tract and pelvic structures. This will assist in ruling out other diagnoses and assessing the presence of extrauterine extension.

Management

Diagnostic Evaluation

- Office endometrial biopsy is very accurate (>90% sensitive) in detecting endometrial carcinoma. Patients with a nondiagnostic office biopsy or negative biopsies in the context of high clinical suspicion should be further evaluated with hysteroscopy and dilatation and curettage (D&C).
- Initial evaluation usually includes investigation of blood counts, liver and renal function, and radiologic imaging as needed to evaluate for suspected advanced

disease. This should include, at minimum, a chest radiograph. When elevated, CA-125 may suggest extrauterine disease and assist in evaluating response to treatment.

Treatment

- All patients who are medically fit should undergo surgical exploration with complete staging. The surgical staging procedure includes pelvic washings for cytologic evaluation, evaluation of peritoneal surfaces with directed biopsies as indicated, extrafascial hysterectomy with bilateral salpingo-oophorectomy, and pelvic and para-aortic lymph node dissection. Nodal dissection can be omitted in cases of well-differentiated adenocarcinoma without myometrial invasion. Laparoscopic procedures are becoming increasingly common for the initial surgical staging and treatment of endometrial cancer.
- Adjuvant treatment with radiation and/or cytotoxic chemotherapy is indicated for extrauterine disease or those with high-risk clinicopathologic features (high grade, deep myometrial invasion, and/or lymph-vascular space invasion).
- The use of adjuvant radiotherapy in patients with early-stage endometrial cancer has not been proven to improve survival but may play a role in preventing local recurrences, which can have an important impact on the quality of life of these patients. Radiation modalities include the use of vaginal brachytherapy, external radiotherapy, and intensity modulated radiotherapy.
- Many cytotoxic chemotherapeutic agents have been evaluated in patients with endometrial cancer. The objective response rates to several cytotoxic agents have varied widely. Platinum compounds (cisplatin and carboplatin), taxanes (paclitaxel), and doxorubicin are among the most active agents and are commonly used alone or in combination for the treatment of advanced cases, with response rates ranging from 20% to >40%. Other cytotoxic agents such as topotecan, pegylated liposomal doxorubicin, and gemcitabine are also used in the advanced and recurrent setting. Most recently, there has been an increasing interest in the use of biologic noncytotoxic agents such as bevacizumab and tyrosine kinase inhibitors in this disease.
- Hormonal manipulation with high-dose progestins approaches response rates of 20% in the presence of estrogen and progesterone receptors. This approach is often used for patients with advanced or recurrent disease whose tumors tested positive for these receptors (most commonly well- or moderately differentiated tumors) or in those with contraindication for cytotoxic chemotherapy or radiation.

Prognosis

- Early diagnosis in patients presenting with early symptoms accounts for high cure rates in patients with endometrial cancer. In general, long-term survivorship exceeds 75%. Patients with localized disease and well-differentiated tumors are usually cured by hysterectomy and bilateral salpingo-oophorectomy alone.
- Several factors are associated with prognosis in patients with endometrial cancer. These include histologic type, age at diagnosis, tumor grade and stage, depth of myometrial invasion, and presence of lymph-vascular invasion. Overall, the survival by Federation of Gynecology and Obstetrics (FIGO) stage in endometrial cancer approaches 85% for stage I, 75% for stage II, 45% for stage III, and 25% for stage IV disease. However, these figures can vary considerably depending on tumor grade, histologic type, and other clinicopathologic variables.

GESTATIONAL TROPHOBLASTIC DISEASE

This entity encompasses a spectrum of pathologic conditions derived from placental tissues.

Hydatidiform Moles

Epidemiology
In the United States, these conditions are diagnosed in ~1 in 1500 pregnancies.

Classification
- **Complete moles** are tumors characterized by edematous chorionic villi with variable degrees of trophoblastic proliferation. No fetal tissue is identified. Most commonly they have a 46,XX karyotype resulting from duplication of the paternal haploid chromosomal complement. Approximately 5% of cases have a Y chromosome (46,XY) derived from double sperm fertilization. The uterine size is typically greater than expected for gestational age and it is often possible to identify ovarian theca lutein cysts as a result of ovarian stimulation by large amounts of hCG. The risk of postmolar gestational trophoblastic neoplasia (GTN) in cases of complete moles is ~15% to 20%.
- **Partial or incomplete moles** have variable and usually just focal villous edema. Trophoblastic proliferation is mild and usually coexists with a fetus or fetal tissues. Most commonly they have a triploid (69,XXX or XXY) chromosomal complement derived from one maternal and two paternal haploid sets of chromosomes. Most cases present as a missed abortion, with uterine size less than that expected for gestational age. The risk of postmolar GTN in cases of partial moles is generally <5%.

Clinical Presentation
Patients with complete moles usually present in early pregnancy with an abnormally elevated hCG. Clinical presentation also includes first-trimester bleeding (95%), excessive uterine enlargement (50%), and medical complications (10% to 25%) such as hyperemesis gravidarum, early-onset pre-eclampsia, and hyperthyroidism. These systemic manifestations are mainly seen in cases with uterine enlargement greater than 14- to 16-week size. Incomplete moles often present as missed or incomplete abortions and incidental diagnosis is made upon histologic evaluation of products of conception.

Management
- **Diagnosis.** With the increased use of ultrasound and measurement of hCG levels in early pregnancy, this condition is usually diagnosed in the first trimester.
- **Workup.** Once the diagnosis of molar pregnancy is suspected, patients should be thoroughly evaluated with complete blood counts, coagulation studies, renal and liver function tests, blood type and antibody screen, determination of serum hCG level, and chest radiograph.
- **Treatment.** Treatment is evacuation of the uterine cavity in the operating room by means of dilatation and suction curettage. After evacuation, patients should be monitored with periodic determinations of serum quantitative hCG levels. These should be obtained weekly while hCG is elevated and then monthly for 6 months. The objective of this surveillance program is to identify patients who will develop postmolar GTNs. The hCG curve in these patients will usually demonstrate rising or plateaued levels.
- **Follow-up.** In most cases, these patients will have subsequent normal pregnancies. However, a normal pregnancy during the surveillance period would make identification of GTN by means of hCG follow-up impossible. Therefore, effective contraception should be prescribed to these patients during this surveillance period. Oral contraceptives represent a highly desirable method for the motivated patient. This method does not increase the incidence of postmolar GTN and is usually associated with a cyclic and predictable uterine bleeding pattern.

Prognosis

The risk of GTN ranges from <5% (partial mole) to 20% (complete mole). After a molar pregnancy, a woman has a 10-fold increased risk of a second hydatidiform mole (1% to 2%). Therefore, early obstetric ultrasound should be recommended in all subsequent pregnancies.

Gestational Trophoblastic Neoplasia

Introduction

The term gestational trophoblastic neoplasia (GTN) or gestational trophoblastic tumor (GTT) refers to various histologic entities that have the ability to invade locally and/or metastasize. These conditions include persistent or invasive hydatidiform moles, placental site trophoblastic tumors, and choriocarcinomas. GTN may develop after a normal pregnancy, after a molar pregnancy, or after an abortion or, alternatively, may present primarily.

Diagnosis

- Most cases will be diagnosed as a result of routine hCG level surveillance after uterine evacuation following a molar pregnancy or a missed/incomplete abortion. Patients with locally invasive persistent or recurrent disease often report vaginal bleeding. Diagnosis in these cases is usually clinical. D&C is generally avoided to prevent potential uterine perforations.
- Most patients with metastatic disease will have pulmonary involvement (80%). Other relatively common metastatic sites include the vagina (30%), liver, brain, spleen, and/or kidneys (≤10%). Biopsy of metastatic lesions should be avoided to avoid risk of uncontrollable hemorrhage.

Workup

Evaluation should include complete blood counts, coagulation studies, renal and liver function tests, pretreatment determination of serum hCG level, and radiographic survey to assess for metastatic disease in the head, chest, abdomen, and pelvis (usually CT scan and/or MRI).

Treatment

- After radiographic studies and clinical determination of risk category (based on age, type of antecedent pregnancy, time interval from index pregnancy, hCG levels, largest tumor size, site and number of metastases, and history of previous failed chemotherapy), patients are assigned a stage and a risk score.
- Almost all patients with nonmetastatic GTN can be cured without hysterectomy. These cases are usually treated with single-agent chemotherapy (methotrexate or, less commonly, actinomycin D). In patients without a desire for future fertility, pretreatment hysterectomy will reduce the amount of chemotherapy required to induce remission.
- Patients with low-risk metastatic GTN can also be treated with single-agent chemotherapy. Hysterectomy may also reduce the number of chemotherapy cycles in these patients. Approximately 40% of low-risk metastatic cases will fail single-agent treatment and require additional multiagent treatment to achieve remission.
- Patients with high-risk metastatic disease or those who have failed single-agent treatment will require multiagent chemotherapy. The most effective and frequently used multiagent regimen involves weekly administration of etoposide, methotrexate, and actinomycin D, alternating with cyclophosphamide and vincristine (EMA/CO). Therapy with methotrexate, actinomycin D, and chlorambucil or cyclophosphamide (MAC) was the standard of care for many years prior to widespread use of

EMA/CO. Salvage regimens usually include combinations with etoposide, cisplatin, and other agents. Occasionally, patients with high-risk metastatic disease will require multimodal treatment, incorporating surgical excision of metastatic lesions and radiotherapy.

• Surveillance of hCG is required during treatment. Chemotherapy is usually continued until after normalization of hCG levels.

Follow-up

Once complete remission is achieved, contraception is recommended and periodic hCG levels should be followed strictly for 12 to 24 months.

Prognosis

GTN is exquisitely sensitive to chemotherapy and even patients with widespread disease can be cured. Cure rates exceed 95% in patients with nonmetastatic disease. Even in high-risk metastatic cases, multimodal treatment results in cure rates up to 75%.

KEY POINTS TO REMEMBER

• Invasive carcinoma of the cervix is preventable with routine screening for dysplasia.
• Concurrent chemotherapy and radiation improve survival in patients with locally advanced cervical cancer.
• Following surgical staging and cytoreduction for ovarian cancer, intraperitoneal cisplatin with intravenous paclitaxel improves disease-free and overall survival.
• GTN is treated with single-agent chemotherapy in the nonmetastatic setting but may require combination chemotherapy in high-risk metastatic disease or if the disease does not respond to single-agent chemotherapy.

REFERENCES AND SUGGESTED READINGS

Fleming GF. Systemic chemotherapy for uterine carcinoma: metastatic and adjuvant. *J Clin Oncol.* 2007;25:2883–2990.

Garner EI, Goldstein DP, Feltmate CM, et al. Gestational trophoblastic disease. *Clin Obstet Gynecol.* 2007;50(1):112–122.

Long HJ. Management of metastatic cervical cancer: review of the literature. *J Clin Oncol.* 2007;25:2966–2974.

Rao G, Crispens M, Rothenberg ML. Intraperitoneal chemotherapy for ovarian cancer: overview and perspective. *J Clin Oncol.* 2007;25:2867–2872.

Intracranial Tumors

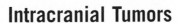

28

Coy Heldermon

INTRODUCTION

Epidemiology

Intracranial lesions are rare malignancies—the thirteenth most common in frequency among tumors in adult patients. Primary intracranial tumors have an incidence of 11.5 per 100,000, with ~20,000 people diagnosed and 13,000 deaths in the United States each year. Metastases to the brain are more common, with one estimate that >100,000 patients per year die from a systemic cancer that has metastasized to the brain.

Classification

Four types of primary intracranial tumors are considered in this chapter: glial tumors (oligodendrogliomas and astrocytic tumors), ependymomas, meningiomas, and primary CNS lymphomas. These constitute the majority of primary intracranial tumors. Metastatic tumors from a primary systemic cancer are also discussed. The most common parenchymal metastases are from primary lung cancer, breast cancer, renal cell cancer, lymphoma, and melanoma. Dural metastases are seen most commonly with breast or prostate cancer.

Causes

Risk Factors

Ionizing radiation is currently the only known unequivocal risk factor for developing a glial or meningeal neoplasm. Irradiation of the cranium, even at low doses, can increase the incidence of meningiomas by a factor of 10 and the incidence of glial tumors by a factor of 3 to 7. Other potential risks, such as use of cellular phones, exposure to high-tension power wires, head trauma, and exposure to nitrosourea compounds, have provided conflicting and unconvincing data and currently are not considered to be risk factors. It is rare for these neoplasms to run in families unless there is an inherited mutation.

Cytogenetics

The allelic loss of chromosome 1p or 19q is associated with several primary CNS tumors and the presence of either of these losses provides favorable prognostic information regarding sensitivity to chemotherapy.

Management

Management of these tumors often involves a multidisciplinary approach involving the neurosurgeon, neuro-oncologist, radiation oncologist, and neurologist, among others. Rehabilitation efforts similarly may be multidisciplinary and involve rehabilitation specialists, physical and occupational therapists, and nurses.

ASTROCYTIC TUMORS

Epidemiology

The epidemiology of astrocytic tumors depends on their histologic grade. Low-grade (grades I and II) astrocytomas are typically found in children and young adults. The peak incidence in adults occurs in the third to fourth decade of life. Malignant astrocytomas (grade III) typically present in the fourth or fifth decade, and glioblastoma multiforme (GBM) usually presents in the sixth or seventh decade. Malignant astrocytoma and GBM are the most common glial tumors, with an annual incidence of 3 or 4 per 100,000 population. Of these, 80% are GBMs. GBMs may be either primary or secondary (meaning the GBM has arisen from a tumor that was initially a low-grade astrocytoma). These secondary GBMs tend to occur in younger adults, typically ≤45 years. The male-to-female ratio of malignant astrocytic tumors is 3:2.

Clinical Presentation

Presentation of these tumors depends on their grade. Low-grade astrocytic tumors present with seizure in ~90% of cases. Typically, the seizures are focal but they may become generalized and cause loss of consciousness. Headache is found in 40% of patients. In general, the headache is worse in the morning and improves in a few hours, usually without treatment. On occasion, headache can be unilateral and throbbing, mimicking a migraine or even a cluster headache. Symptoms such as hemiparesis and mental status changes are found in 15% and 10% of patients, respectively. These symptoms reflect the location of the tumor. Malignant astrocytic tumors, on the other hand, present with seizure 15% to 25% of the time and present with headache 50% of the time. These tumors are much more likely to present with focal neurologic deficits such as hemiparesis, seen in 30% to 50% of patients, and mental status abnormalities, seen in 40% to 60% of patients.

Management

Diagnosis

The diagnosis of the tumors is usually suggested by MRI. Low-grade astrocytoma is usually seen as a diffuse, nonenhancing mass that typically has a local mass effect and evidence of cortical infiltration with abnormal signal, reaching the surface of the brain. The radiologic borders of these tumors are usually distinct, with no surrounding edema. High-grade astrocytomas have an irregular contrast enhancement, which is often ringlike. These lesions are usually associated with edema, and the mass effect can be severe enough to cause herniation. Pathologic diagnosis of these tumors can be done by stereotactic biopsy or surgical excision of the lesion. Stereotactic biopsy will provide the diagnosis of an astrocytoma but will not provide enough information to determine the grade of the tumor, because astrocytic tumors are histologically variable from region to region.

Grading

These tumors are graded by the World Health Organization's four-tiered grading system. The criteria used to grade these tumors include the following features: nuclear atypia, mitotic activity, endothelial proliferation, and necrosis.

- Grade I: absence of all features
- Grade II: any one feature
- Grade III: any two features (malignant astrocytoma)
- Grade IV: any three features (GBM)

Treatment

- Therapy of these tumors involves surgical debulking of the tumor and perhaps excision of the entire tumor if the tumor does not involve critical structures such as the language areas. With low-grade lesions, the next step in treatment is typically irradiation if the tumor is not completely resected or the patient is over 45 years of age. In younger patients with low-grade tumors that are completely resected, observation is also appropriate. Radiation may be done immediately after surgery or may be deferred until there is radiographic evidence of tumor progression. Studies at this time have not shown a difference in survival benefit between immediate and delayed irradiation. Many physicians will wait to start radiation to provide another treatment option at the time of progression. Chemotherapy is also a treatment option in the recurrent setting.

- Therapy of malignant astrocytoma and GBM is identical. The initial step is to surgically excise the tumor. Every effort should be made to remove as much tumor as possible, as this is associated with longer survival and improved neurologic function. During surgery, carmustine (BCNU) wafers may be placed for local chemotherapy. This is followed by high-dose irradiation of the involved field with concurrent daily temozolomide. After completion of radiation, the temozolomide is continued with monthly treatments of 5 days' duration.
- Surveillance for recurrence with an MRI is performed at 1 month and then every 3 months for 3 years. At the time of recurrence, if the disease is localized, a second resection and BCNU wafer insertion should be done, if possible. This should be followed by stereotactic radiosurgery, if it has not been used earlier. Chemotherapy with temozolomide or, alternatively, nitrosourea drugs and procarbazine may also be useful.
- Brainstem gliomas are inoperable. These tumors are treated with irradiation. If there is increased intracranial pressure, a shunt may be placed.

Prognosis
Prognosis associated with astrocytomas is determined by their grade. The median survival for adult low-grade astrocytomas is 5 years. Most of these patients die from the progression of their disease to a higher grade. The median survival for malignant astrocytomas is typically ~3 years. The median survival for GBM is typically 1 year.

OLIGODENDROGLIOMAS

Introduction
Background
Oligodendrogliomas are usually low-grade neoplasms and account for <5% of intracranial tumors and ~20% of glial neoplasms. They arise from oligodendroglial cells, which are responsible for axonal myelination. More than one third of these tumors have intermixed astrocytic or ependymal elements and are therefore considered "mixed gliomas."

Epidemiology
Mean age at presentation is 38 to 45 years, with a slight male predominance.

Clinical Presentation
Patients may present with seizure, progressive hemiparesis, or cognitive impairment, depending on tumor location. These tumors are known to have delicate vasculature and hemorrhage easily, and the patient may present with an acute onset of hemiparesis, headache, and/or lethargy.

Management
Diagnosis
Diagnostic evaluation usually begins with an MRI. The radiologic hallmarks differentiating this tumor from an astrocytoma are lack of contrast enhancement and calcification of the tumor. Biopsy, as in astrocytoma, is necessary for definitive diagnosis, and excisional

biopsy is preferred to stereotactic biopsy. Exam by light microscopy shows oligoden-droglioma cells that may have regular and rounded nuclei, with some nuclei having a halo-like appearance (sometimes termed *fried egg appearance*). There are currently no immuno-histochemical stains or markers that definitively establish the diagnosis.

Treatment

As is seen with astrocytomas, therapy may not be necessary at initial presentation if the patient is asymptomatic and seizures are adequately controlled. Therapy of these tumors usually begins with the excisional biopsy performed to diagnose these tumors. After surgery, observation or focal irradiation and chemotherapy are performed. The chemotherapy regimen includes procarbazine, lomustine, and vincristine (PCV regimen) or temozolomide. Studies have shown that 66% of these tumors respond to therapy. Chemotherapy is not curative, but it can induce sustained remissions. Management should be individualized, and there is some evidence that **1p and 19q loss in the tumor is associated with increased survival.**

Prognosis

The median survival for patients with low-grade oligodendroglioma is currently 10 years and that for anaplastic oligodendroglioma is 3 to 5 years. This long survival is attributed to earlier diagnosis of these tumors with MRI and to their chemosensitivity. Most oligo-dendrogliomas progress by becoming malignant.

EPENDYMOMAS

Introduction

Background

Histologically, ependymomas arise from the ependymal cells, which are normally lining the ventricular chambers and the central canal of the spinal cord. Most are histologically benign. Usually they are classified as either high or low grade. These tumors may metasta-size via cerebrospinal fluid (CSF) pathways. Spinal cord metastases that arise from a brain lesion are known as "drop metastases." The overall risk of seeding is ~10%, and the greatest risk occurs with high-grade infratentorial lesions.

Epidemiology

Ependymomas have a bimodal incidence, with an early major peak at 5 years and a late minor peak at the median age of 34 years. They account for 5% of intracranial tumors in the adult population. There is a 3:2 male predominance.

Clinical Presentation

Clinical presentation depends on the location of the tumor. Most adult tumors occur in supra- and infratentorial regions. They are also frequently seen in the spinal canal, especially the lumbosacral region. The supra- and infratentorial lesions may lead to symptoms of increased intracranial pressure or focal neurologic deficits and seizures. Ataxia, vertigo, and neck stiffness are common presenting symptoms with infratentorial lesions.

Management

Diagnosis

Extent of disease is assessed with an MRI of the brain and spinal cord. More than 50% of these tumors will have calcification.

Treatment

Therapy is surgical excision followed by observation if completely resected or irradiation if not completely resected. Gross total resection is the best determinant of outcome. Steroids may be given both before and after surgery to help decrease edema and other complications. Targeting only the local site with methods such as high-fractionation radiotherapy and stereotactic radiosurgery has shown promise in treating the tumor and limiting some of the complications seen. There is no definitive role for chemotherapy at this time. Evidence of dissemination, as determined by MRI, positive CSF cytology, or myelographic findings, warrants additional radiation of the spinal axis. The dose and extent of irradiation are also determined by the histologic grade, with anaplastic lesions generally receiving more intensive regimens.

Prognosis
Prognosis for these patients is excellent after treatment if the tumor is completely resected. The 5-year disease-free survival is >80%. Ten-year survival rates range from 40% to 60%. Age is the most important prognostic factor with younger patients having a worse outcome.

Follow-up
Patients should be followed by MRI, as the recurrence rate is significant.

MENINGIOMA

Introduction
Background
Meningiomas are extra-axial primary brain tumors. They are of leptomeningeal origin, arising from arachnoid cap cells. They account for nearly 20% of intracranial neoplasms.

Epidemiology
The annual incidence of meningiomas is ~7.8 per 100,000, although most are asymptomatic and discovered incidentally at autopsy. The incidence of symptomatic tumors is ~2 in 100,000 and they occur more frequently in women than men. They are primarily adult tumors, with a peak occurrence at age 45 years. There is an association with breast cancer, neurofibromatosis, and a history of cranial irradiation.

Classification
They typically are classified as one of four histologic patterns: meningothelial, transitional, fibrous, and angioblastic. The first three subtypes account for the majority of the meningiomas and have benign behavior. The angioblastic subtype is the least common but most aggressive form. Malignancy is determined by the amount of brain invasion, increased and atypical mitotic figures, increased cellularity, a papillary histologic pattern, and distant metastases. Malignant meningiomas account for between 1% and 10% of cases. Metastatic disease is seen in <0.1% of cases. Radiation-induced meningiomas are more commonly atypical or malignant. All meningiomas are characterized by the loss of chromosome 22q, which is associated with loss or mutation of the NF-2 gene.

Presentation
Meningiomas can arise virtually anywhere along the leptomeninges. Ninety percent are intracranial, and 90% of these are supratentorial. The three most common sites are adjacent to the superior sagittal sinus, over the cerebral convexities, and along the sphenoid ridge. These three sites account for 60% of intracranial meningiomas. Clinical presentation of meningiomas varies greatly depending on where they arise. Focal neurologic deficits are common, as are symptoms of increased intracranial pressure. Seizures are particularly common, occurring in >50% of patients. Many are found incidentally on CT or MRI.

Management

Diagnosis
Diagnosis of these tumors is suggested by MRI. They have a characteristic appearance as well as circumscribed, extra-axial, homogeneously enhancing, dural-based masses. Peritumoral edema and mass effect are common. Twenty percent have calcification.

Treatment
Surgical resection of these tumors is considered curative in patients with total resection. Tumors at the base of the skull are usually unresectable, because they are intertwined with vital structures. Stereotactic radiosurgery is another option in patients with a tumor that is <3 cm in diameter. At the time of recurrence, a second resection should be performed, followed by external-beam irradiation.

Prognosis
Meningiomas have an excellent prognosis. Disease-free survival at 10 years is 80% to 90% for all meningiomas. If the tumor is partially resected, the 10-year progression-free survival is 50% to 70%. Nearly 65% of malignant meningiomas will recur in 5 years, and nearly 80% will recur in 10 years. Patients who are younger, do not have CNS invasion, and were able to have more extensive resection do better overall.

Follow-up
All patients should be followed closely for recurrence.

PRIMARY CENTRAL NERVOUS SYSTEM LYMPHOMA

Introduction

Background
B cell malignancies of intermediate- to high-grade, usually diffuse, and large-cell subtype may present within the CNS without any evidence of systemic lymphoma. They represent 1% to 3% of intracranial tumors.

Epidemiology
Patients with congenital or acquired immunosuppression have a markedly increased risk of primary CNS lymphoma. The incidence of primary CNS lymphoma peaks in the sixth to seventh decades, with a male:female ratio of 2:1. There are no environmental or behavioral risk factors that are associated with the development of this disease. In immunocompromised patients, the risk increases 100- to 1000-fold. This increase is believed to most likely be secondary to infection with Epstein-Barr or other lymphatic viruses, which have been speculated to be possible transforming events.

Clinical Presentation

These lymphomas are solitary in ~40% of patients on presentation, but they typically become multifocal in most patients. They most commonly present with behavioral or cognitive changes, seen in approximately two thirds of patients. Hemiparesis, aphasia, and visual field deficits are seen in ~50% of patients and seizures in 15% to 20%. Approximately 15% will develop uveitis, sometimes preceding cerebral symptoms by months.

Management

Diagnosis
These tumors are typically diagnosed with the use of MRI. They usually are periventricular in location and have a homogeneous pattern of enhancement. Approximately 25% to 50% of patients will also have cells identified in the CSF. Stereotactic biopsy is necessary

for tissue diagnosis. Further workup should also include a slit-lamp eye exam, CSF cytology with cell count and protein assessment, spinal MRI, chest x-ray, HIV test, blood cell count, and complete metabolic panel to assess for other sites of disease.

Treatment

Unlike other intracranial tumors, there is no role for surgery other than a stereotactic biopsy in primary CNS lymphoma treatment. Treatment usually includes high-dose methotrexate, which is associated with complete response rates of 50% to 80%. Addition of radiation after chemotherapy has been beneficial. The radiation ports should include the orbits if retinal or vitreous disease is present and also the spinal axis if CSF cytology findings suggest meningeal disease.

Prognosis

Prognosis is dependent on treatment regimen. Steroids may be given for symptom palliation after a biopsy is obtained. Radiation alone usually results in a median survival of 12 to 18 months but is not recommended for patients older than 60 years. When chemotherapy is used before radiation, the median survival improves to 42 months, with 25% of patients alive at 5 years. Important indicators of poor prognosis include nonambulatory performance status and age >60 years. Additional factors that have been associated with a poor prognosis include the presence of multiple neurologic deficits, elevated CSF protein, and nonhemispheric location.

METASTATIC TUMORS OF THE CENTRAL NERVOUS SYSTEM

Introduction

Background

Metastatic lesions to the brain typically occur via hematogenous spread and are 10 times as common as primary CNS tumors. There typically is a predilection for the gray matter-white matter junction in which cerebral blood flow is greatest. Spinal involvement may be secondary to spread from the primary site to the vertebral body, with subsequent compression of the spinal cord, retrograde spread via the vertebral venous plexus, or direct invasion of the epidural space via the intervertebral foramen. Alternatively, multifocal spread to the meninges may occur. Twenty percent of cancer patients will develop brain metastases, and 10% will develop spinal metastases. Refer to Chapter 35 for more information regarding spinal cord compression.

The lung is the most common origin of brain metastases. Other sources include breast (especially ductal carcinoma), lymphoma, GI malignancies, melanoma, germ cell tumors, and thyroid cancer.

Clinical Presentation

Metastatic tumors present with the *same clinical features* common to any intracranial mass but occur with a *much more rapid rate of progression*. Focal deficits, seizures, and symptoms of increased intracranial pressure are the usual presenting symptoms. The rapid progression is believed to be secondary to the development of cerebral edema, which is usually associated with metastatic lesions.

Management

Diagnosis

Diagnosis of these lesions is suggested by their appearance on MRI or CT using contrast. Ring enhancing or diffusely enhancing lesions, typically surrounded by a zone of edema disproportionate to the size of the lesion, are most commonly seen. MRI is also useful and is more sensitive in identifying multiple lesions. Meningeal involvement requires both brain and spinal imaging, where hydrocephalus or more diffuse enhancement may be seen. CSF with positive cytology is diagnostic, and an elevated CSF protein level is suggestive of meningeal disease. These cancers are typically considered incurable with few exceptions.

Treatment

Therapy is palliative in nature. High-dose glucocorticosteroids will frequently provide a rapid improvement in symptoms as the surrounding edema decreases. Improvement occurs within 6 to 24 hours and is sustained with continuous therapy. Anticonvulsants are administered empirically, as one third of patients will develop seizures. Whole-brain radiation therapy is the primary treatment mode for focal brain metastases. For those patients who have a single lesion in the brain, surgical excision or gamma-knife radiation may be used as a palliative measure. Surgical excision is typically followed by whole-brain irradiation. For leptomeningeal disease, radiation is limited to symptomatic sites and intrathecal chemotherapy is initially administered weekly, then monthly after four treatments. Methotrexate is the most often used regimen but cytarabine and thiotepa are other options. In primary cancers that are chemotherapy responsive, systemic chemotherapy may provide some improvement, although there is typically less of a response than seen in the primary tumor.

Prognosis

Survival in untreated brain metastases is typically 1 month. Survival improves to a median of 3 to 6 months with the use of steroids and radiation. If the tumor is amenable to surgical excision, the survival may improve to a median of 40 weeks.

KEY POINTS TO REMEMBER

- Metastases to the CNS are far more common than primary CNS lesions in adults. The most common primary CNS lesions are astrocytic tumors.
- There are currently no convincing data that cellular phones or power lines cause CNS tumors.
- CNS lymphoma is the only primary CNS malignancy that does not require surgical excision.
- Metastasis to the CNS is associated with an extremely poor short-term survival.

REFERENCES AND SUGGESTED READINGS

Bigner DD, McLendon RE, Bruner JM, eds. *Russell and Rubinstein's Pathology of Tumors of the Nervous System.* New York: Oxford University Press; 1998.

Carincross G, Macdonald D, Ludwin S, et al. Chemotherapy for anaplastic oligodendroglioma. *J Clin Oncol.* 1994;12:2013–2021.

DeAngelis L. Medical progress: brain tumors. *N Engl J Med.* 2001;344(2):114–123.

Galanis E, Buckner J. Chemotherapy of brain tumors. *Curr Opin Neurol.* 2000; 13(6):619–625.

Landis SH, Murray T, Bolden S, et al. Cancer statistics, 1999. *CA Cancer J Clin.* 1999; 49:8–31.

Legler JM, Ries LA, Smith MA, et al. Brain and other central nervous system cancers: recent trends in incidence and mortality. *J Natl Cancer Inst.* 1999;91:1382–1390.

Lindegaard KF, Mork SJ, Eide GE, et al. Statistical analysis of clinicopathological features, radiotherapy, and survival in 170 cases of oligodendroglioma. *J Neurosurg.* 1987; 67:224–230.

Murphy G, Lawrence W, Raymond EL, eds. *American Cancer Society Textbook of Clinical Oncology*. Atlanta, GA: American Cancer Society; 1995.

Perry JR, Louis DN, Cairncross MD. Current treatment of oligodendrogliomas. *Arch Neurol.* 1999;56:434–436.

Pollack IF, et al. Prognostic factors in the diagnosis and treatment of primary central nervous system lymphoma. *Cancer.* 1989;63(5):939–947.

Van den Bent MJ. New perspectives for the diagnosis and treatment of oligodendroglioma. *Expert Rev Anticancer Ther.* 2001;1:348–356.

Van den Bent MJ, Taphoorn MJ, Brandes AA, et al. Phase II study of first line chemotherapy with temozolomide in recurrent oligodendroglial tumors: the European Organization for Research and Treatment of Cancer Brain Tumor Group Study 26791. *J Clin Oncol.* 2003;21:2525–2528.

Leukemias

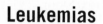

Mike G. Martin and John S. Welch

INTRODUCTION

Leukemia is the result of somatically acquired genetic mutations leading to the dysregulation and clonal expansion of myeloid and/or lymphoid progenitor cells. The accumulation of neoplastic cells, both in the bone marrow and in the peripheral tissues, manifests as cytopenias with associated complications, elevation of the total WBC count, and dysfunction of the various involved organs. The diagnosis is typically suspected based on an abnormal CBC and peripheral smear and then confirmed on bone marrow biopsy. The prognosis and treatment depend on the age of the patient, accurate determination of the type of the leukemia, and cytogenetics and molecular markers.

ACUTE MYELOGENOUS LEUKEMIA

Introduction

The acute leukemias are the result of abnormal clonal proliferation of mutated progenitor cells. The mutations cause a block in the maturation process, leading to an accumulation of immature cells. The expansion of the abnormal clone leads to suppression of the other elements in the marrow, often producing clinical bone marrow failure and making the patient gravely ill. The clinical course of untreated acute leukemia is very brief, with patients succumbing in days to weeks from the complications of marrow failure. Therapy involves intensive chemotherapy regimens, prolonged hospitalizations, and, potentially, stem cell transplantation.

Acute myelogenous leukemia (AML) results from the abnormal proliferation of a myeloid hematopoietic progenitor cell and accounts for 80% of adult acute leukemias. The median age at diagnosis is 67 years old. The American Cancer Society estimated that 11,930 men and women would be diagnosed with AML in 2006 and that 9040 persons would die from it. Radiation, previous chemotherapy with alkylating agents or topoisomerase inhibitors, myelodysplasia, myeloproliferative disorders, aplastic anemia, and exposure to benzene are known **risk factors** for the development of AML. Higher risk for AML is seen in people with Down (particularly AML-M7), Turner, and Klinefelter syndromes. In most cases, no risk factors are clearly defined.

Classification

The French-American-British (FAB) group identifies nine subtypes of AML that are based on morphology and staining (Table 29-1). They indicate the myeloid lineage and the degree of differentiation. Cytogenetic evaluation is crucial, as it helps to determine treatment and prognosis (Table 29-2). For example, the M3 subtype (acute promyelocytic leukemia; APL) is associated with the translocation 15;17, a distinct clinical phenotype (DIC), a good

TABLE 29-1 ACUTE MYELOGENOUS LEUKEMIA, FAB CLASSIFICATION

Subtype	Name	Frequency (%)	Peroxidase/ SB/NP[a]
M0	Myeloblastic with minimal differentiation	<5	–/–/–
M1	Myeloblastic without maturation	20	+/+/–
M2	Myeloblastic with maturation	25	+/+/–
M3	Promyelocytic (APL)	10	+/+/–
M4	Myelomonocytic	20	+/+/+
M4Eo	Myelomonocytic with abnormal eosinophils	5–10	+/+/+
M5	Monocytic	20	–/–/+
M6	Erythroleukemia	5	+/+/–
M7	Megakaryoblastic	<5	–/–/+

+, positive; −, negative.
[a]Myeloperoxidase, Sudan black (SB), and nonspecific esterase (NE) stains.
Adapted from DeVita VT, Hellman S, Rosenberg S. *Cancer: Principles and Practice of Oncology*. 6th ed. Philadelphia: Lippincott Williams & Wilkins; 2001.

prognosis, and tailored therapy. M7 is associated with a poor clinical outcome in the absence of transplantation. The World Health Organization (WHO) has developed a classification system of AML based not only on morphologic findings but also on genetic and clinical findings (Table 29-3). In the WHO system, AML is defined by >20% myeloblasts in the bone marrow aspirate. Patients with clonal cytogenetic abnormalities such as t(8;21),

TABLE 29-2 CYTOGENETIC ABNORMALITIES IN ACUTE MYELOID LEUKEMIA AND ASSOCIATED PROGNOSIS

Risk Group	Cytogenetic Findings	Preferred Consolidation Strategy
Favorable	t(15;17), t(8;21), inv(16)	Chemotherapy
Intermediate	Normal or ≤2 nonspecific chromosomal aberrations	Chemotherapy OR allogeneic transplant
Unfavorable	Complex karyotype (defined as ≥3 abnormalities, excluding the favorable-risk cytogenetics) inv(3), t(6;9), t(6;11), t(11;19) del(5q) −5, −7, +8	Allogeneic transplant

Adapted from Mrozek K, Bloomfield CD. Chromosome aberrations, gene mutations and expression changes, and prognosis in adult acute myeloid leukemia. *Hematol Am Soc Hematol Educ Program*. 2006:169–177.

TABLE 29-3	WHO CLASSIFICATION OF ACUTE MYELOID LEUKEMIA (SIMPLIFIED)

I: AML with recurrent genetic abnormalities
II: AML with multilineage dysplasia (MDS-related)
III: AML and MDS, therapy related (from alkylator/topoisomerase II inhibitors)
IV: AML, not otherwise categorized

MDS, myelodysplastic syndrome.
Adapted from Vardiman JW, Harris NL, Brunning RD. The World Health Organization (WHO) classification of the myeloid neoplasms. *Blood.* 2002;100(7):2292–2302.

inv(16), and t(15;17) have AML regardless of the blast percentage. This classification is meant to better highlight biologic behavior and response to therapy.

Presentation

Marked cytopenias from leukemic infiltration of the marrow result in diverse presentations, including fatigue, pallor, and dyspnea on exertion from anemia; hemorrhage from thrombocytopenia; and fevers and infection from neutropenia. Extramedullary tissue invasion by leukemic cells (most commonly with AML-M5) may result in hepatomegaly, splenomegaly, lymphadenopathy, rashes (leukemia cutis), gingival hypertrophy, CNS dysfunction and cranial neuropathies, intestinal involvement, lytic bony lesions, or even establishment of infiltrative masses (granulocytic sarcomas or chloromas). With myeloblast counts >50,000, **leukostasis** may occur, resulting in dyspnea from pulmonary infiltrates or CNS dysfunction (ranging from somnolence to cerebral ischemia). Spontaneous tumor lysis syndrome may cause hyperuricemia, hyperphosphatemia, hypocalcemia, or hyperkalemia and renal failure. Patients may also present with disseminated intravascular coagulation (DIC; with excessive bleeding), which is more commonly seen in the M3 and M5 subtypes.

Management

Workup
Workup should include the following.

- CBC: Pancytopenia or leukocytosis may be present.
- Coagulation profile: Determine International Normalized Ratio, prothrombin time, partial thromboplastin time, D-dimer, and fibrinogen to look for DIC.
- Electrolytes: Check for hyperkalemia, hypocalcemia, hyperphosphatemia, or hyperuricemia as a result of tumor lysis.
- Lactate dehydrogenase (LDH)
- Peripheral smear: Leukemic myeloblasts on Wright-Giemsa stain of the peripheral blood and bone marrow aspirate demonstrate large nuclei with scant cytoplasm and may contain Auer rods (eosinophilic needlelike inclusions).
- Lumbar puncture: This should be done if neurologic symptoms are present.
- **Bone marrow aspirate and biopsy,** evaluated for the following.
  - Morphology and histochemical staining
  - Flow cytometry, to distinguish AMLs from lymphoid and to determine the subtype of AML
  - Cytogenetics, which is critical in the initial work up for AML since it provides a wealth of prognostic information and helps to guide therapy

Treatment

Treatment is divided into two phases: **induction** and **consolidation**. The goal is to achieve remission, defined as <5% blasts in the bone marrow and recovery of peripheral blood counts.

- **Induction** chemotherapy consists of 7 days of cytarabine (Ara-C) and 3 days of an anthracycline: daunorubicin or idarubicin ("7+3" regimen). Complete remission can be obtained in approximately 70% to 80% of patients <60 years and in ~50% of older patients. Patients are generally admitted to the hospital during induction for nearly a month, require frequent blood and platelet transfusions, and often have febrile neutropenia.
- **Consolidation** therapy is essential to prevent relapse and is guided by cytogenetics, age, and patient comorbidities. Two therapeutic options are available: allogeneic bone marrow transplantation or further chemotherapy with high-dose cytarabine or other regimens. Autologous transplants offer little to no benefit over chemotherapy.
- For **promyelocytic** (M3) **leukemia**, *all-trans retinoic acid* (ATRA) is given with induction chemotherapy. ATRA ameliorates the coagulopathy associated with M3 but is also associated with the potentially dangerous APL differentiation syndrome. Maintenance therapy with lower-dose ATRA is then necessary. Recent data show that arsenic trioxide as consolidation decreases risk of relapse and improves overall survival. In relapse, salvage therapy with arsenic trioxide has shown considerable promise.
- In the case of **relapse,** patients should be salvaged with intensive chemotherapy and then considered for allogeneic bone marrow transplantation. Patients who are not transplant candidates, due to age or comorbidities, should be considered for treatment on clinical trials.

Prognosis

Leukemia can typically be divided into good, poor, and intermediate prognostic groups. These groups help guide the decision of the most appropriate consolidation therapy (Table 29-2). *Good-prognosis* leukemias are those with favorable cytogenetics: translocation (15;17) (associated with M3 AML), translocation (8;21) (associated with M2 AML), and inversion 16 (associated with M4 AML with eosinophilia). These patients are typically offered induction therapy followed by chemotherapy-based consolidation, as they have a relatively high rate of cure by this strategy (~60% to 70%). *Poor prognostic indicators* include age >60 years; AML secondary to myelodysplastic syndrome or antecedent hematologic disorder; deletion of 5q, 7q, or trisomy 8; and lack of the favorable cytogenetics noted earlier. Patients with poor-prognosis leukemia have a high rate of relapse and should be considered for allogeneic bone marrow transplant in first remission. Patients with normal cytogenetics fall into an intermediate risk group, and management should be individualized after remission. New molecular prognostic markers such as mutations in the FLT-3, NPM, and MLL genes may help guide therapy in this group. Clinical trials are always ongoing, and whenever appropriate, patients in all groups should be considered for participation. Since 1970, the 5-year survival rate has increased from 15% to 40% with advances in antileukemic and supportive therapies (i.e., antibiotics, antifungals, improvement in transfusion medicine).

Complications

Leukostasis may cause symptoms that require emergent cytoreduction with hydroxyurea and/or leukapheresis. Tumor lysis syndrome, fever, and neutropenia are all concerns as well (see Chap. 35). Cytopenias should be supported with transfusions, and coagulopathy should be monitored for and corrected. Prospective trials have identified $10,000/\mu L$ as a relatively safe transfusion threshold for platelets during inpatient induction chemotherapy. If the patient has received a bone marrow transplant, he or she should be followed closely for symptoms of opportunistic infections and graft-versus-host disease (see Chap. 31).

ACUTE LYMPHOBLASTIC LEUKEMIA

Introduction

Acute lymphoblastic leukemia (ALL) results from the abnormal proliferation of a lymphoid hematopoietic progenitor cell. The American Cancer Society estimated that 3930 men and women would be diagnosed with ALL in 2006 and that 1490 persons would die from it. It accounts for 80% of childhood leukemias and 20% of adult acute leukemias. The median age at diagnosis is 13 years old, with 39% of cases being diagnosed in patients older than 20 years. People with Down syndrome are at a higher risk for developing ALL. This section deals only with adult ALL, which has a worse prognosis than childhood ALL.

Classification

Classification is based on morphologic (FAB system) and immunophenotypic information (Table 29-4).

Presentation

The clinical phenotype of ALL is very similar to that of AML. Patients present with malaise, fatigue, dyspnea, and bone pain. Patients also typically have signs of marrow failure such as bleeding, bruising, fever, and infection. Much more commonly than in AML, in up to 10% of patients, the CNS may be involved at presentation, manifesting as headache and/or cranial nerve palsies. Leukostasis may also be present. Hepatosplenomegaly and lymphadenopathy can be seen. ALL can be associated with an anterior mediastinal mass (in T-cell subtypes) or large abdominal lymph nodes (in B-cell subtypes).

Management

Workup

Basic workup is similar to that for AML. A peripheral smear will usually demonstrate the presence of circulating blasts. Bone marrow will be hypercellular, with >30% blasts. Cytoplasmic granules and Auer rods should be absent. However, it can be extremely difficult to diagnose ALL on clinical and morphologic grounds alone. Immunophenotyping is often necessary to distinguish ALL from AML. Thirty percent of adult ALL patients exhibit the Philadelphia chromosome t(9;22), as seen in chronic myelogenous leukemia (CML).

TABLE 29-4	ACUTE LYMPHOBLASTIC LEUKEMIA, IMMUNOTYPE, AND FAB CLASSIFICATION		
Immuno-Type	Frequency (%)	FAB Subtype	Staining
Pre-B cell	75	L1, L2	+TdT, + CALLA, B-cell markers (CD19, CD20)
T cell	20	L1, L2	+TdT, −CALLA, +acid phosphatase, +T cell markers (CD2, CD7, CD5)
B cell	5	L3	−TdT, +surface IgG

CALLA, common acute lymphoblastic leukemia antigen; TdT, terminal deoxynucleotidyl transferase.

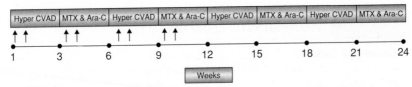

FIGURE 29-1. Schema of hyper-CVAD (cyclophosphamide, vincristine, dexamethasone, and doxorubicin alternating with high-dose methotrexate and cytarabine with incorporated intrathecal therapy). Arrows indicate intrathecal chemotherapy administrations. (Adapted from Thomas DA, et al. Outcome with the hyper-CVAD regimens in lymphoblastic lymphoma. *Blood.* 2004;104:1624–1630.)

Treatment

Therapy for ALL consists of multiple phases.

- **Induction chemotherapy** typically consists of vincristine, a steroid, and an anthracycline. Some protocols include L-asparaginase as well. One regimen is hyper-CVAD (cyclophosphamide, vincristine, dexamethasone, and doxorubicin alternating with high-dose methotrexate and cytarabine with incorporated intrathecal therapy) (Fig. 29-1). These multiagent protocols carry the burden of profound myelosuppression, and patients must be followed for infectious and cytopenic complications. Induction mortality rates range from 3% to 20% but these regimens boast complete remission rates of 65% to 90%. The BCR-ABL tyrosine kinase inhibitor imatinib has been incorporated into induction regimens in patients who harbor the Philadelphia chromosome (t(9;22)).

- **CNS prophylaxis** is an important component of therapy for ALL, as it has a high incidence of recurrence in the CNS. Regimens typically consist of intrathecal methotrexate and cytarabine.

- **Maintenance therapy** is typically continued for 2 years, often with mercaptopurine, prednisone, vincristine, and methotrexate (the so-called POMP regimen).

- **Relapse**, unfortunately, is common in adult ALL. Salvage chemotherapy regimens are able to induce a second complete remission in ~30% to 70% of persons, and when they are consolidated with allogeneic stem cell transplantation about 40% of patients will be alive at 4 years.

Prognosis

Although 60% to 90% of patients can expect to undergo a complete remission with induction chemotherapy, the majority of patients will relapse. Patients who are younger and have good prognostic indicators have a cure rate of 50% to 70%. Those who are older and have poor prognostic indicators have a cure rate of only 10% to 30%. Adverse risk factors are summarized in Table 29-5.

CHRONIC MYELOGENOUS LEUKEMIA

Introduction

CML accounts for 14% of all leukemias and 20% of adult leukemias, with an annual incidence of 1.6 cases per 100,000 adults. Since the advent of imatinib, the annual mortality has decreased to 1% to 2%. The median age at presentation is 65, and incidence increases with age. The etiology is unclear; no correlation with monozygotic twins, geography, ethnicity, or economic status has been observed. However, a significantly higher

TABLE 29-5	ADVERSE PROGNOSTIC FACTORS IN ADULT ACUTE LYMPHOBLASTIC LEUKEMIA (ALL)
Adverse Risk Factor	
Age	>60 years old
WBC at presentation	>50,000
Prolonged time to complete remission	>4–6 weeks
Adverse cytogenetics	Hypodiploidy t(9;22) t(4;11) Trisomy 8

incidence of CML has been noted in survivors of the atomic disasters at Nagasaki and Hiroshima, in radiologists, and in patients treated with radiation to the spine for ankylosing spondylitis.

Causes

Pathophysiology

Historically, CML was the first disease in which a specific chromosomal abnormality was linked to the pathogenesis of the disease: the foreshortened chromosome 22, named the Philadelphia (Ph) chromosome. Subsequently the BCR-ABL fusion gene resulting from the common t(9;22) translocation has been noted in almost all patients with CML and is now considered pathognomonic. This fusion results in constitutive tyrosine kinase activity of ABL and thus dysregulated activity of multiple signal-transduction pathways controlling cell proliferation and apoptosis.

Blast-phase CML is characterized by **cytogenetic evolution** in nearly 70% of patients. The most common chromosomal abnormalities are trisomy 8, in 30% to 40% of patients, additional Ph chromosome, in 20% to 30%, and isochromosome 17, in 15% to 20%. Corresponding mutations in p53 are also seen in 20% to 30% of patients, amplification of c-myc in 20%, and, less commonly, mutations and deletions of ras, Rb, or p16. As with de novo AML, complex cytogenetics are associated with decreased response rates and survival.

Natural History

The natural history of CML is a triphasic process. Most patients present in **chronic phase**, characterized by an asymptomatic accumulation of differentiated myeloid cells in the bone marrow, spleen, and peripheral blood. CML usually progresses through a transient **accelerated phase**, lasting 4 to 6 months, and then inevitably to **blast phase**, an incurable acute leukemia that is fatal within 3 to 6 months. In the 2 years after initial diagnosis of CML, 5% to 15% of untreated patients will enter blast crisis. In subsequent years, the annual rate of progression increases to 20% to 25%, with progression commonly occurring between 3 and 6 years after diagnosis.

The definition of accelerated-phase CML relies on several clinical and laboratory features and is characterized by increasing arrest of maturation. Current WHO criteria include at least one of the following: 10% to 19% blasts in peripheral blood or bone marrow, ≥20% peripheral basophils, thrombocytopenia <100,000/μL and lack of response to therapy, increasing spleen size and increasing WBC unresponsive to therapy, and cytogenetic evidence of clonal evolution. Once either accelerated phase or blast crisis occurs, the success of any therapy declines dramatically.

Presentation

In most patients, CML is diagnosed incidentally. Symptomatic constellations typically result from concurrent anemia and splenomegaly: fatigue, early satiety, and sensation of abdominal fullness but may also include weight loss, bleeding, and bruising in advanced disease. Leukocytosis with a myeloid shift is universal. In contrast to cases of acute leukemia, in which an arrest in maturation is the rule, **granulocytes at all stages of maturation** are observed on the peripheral smear. Anemia and thrombocytosis are common, while basophilia (>7%) occurs in only 10% to 15% of patients.

Management

Diagnosis

Leukocyte alkaline phosphatase (LAP) activity is usually reduced but can be increased with infections, stress, on achievement of remission, or on progression to blast phase. The diagnosis is confirmed by the detection of the **Ph chromosome t(9;22)(q34.1;q11.21)**. In 5% of patients a BCR-ABL fusion can be detected without classic Ph chromosomal cytogenetics, and rarely translocations can involve three or more chromosomes. The bone marrow is typically hypercellular and devoid of fat. All stages of myeloid differentiation are present and megakaryocytes may be increased, suggesting that chronic-phase CML is a disease of discordant maturation, where a delay in myeloid maturation results in increased myeloid cell mass.

Treatment

Chronic-Phase Chronic Myelogenous Leukemia. Imatinib mesylate (Gleevec) revolutionized the treatment of CML with its phase I trial in 2001. Imatinib is a targeted tyrosine kinase inhibitor, which antagonizes the activity of the ABL tyrosine kinase, as well as c-Kit and platelet-derived growth factors alpha and beta. At nanomolar concentrations imatinib binds to the inactive conformation of the BCR-ABL ATP-binding pocket, resulting in competitive inhibition of BCR-ABL and growth inhibition of BCR-ABL-positive bone marrow progenitor cells.

Side effects of imatinib mesylate are generally mild but include hematologic suppression (neutropenia, thrombocytopenia, and anemia), constitutional symptoms (diarrhea, edema, and rash), and rare organ damage (elevated transaminases, hypophosphatemia, and potentially cardiotoxicity). These can usually be managed with growth factors or dose reduction but occasionally require discontinuation, either briefly or permanently.

Although a few case reports are emerging of patients with continued complete cytogenetic response after imatinib withdrawal, relapse is common, and we recommend lifelong maintenance therapy at this time.

Increased risk of progression to accelerated and blast phase has been demonstrated if imatinib does not help patients achieve specific **clinical goals**. These currently include the following, from the time a patient starts imatinib.

- 3 months: **complete hematologic response** with normal peripheral counts and a >1 log reduction in BCR-ABL transcripts by quantitative PCR (qPCR)
- 6 months: **cytogenetic response** with <35% Ph chromosome-positive bone marrow cells
- 12 months: **complete cytogenetic response** with undetectable Ph chromosome
- 18 months: **major molecular remission** with a 3 log reduction by qPCR of peripheral BCR-ABL

Failure to reach any of these goals warrants close follow-up, ABL tyrosine kinase domain mutation analysis, dose escalation, or change to second-line tyrosine kinase inhibitor and consideration of hematopoietic stem cell transplant.

Follow-up during initial treatment requires CBC monthly, peripheral BCR-ABL qPCR every 3 months, and bone marrow biopsy every 6 months until major molecular remission is achieved. Once molecular remission is documented, BCR-ABL transcripts should still be followed every 3 months, with an annual bone marrow exam for cytogenetics. Rising BCR-ABL transcripts should be quickly re-evaluated and treatment altered accordingly.

Resistance to imatinib has been noted in 2% to 4% of patients annually for the first 3 years of imatinib therapy and may decrease thereafter. Point mutations in the SH1 kinase domain are commonly associated with resistance. These mutations either decrease the affinity for imatinib binding in the ATP-binding pocket or shift the kinetics of BCR-ABL to prefer the active conformation, to which imatinib will not bind. More than 50 distinct mutations have been documented in 42% to 90% of resistant cases, with increasing prevalence in accelerated phase and blast crisis.

Imatinib resistance can be overcome with either increasing doses or a second-line tyrosine kinase inhibitor such as dasatinib. Dasatinib inhibits BCR-ABL in either active or inactive conformation, providing sensitivity to most imatinib-resistant point mutations with the exception of T315I, which confers a high degree of resistance to both drugs. Mutational analysis is thus critical in determining the treatment choice after resistance is noted. Multiple novel multitarget kinase inhibitors are in development, which promise improved response against imatinib-resistant BCR-ABL.

While effective, **chemotherapy** is second-line to the well-tolerated tyrosine kinase inhibitors. Hydroxyurea, busulfan, and interferon-alpha have been used with some success. However, interferon-alpha therapy has significant side effects including flulike symptoms, anorexia, weight loss, depression, autoimmune disorders, thrombocytopenia, alopecia, rashes, and neuropathies, resulting in discontinuation in about a fifth of patients.

Allogeneic hematopoietic stem cell transplant from either related or unrelated donors remains the only known curative therapy for CML. Transplantation from a matched sibling donor during chronic phase is associated with a 10-year survival of 50% to 70%, but this decreases to 20% to 40% and <20% in accelerated and blast phase, respectively. Results of transplantation from unrelated donors are somewhat less impressive but are improving with better matching strategies and supportive care. Most CML patients transplanted in chronic phase are cured of their disease, although transplant-related morbidity and mortality remain a significant problem. Given the high response rates to tyrosine kinase inhibitors, their initial use is still recommended.

Accelerated and Blast-Phase Chronic Myelogenous Leukemia. Despite significant advances in the treatment of chronic phase CML, accelerated and blast-phase CML (BP-CML) are typically progressive, and there is no successful standard therapy. Imatinib has been shown to improve survival in accelerated phase at higher doses (600 to 800 mg), but responses are often short-lived.

Treatment of BP-CML remains a challenge, with survival of only 2 to 4 months in nonresponders. Treatment is dictated by hematologic features. Myeloid features are seen in 50% of patients, lymphoid in 25%, and undifferentiated in 25%. Typical AML induction chemotherapy is used for BP-CML with myeloid features and ALL induction chemotherapy for lymphoid features. Each has a response rate of only 30%. Transplant during BP-CML remains the only curative options, but it is associated with a nearly 80% risk of relapse and a 5-year survival of only ~5%.

CHRONIC LYMPHOCYTIC LEUKEMIA

Introduction

Chronic lymphocytic leukemia (CLL) is the most common form of leukemia in adults, accounting for ~30% of adult leukemia in Western countries. Approximately 10,000 new cases are diagnosed annually, and 4700 deaths are attributed to CLL in the United States each year. According to the SEER cancer database, from 2000 to 2003 the median age at presentation was 72 years, and only 13% of patients were <55 years old at the time of diagnosis. Nearly 4% of elderly individuals have a monoclonal lymphocytosis, although most of these do not progress to CLL. The age-adjusted incidence rate for CLL was 3.8 per 100,000 per year, with a ~2:1 male:female ratio. Patients with a history of immunodeficiency syndromes are more prone to the development of CLL. There are no clear environmental or occupational risk factors that predispose to CLL, and patients who are exposed to radiation do not appear to have an increased frequency of CLL.

Causes

Pathophysiology
CLL is an accumulation of malignant, immunologically incompetent, but mature B-cell lymphocytes. The malignant cells of CLL express high levels of the antiapoptotic protein, bcl-2, and express common B-cell antigens CD19, CD20, and CD23. Of note, CD5 antigen, a T-cell antigen, is found in all cases of CLL. A Coombs-positive, warm antibody, hemolytic anemia occurs in 10% of patients, and an immune thrombocytopenia occurs in ~5% of patients. In 5% of patients, **Richter syndrome** develops, which is a malignant transformation to diffuse large B-cell lymphoma.

Differential Diagnosis
It is important to consider benign causes of lymphocytosis, including Epstein-Barr virus mononucleosis, chronic infections, autoimmune diseases, drug and allergic reactions, thyrotoxicosis, adrenal insufficiency, and postsplenectomy. The other possible malignancies to consider are hairy cell leukemia (HCL), cutaneous T-cell lymphoma, other indolent non-Hodgkin lymphomas (mantle cell, follicular, lymphoplasmacytic), and large granular lymphocytic leukemia.

Presentation

Many patients are discovered by routine CBC and are asymptomatic. However, chronic fatigue is one of the more common initial complaints. With bone marrow involvement, patients may develop severe fatigue, anemia, bruising, weight loss, and fever. On physical exam, marked splenomegaly, hepatomegaly, and lymphadenopathy can be present. With advancing immunodeficiency, herpes zoster infections, *Pneumocystis jiroveci* pneumonia, and bacterial infections become more frequent.

Management

Diagnosis
A CBC with differential reveals an absolute lymphocytosis, with >95% small lymphocytes. A blood smear should show mature lymphocytes. The classic smudge cell is nonspecific, but more than 30% smudging has been suggested as a poor prognostic marker. Anemia and/or thrombocytopenia may be present from bone marrow infiltration or from an autoimmune phenomenon. It is important to assess renal and hepatic function, LDH, uric acid, beta-2-microglobulin, Coombs antiglobulin, serum protein electrophoresis, quantitative immunoglobulins, chest radiograph, and CT scan of the chest, abdomen, and pelvis. Patients with CLL typically have at least 30% lymphocytes in the bone marrow. A bone marrow biopsy should be obtained for cytogenetics.

The essential diagnostic criteria for CLL identified by the CLL international working group include an absolute lymphocytosis of >5000/μL with a typical morphology, a bone marrow infiltrated with small lymphocytes accounting for >30% of nucleated cells, and a typical immunophenotype (CD5$^+$, CD23$^+$, CD10$^-$, CD19$^+$, CD20^{+dim}, CyclinD1$^-$, CD43$^\pm$) (Table 29-6).

TABLE 29-6	IMMUNOPHENOTYPIC FEATURES OF MALIGNANT CONDITIONS AFFECTING MATURE B LYMPHOCYTES
Disorder	**Common Immunophenotype**
CLL	DR+, CD19+, CD20+, CD5+, CD22−, CD23+, CD10−, weak sIg
Prolymphocytic leukemia	DR+, CD19+, CD20+, CD5−, CD22+, CD23−, CD10−, bright sIg
Mantle cell lymphoma	DR+, CD19+, CD20+, CD5+, CD22+, CD23−, CD10−, moderate sIg
Follicular lymphoma	DR+, CD19+, CD20+, CD5−, CD22+, CD23−, CD10+, bright sIg
Hairy cell leukemia	DR+, CD19+, CD20+, CD5−, CD22+, CD23−, CD10−, CD11c+, bright sIg

CLL, chronic lymphocytic leukemia; sIg, surface immunoglobulin.

Classification of CLL is based on the extent of systemic infiltration of lymphocytes. This helps to determine the prognosis and initiation of treatment (Table 29-7). Molecular and cytogenetic markers have become increasingly useful for prognostication. Cytogenetic markers have been noted to predict overall progression of disease and response to therapy. Important molecular markers include ZAP70 and IgVH (immunoglobulin heavy chain variable region) gene rearrangements.

TABLE 29-7	CHRONIC LYMPHOCYTIC LEUKEMIA STAGING AND MOLECULAR PROGNOSTICS

Rai
- Stage 0: lymphocytosis
- Stage 1: lymphadenopathy
- Stage 2: splenomegaly
- Stage 3: Hgb <11 g/dL
- Stage 4: Platelets <100,000/μL

High-risk molecular markers
- Elevated β2, LDH, sCD23
- CD38+ in >30% lymphocytes
- ZAP70+ in >30% lymphocytes
- Germline IgVH

Low risk: overall survival, 7–10 years
- Rai 0-1
- Binet A
- Deletion 13q
- Doubling time >12 months

Binet
- Stage A: lymphocytosis
- Stage B: lymphadenopathy in >3 areas
- Stage C: Hgb <10 g/dL or platelets <100,000/μL

Good-risk cytogenetics
- Deletion 13q

High-risk cytogenetics
- 14q rearrangement
- 11q rearrangement
- Deletion 17p
- Trisomy 12

High risk: overall survival, 2–5 years
- Rai 3-4
- Binet C
- Molecular or cytogenetic changes noted
- Doubling time <12 months

Hgb, hemoglobin; LDH, lactate dehydrogenase.

Treatment

It is not necessary to initiate therapy early in the course of CLL. However, CLL patients may be immunocompromised, and fever or any other signs of infection need to be evaluated promptly. **Indications for therapy** include eligibility for a clinical trial, symptoms (fevers, sweats, weight loss), obstructive or advancing lymphadenopathy, hepatosplenomegaly, stage III or IV disease, rapid elevation in lymphocyte count with a doubling time <6 months, and complications including immune hemolysis, thrombocytopenia, infections, threatened organ function, and transformation. Conventional treatment is given to control these symptoms, although it has not typically improved overall survival. Newer monoclonal antibodies are demonstrating improved response rates and may improve overall survival.

Current therapies include purine analogues (fludarabine and cladribine), monoclonal antibodies against CD20 (rituximab) and CD52 (alemtuzumab), radiation, and alkylating agents (chlorambucil and cyclophosphamide).

Randomized clinical trials have established higher complete remission rates and progression-free survival intervals for fludarabine over alkylating agents, and for combination therapies such as FC (fludarabine, cyclophosphamide) over fludarabine alone; however, no difference in overall survival has been demonstrated. We currently utilize combination fludarabine-rituximab (FR) as our standard front-line therapy for CLL patients and reserve oral chlorambucil and prednisone for patients with poor performance status not related to disease. Treatment is typically four to eight cycles aimed at symptom management. With elevated leukocyte counts, consideration of tumor lysis risk and prevention is important prior to therapeutic intervention. In addition, patients treated with purine analogues should be considered for prophylaxis against *Pneumocystis* and varicella zoster.

Refractory and relapsed disease may be treated with retreatment of prior agents, if relapse is >12 months, or with further combination therapy. FCR (fludarabine, cyclophosphamide, rituximab) and PCR (pentostatin, cyclophosphamide, rituximab) have both shown response rates of 30% to 60% in fludarabine-pretreated populations. Alemtuzumab is showing increasing promise as a single or combined agent in refractory disease.

Autologous and allogeneic bone marrow transplantations are being explored as treatment options. Improved results have been noted with nonmyeloablative therapies. Young patients with high-risk disease should be considered for this therapy.

Complications

Autoimmune hemolytic anemia (AIHA) and autoimmune thrombocytopenia occur more frequently in advanced-stage patients and those with unmutated-IgVH. These complications should be evaluated with reticulocyte count, haptoglobin, LDH, and Coombs assay. The results should be interpreted in context of other features, as the reticulocyte count may be low due to bone marrow suppression or infiltration, the LDH may be elevated due to the disease, not hemolysis, and treatments such as fludarabine may induce AIHA by themselves. Treatment is typical of other AIHA and autoimmune thrombocytopenia processes with prednisone or equivalent glucocorticoid at a dose of 1 mg/kg/day, tapered after control of blood counts. Splenectomy may be needed if the blood counts do not improve on steroids. Local irradiation or splenectomy can control the effects of hypersplenism.

Infection can result from hypogammaglobulinemia, T-cell dysfunction, and decreased phagocytic function. Hypogammaglobulinemic patients with recurrent infections should be treated with intravenous immunoglobulin, 400 mg/kg IV, every 3 to 4 weeks (goal IgG trough, ~500 mg/dL), which reduces serious bacterial infection rates without altering overall survival. Patients treated with fludarabine or alemtuzumab develop therapy-related T-cell immune defects and are at a significantly increased risk of cytomegalovirus (CMV) reactivation, *Pneumocystis*, varicella zoster, herpes viruses, *Listeria*, and other opportunistic infections. Prophylaxis against *Pneumocystis*, herpes simplex virus, and varicella zoster virus, as well as monitoring for CMV reactivation should be considered when treating CLL patients with these agents.

Prognosis

Diffuse marrow involvement, rapidly increasing lymphocyte counts, and initial lymphocytosis of >50,000/μL indicate a poor prognosis for an individual patient with early-stage disease. Anemia and thrombocytopenia correspond with decreased median survival time. Overall, CLL is an indolent disease, and in the case of stages 0, I, and II, median survivals of >10 years are reported. Thus, these patients may die of other conditions rather than from CLL. However, if a patient presents with advanced disease, the course may be rapid, with a median survival of months to years. It is unclear whether cytotoxic therapy actually improves survival, although it can effectively palliate disease-related symptoms. Improved supportive care and infection therapy have improved survival and quality of life.

HAIRY CELL LEUKEMIA

Introduction

Hairy cell leukemia is a chronic B-cell leukemia, accounting for only 2% to 3% of all leukemias, usually affecting men >55 years old.

Presentation

Most patients present with malaise and fatigue. On physical exam, splenomegaly and hepatomegaly are evident in 95% and 40%, respectively. With more advanced disease, pancytopenia develops, and patients may present with bleeding or recurrent infections (bacterial, viral, fungal, or atypical mycobacterial).

Management

Diagnosis

A peripheral smear and bone marrow reveal the pathognomonic mononuclear cells. These cells have characteristic irregular hairlike projections around the border of the cytoplasm. CBC frequently shows anemia and thrombocytopenia and, less frequently, granulocytopenia. Although bone marrow aspiration is frequently unsuccessful, the biopsy may show the characteristic hairy cells. Immune studies are CD19, CD20, and, typically, CD103 positive. Also, hairy cells are TRAP (tartrate-resistant acid phosphatase) positive. Hairy cell leukemia is differentiated from CLL, lymphomas, and monocytic leukemia based on the characteristic cell morphology, TRAP test, and immune phenotype. There is no formal staging system.

Treatment

As with other chronic leukemias and lymphomas, early treatment does not improve overall outcome. The decision to treat is based on the development of cytopenias (hemoglobin, <10 g/dL, absolute neutrophil count, <1000/μL; platelets, <100,000/μL) and recurrent infections. Several treatment options are available (Table 29-8). Typically, cladribine or pentostatin is used. However, both of these agents induce significant and prolonged immunosuppression, which may last up to 54 months. Prophylaxis for herpes simplex virus and *Pneumocystis*, especially if concurrent steroids are used, is advised.

Prognosis

Before treatment, median survival was between 5 and 10 years. Survival has markedly improved with current therapies, as most untreated and pretreated patients have excellent response rates to cladribine or pentostatin (85% to 97% ORR), with 4-year survival rates of up to 96%.

TABLE 29-8	THERAPEUTIC OPTIONS FOR HAIRY CELL LEUKEMIA
Therapy	**Comment**
Cladribine	First-line agent, 7-day IV infusion with >90% response rate. Risk of myelosuppression
Interferon-alpha	Given for 1 year, >90% response rate
Pentostatin	Given for 3–6 months, many patients have a complete response. Complicated by neurotoxicity and skin rash
Splenectomy	Achieves a 75% response rate

KEY POINTS TO REMEMBER

- The leukemias are malignant proliferations of WBCs circulating in the blood. An accurate determination of the type and staging of the leukemia is essential for proper treatment and determination of prognosis.
- Acute leukemias are proliferations of immature cells that are rapidly progressive, whereas chronic leukemias tend to be more indolent and have a longer course, with mature circulating cells.
- It can be extremely difficult to distinguish ALL from AML on clinical and morphologic grounds alone, and flow cytometry is needed for accurate diagnosis.
- As a general rule, ALLs are childhood diseases, and AMLs are adult diseases. ALL in adults typically confers a worse prognosis.
- In promyelocytic (M3) leukemia, ATRA is given with induction chemotherapy to help manage DIC.
- "Good-prognosis" AMLs include those with t(15;17) (M3 or APL), t(8;21), and inversion 16. They can often be cured without stem cell transplant.
- CNS prophylaxis is an important component of therapy for ALL, as it has a high incidence of recurrence in the CNS.
- CML is characterized by Philadelphia t(9:22) and is treated with tyrosine kinase inhibitors.
- Once CML progresses to cytogenetically complex accelerated and blast phase, response rates and outcomes decline significantly.
- CLL treatment is based on risk factors and symptom management. Early therapy does not improve overall outcome.

REFERENCES AND SUGGESTED READINGS

Baccarani M, Saglio G, Goldman J, et al. Evolving concepts in the management of chronic myeloid leukemia: recommendations from an expert panel on behalf of the European LeukemiaNet. *Blood.* 2006;108:1809–1820.

Byrd JC, Lin TS, Grever MR. Treatment of relapsed chronic lymphocytic leukemia: old and new therapies. *Semin Oncol.* 2006;33:210–219.

Casciato DA, Lowitz BB. *Manual of Clinical Oncology.* 4th ed. Philadelphia: Lippincott Williams & Williams; 2000.

Cassileth PA, Harrington DP. Chemotherapy compared with autologous or allogeneic bone marrow transplantation in the management of acute myeloid leukemia in first remission. *N Engl J Med.* 1998;339:1649–1656.

Densmore JJ, Camitta BM, Williams ME. Acute lymphoblastic leukemia and lymphoblastic lymphoma. In: *American Society of Hematology Self-Assessment Program.* 2nd ed. Cambridge, MA: Blackwell; 2006.

DeVita VT, Hellman S, Rosenberg S. *Cancer: Principles and Practice of Oncology.* 6th ed. Philadelphia: Lippincott Williams & Wilkins; 2001.

Kantarjian HM, O'Brien S, Smith TL, et al. Results of treatment with Hyper-CVAD, a dose-intensive regimen, in adult acute lymphocytic leukemia. *J Clin Oncol.* 2000;18:547–561.

Rebulla P, Finazzi G, Marangoni F, et al. The threshold for prophylactic platelet transfusions in adults with acute myeloid leukemia. *N Engl J Med.* 1997;337:1870–1875.

Tallman MS, Nabhan C, Camitta BM. Acute myeloid leukemia. In: *American Society of Hematology Self-Assessment Program.* 2nd ed. Cambridge, MA: Blackwell; 2006.

Vardiman JW, Harris NL, Brunning RD. The World Health Organization (WHO) classification of the myeloid neoplasms. *Blood.* 2002;100(7):2292–2302.

Lymphoma

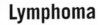

30

Todd A. Fehniger

Introduction

Lymphoma refers to the malignant transformation of lymphocytes (T cells, B cells, or NK cells). As a disease entity, it has an extraordinarily heterogeneous natural history and prognosis. This heterogeneity derives from the varied pathways leading to lymphoma, including the transformation of different lymphocyte types, at different developmental or differentiation stages, and through multiple molecular pathways. This complexity is exemplified by the >30 subtypes of lymphoma that are included in the current World Health Organization (WHO) classification, which divides lymphoma into subtypes based on the cell of origin, immunophenotype, morphologic appearance, and molecular pathophysiology. Hodgkin lymphoma (HL) is distinct from non-Hodgkin lymphoma (NHL). This chapter begins with the evaluation of suspected lymphoma, reviews lymphoma classification, epidemiology, and general diagnostic principles, and then describes the staging, prognosis, and treatment approaches to HL and common NHLs.

CLASSIFICATION

Lymphoma is currently classified based on the WHO classification of hematologic malignancies (Tables 30-1 and 30-2). Lymphoma is divided into HL and NHL variants and then subtyped into specific diagnoses. From a clinical perspective, NHLs are divided into indolent (low grade), aggressive (intermediate grade), and very aggressive (high grade) categories based on natural history, overall prognosis, and treatment approach.

EPIDEMIOLOGY

Overall, lymphoma is the fifth most common malignancy in the United States. There are about 7500 new cases of HL and 1500 deaths from HL annually. HL has a bimodal age-incidence curve, with a peak at age 30 and a second peak at age >50 years. In contrast, there are about 60,000 new cases of NHL and 15,000 deaths from NHL each year. The most common type of aggressive lymphoma is diffuse large B cell lymphoma (DLBCL), and the most common indolent lymphoma is follicular lymphoma (FL), together accounting for >50% of lymphoma diagnoses (Fig. 30-1). Risk factors for specific lymphoma subtypes include defined infectious pathogens (EBV, HTLV-1, HIV-1 [see Chap. 32], HHV-6, *H. pylori*), but in general, it remains unclear to what extent environmental or other exposures contribute to the development of lymphoma.

TABLE 30-1 · WHO CLASSIFICATION OF HODGKIN LYMPHOMA

Classical Hodgkin lymphoma (cHL)
  Nodular sclerosis cHL
  Mixed cellularity cHL
  Lymphocyte-rich cHL
  Lymphocyte-deplete cHL

Nodular lymphocyte-predominant Hodgkin
  lymphoma (NLPHL)

From Jaffe ES, Harris NL, Stein H, et al. Pathology and genetics of tumours of haematopoietic and lymphoid tissues. In: *World Health Organization Classification of Tumours.* Lyon, France: IARC Press; 2001, with permission.

TABLE 30-2 · WHO CLASSIFICATION OF NON-HODGKIN LYMPHOMA

Indolent	Aggressive	Highly Aggressive
B cell		
Follicular (grades I–IIIa)	Diffuse large B cell	Pre-B lymphoblastic
Small lymphocytic	Mediastinal (thymic)	Burkitt and Burkitt-like

Marginal zone
  Splenic MZL
  MALT MZL
  Nodal MZL
  Extranodal MZL
	Intravascular
	Mantle cell
	Follicular (grade IIIb)
	Primary effusion	

Lymphoplasmacytic		
T cell/NK cell		

Mycosis fungoides
Sezary syndrome
Primary cutaneous
  ALCL
	Anaplastic large cell
	Peripheral T cell NOS
	Angioimmunoblastic T cell
	Adult T cell
	Subcutaneous panniculitis-like
	  T cell
	Blastic NK cell lymphoma
	Extranodal NK/T cell, nasal type
	Enteropathy-type T cell
	Hepatosplenic T cell
		Pre-T lymphoblastic

ALCL, anaplastic large-cell lymphoma; MALT, extranodal MZL of mucosa-associated lymphoid tissue; MZL, marginal-zone lymphoma; NK, natural killer; NOS, not otherwise specified; WHO, World Health Organization. Diseases not included are reviewed in Chapters 13 and 29.

From Jaffe ES, Harris NL, Stein H, et al. Pathology and genetics of tumours of haematopoietic and lymphoid tissues. *World Health Organization Classification of Tumours.* Lyon, France: IARC Press; 2001, with permission.

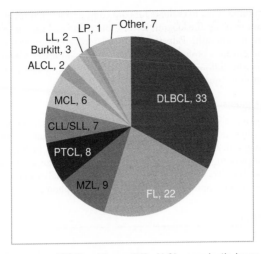

FIGURE 30-1. Frequency of NHL subtypes (%). ALCL, anaplastic large-cell lymphoma; CLL/SLL, chronic lymphocytic leukemia/small lymphocytic lymphoma; DLBCL, diffuse large B cell lymphoma; FL, follicular lymphoma; LL, lymphoblastic lymphoma; LP, lymphoplasmacytic lymphoma; MCL, mantle cell lymphoma; MZL, marginal-zone lymphoma; PTCL, peripheral T cell lymphoma. (Modified from Jaffe ES, Harris NL, Stein H, et al. Pathology and genetics of tumours of haematopoietic and lymphoid tissues. In: *World Health Organization Classification of Tumours.* Lyon, France: IARC Press; 2001, and A clinical evaluation of the International Lymphoma Study Group classification of non-Hodgkin's lymphoma. The Non-Hodgkin's Lymphoma Classification Project. *Blood.* 1997;89(11):3909–3918.)

PRESENTATION

History

Painless lymphadenopathy is the most frequent complaint of lymphoma patients. Defining the time of presentation and pace of lymph node enlargement provides clues to an indolent or aggressive character. Systemic **B symptoms** due to lymphoma include fever ($\geq 38.5°C$), drenching night sweats, and weight loss ($\geq 10\%$ of body weight over 6 months) and are used in lymphoma staging. Other symptoms reported by lymphoma patients include pruritus, fatigue, abdominal pain (enlarged spleen, liver, or bulky lymph node mass), bone pain (bone destruction or diffuse marrow involvement), neuropathic pain (nerve root compression, nerve infiltration, meningeal involvement, cord compression), and back pain (retroperitoneal lymph node involvement). Rare symptoms associated with HL include pain in enlarged lymph nodes after alcohol ingestion and periodic fever. In some cases, lymphoma presents at an extranodal site and may cause symptoms depending on the organ(s) involved. Determining the patient's performance status is also important for prognosis and treatment decisions.

Physical Exam

The physical exam is focused on identifying the number, size, and characteristics of palpable lymph nodes (cervical, submental, supraclavicular, infraclavicular, axillary, epitrochlear, inguinal, femoral), Waldeyer ring (tonsils, oropharynx), and enlargement of the liver or spleen. A complete neurological exam is warranted in patients presenting with back pain or neurologic symptoms (i.e., to evaluate for cord compression). During the physical exam it is also important to be on the lookout for possible extranodal sites of involvement (e.g., thyroid enlargement, skin rash). Palpation of an enlarged spleen or liver may be facilitated by deep palpation during a prolonged inspiration/expiration cycle. Massive splenomegaly may extend across the abdomen or into the pelvis, resulting in the splenic border being outside of the left upper quadrant.

Differential Diagnosis

The differential diagnosis of lymphoma typically includes other causes of lymphadenopathy: metastatic malignancies or infectious, autoimmune, and rheumatologic disorders. For patients presenting with isolated splenomegaly, other etiologies include infection, portal hypertension (congestion), storage diseases, metastatic tumors, autoimmune disorders, and myeloproliferative disorders (see Chap. 9). The main differential diagnoses of isolated massive splenomegaly are myeloproliferative disorders and lymphoma.

MANAGEMENT

Diagnosis

When lymphoma is suspected based on lymphadenopathy, an **excisional or incisional biopsy** is critical to obtain generous amounts of tissue for morphologic review of the lymph node architecture, immunostains (immunohistochemistry or flow cytometry), and ancillary genetic tests. If multiple peripheral lymph nodes are enlarged, the biopsy should be obtained from the largest accessible lymph node group. In general, smaller inguinal lymph nodes should be avoided if possible, as they may yield false negatives due to enlargement from common infections or inflammation in the lower extremities. If there are no peripheral lymph nodes accessible for surgical biopsy, the next option is core needle biopsy and fine-needle aspiration under ultrasound or CT guidance. In some cases, invasive procedures such as bronchoscopy, upper endoscopy, mediastinoscopy, and laparoscopy may be required. If a patient has isolated splenomegaly, splenectomy is usually recommended over a splenic needle biopsy. Finally, if there are no sites of disease amenable to biopsy, and the patient has abnormal circulating cells or cytopenias, a bone marrow biopsy may yield the diagnosis. Obtaining adequate biopsy material to make a definitive WHO classification diagnosis is important, as this will inform both prognosis and choice of therapy.

Workup

- **Radiographic studies.** In general, the first radiologic test in suspected lymphoma is a **contrast CT scan of the chest, abdomen, and pelvis** (and neck, if clinically involved). Alternatively, the combination of a PET scan with noncontrast CT (PET-CT) may provide a more accurate disease burden assessment. However, it is important to note that false positives and negatives do occur with PET scans, especially in indolent lymphomas. Additional imaging should be directed by the findings on history and physical (H&P) exam, and may include MRI or assessment of the spine (MRI or CT) or another suspected extranodal site.
- **Laboratory and ancillary diagnostic tests.** Lymphoma patients routinely require a CBC with differential, chemistries, lactate dehydrogenase (LDH; NHL), erythrocyte sedimentation rate (ESR; HL), and, in NHL with possible tumor lysis syndrome (e.g., aggressive/highly aggressive subtypes), measurement of uric acid, potassium, calcium, phosphorus, and creatinine. In most patients with lymphoma, a bilateral bone marrow biopsy and aspirate is required for accurate staging. If anthracycline-based chemotherapy is being considered, assessment of left ventricular function with a radionuclide ventriculogram (RVG)/multiple-gated acquisition (MUGA) scan or

two-dimensional echocardiogram is warranted. If CNS involvement is suspected based on clinical findings or a high-risk presentation, lumbar puncture with cytology should be performed.

- **Urgent or emergent presentations.** Due to its varied clinical presentation and multiple potential sites of involvement, several emergent or urgent problems need to be considered by the physician evaluating suspected or diagnosed lymphoma (also see Chap. 35). These include spinal cord compression (epidural mass), superior vena cava syndrome, hyperuricemia/tumor lysis syndrome, ureteral obstruction/hydronephrosis (bulky retroperitoneal or mesenteric disease), autoimmune hemolytic anemia, airway obstruction (bulky mediastinal disease), leptomeningeal lymphomatous involvement or CNS mass effect, hypercalcemia, and hyperviscosity syndrome (lymphoplasmacytic lymphoma).

HODGKIN LYMPHOMA

Pathophysiology

The malignant B cell in HL is the **Hodgkin Reed-Sternberg** (HRS) **cell**, which is a large, bi- or multinucleated cell that contains large nucleoli and expresses the CD30 and CD15 cell surface antigens. HL is defined by the presence of HRS cells located in the appropriate cellular background. Based on pathologic and clinical similarities, the WHO classification groups nodular sclerosis, mixed cellularity, lymphocyte-deplete, and lymphocyte-rich together as classical HL (cHL), whereas nodular lymphocyte-predominant HL is a separate diagnosis (Table 30-1). Nodular lymphocyte-predominant HL accounts for ~5% of HL diagnoses and is characterized by a clonal B cell population that expresses CD45, CD20, and CD79a.

Presentation

HL patients typically present with asymptomatic enlarged lymph nodes, with the disease originating in one lymph node group and spreading in a contiguous pattern. In older patients (>50 years), there may be a "skipped" lymph node segment (e.g., involvement of the cervical, supraclavicular, and portahepatic lymph nodes with skipping of the mediastinum). Alternative presentations include systemic B symptoms, usually indicative of advanced stage disease, and, rarely, symptoms due to extranodal involvement. The most common sites of extranodal involvement in cHL are the spleen, liver, lung, and bone marrow.

Management

Workup

The modified Ann Arbor staging system (Table 30-3) is based on the history of B symptoms, physical examination of lymphadenopathy and hepatosplenomegaly, and imaging of the chest, abdomen, and pelvis (chest x-ray [CXR] and CT, or PET-CT). Laboratory testing includes a CBC with differential, ESR, and chemistry panel. Bone marrow aspirate and biopsy (bilateral) are indicated in patients with advanced (stage III/IV) disease, B symptoms, or cytopenias, but they have a low yield in otherwise asymptomatic early stage (stage I/II) patients.

Prognosis

Stage is the most important determinant of overall prognosis in patients with cHL and guides appropriate therapy. Additional prognostic factors in early-stage disease are not well defined but include B symptoms, elevated ESR (>50), and four or more nodal sites. The **international prognostic score** (IPS; Table 30-4) was developed for patients with advanced-stage cHL and utilizes seven factors to predict outcomes after treatment with

TABLE 30-3	MODIFIED ANN ARBOR STAGING SYSTEM FOR LYMPHOMAS

Stage
I   Single lymph node region or lymphoid structure
II   ≥2 nodal regions on the same side of the diaphragm
III Involvement of lymph nodes on both sides of the diaphragm
IV Involvement of one or more extranodal sites

Modifiers
A   No additional symptoms
B   Presence of fever, drenching sweats, or weight loss
X   Bulky disease (nodal mass >10 cm or more than one third the width of the thorax)
E   Involvement of a single extranodal site contiguous or proximal to a nodal site
S   Splenic involvement

From Lister TA, Crowther D, Sutcliffe SB, et al. Report of a committee convened to discuss the evaluation and staging of patients with Hodgkin's disease: Cotswolds meeting. *J Clin Oncol.* 1989;7(11): 1630–1636.

standard (e.g., ABVD; Table 30-5) chemotherapy regimens. In general, cHL patients are categorized into early (stage I/II, no B symptoms, no bulky disease) and late/advanced (stage III/IV, B symptoms, bulky stage II) groups for treatment stratification. Early clinical trials with PET-CT suggest that patients with a positive scan after two to four cycles of therapy have a worse outcome compared to patients with a negative interim PET-CT.

TABLE 30-4	INTERNATIONAL PROGNOSTIC SCORE (IPS) FOR CLASSICAL HODGKIN LYMPHOMA

IPS Factors
1. Serum albumin <4 g/dL
2. Hemoglobin <10.5 g/dL
3. Male gender
4. Stage IV
5. Age >45 years
6. WBC ≥15,000/μL
7. Lymphocytes <8% of WBC or < 600/μL

Risk Factors	FFP at 5 yr (%)	OS at 5 yr (%)	Patients (%)
0	84	89	7
1	77	90	22
2	67	81	29
3	60	78	23
4	51	61	12
≥5	42	56	7

FFP, freedom from progression; OS, overall survival.
From Hasenclever D, Diehl V. A prognostic score for advanced Hodgkin's disease. International Prognostic Factors Project on Advanced Hodgkin's Disease. *N Engl J Med.* 1998;339(21):1506–1514.

TABLE 30-5	COMMONLY USED CHEMOTHERAPY REGIMENS IN CLASSICAL HODGKIN LYMPHOMA
ABVD	Doxorubicin, bleomycin, vinblastine, dacarbazine
Stanford V	Mechlorethamine, doxorubicin, vinblastine, vincristine, bleomycin, etoposide, prednisone
BEACOPP	Bleomycin, etoposide, doxorubicin, cyclophosphamide, vincristine, procarbazine, prednisone

Treatment
- **Early-stage cHL (stages I/II, no B symptoms, no bulky disease).** The modern treatment of early stage cHL results in very high response rates and long disease-free survival; thus, the focus of clinical investigation is on maintaining excellent disease results while minimizing long-term complications of therapy. Standard treatment approaches include combined modality therapy with **ABVD chemotherapy** (Table 30-5) × 2–4 cycles plus involved field radiotherapy (IFRT) or chemotherapy only with ABVD × 6 cycles. These approaches yield 85% to 95% 5-year disease-free survival rates. Late side effects and complications from radiation include secondary cancers and an elevated risk of coronary artery disease (CAD). Young patients (<30 years), smokers, patients with multiple risk factors for CAD, and patients with a family history of early breast cancer should be counseled on these risks and considered for treatment with chemotherapy alone. Current clinical trials are optimizing combined modality therapy by defining the necessary number of chemotherapy cycles and the dose of radiation.
- **Advanced-stage cHL (stages III/IV, B symptoms, bulky stage II).** Standard treatment of advanced cHL includes systemic chemotherapy with **ABVD** × 6–8 cycles. Consolidative radiotherapy is typically recommended for all patients with bulky (>10-cm) disease. This approach results in 5- and 15-year failure free survival rates of ~60% and ~45%, respectively, and 5- and 15-year overall survival rates of ~75% and ~60%. Alternative regimens include Stanford V (which includes IFRT to the initial sites of tumor bulk >5 cm) and dose-escalated BEACOPP (Table 30-5). Several randomized trials that evaluated high-dose therapy with autologous stem cell transplantation (SCT) for patients in their first complete remission have shown no difference in overall survival compared with standard chemotherapy, indicating that autologous SCT should be reserved for relapsed disease or a clinical trial. Clinical trials are currently comparing different chemotherapy approaches and will also stratify patients for treatment based on prognostic factors.
- **Relapsed cHL.** The approach to patients with relapsed cHL takes into account the primary therapy and duration of remission. Historically, patients with early-stage HL were treated with radiation therapy alone, and these patients are excellent candidates for standard systemic chemotherapy for cHL, which results in long-term disease-free survival in 50% to 80%. Patients who received initial chemotherapy and relapse late (>1 year) after remission may be considered for standard dose chemotherapy, resulting in 30% to 50% long-term disease free survival. Patients who relapse early (<1 year) after remission or those with poor prognostic factors (e.g., stages III/IV at relapse, B symptoms) should be treated with aggressive salvage chemotherapy (e.g., ICE, ESHAP) and be considered for high-dose chemotherapy with autologous SCT, which results in long-term disease-free survival in ~40%. Patients who relapse after autologous SCT should be considered for clinical trials evaluating novel agents and, in appropriate candidates, allogeneic SCT.

Follow-up

During the first 2 years after obtaining a complete remission, routine follow-up includes H&P, CBC, ESR, and comprehensive metabolic panel at 3-month intervals. Imaging is typically performed at 1 and 2 years postremission and as clinically indicated. After 2 years, evaluations (H&P and labs) may be spaced out to every 4 months, every 6 months, and then annually. Additional surveillance is required for patients who received radiation therapy. Thyroid screening tests should be performed annually after 1 year in patients who received radiation involving the neck. Surveillance for solid tumors (cancers of the skin, soft tissue, breast, and lung) should begin 5 to 10 years following therapy and continue for the lifetime of the patient. In all cases, appropriate diagnostic testing should be performed if new findings (e.g., lymphadenopathy) or symptoms arise.

Complications

Short-term adverse effects of chemotherapy depend on the regimen used. For example, ABVD may cause nausea/vomiting, constipation, alopecia, bone marrow suppression, neuropathy, cardiotoxicity, pulmonary toxicity, mucositis, and infection. Long-term side effects of radiation therapy include **secondary malignancies**, which typically occur 2 to 10 years after treatment and include solid cancers of the lung (very high risk in smokers), breast (especially in women radiated when <30 years old), skin (melanoma), and bone/soft tissue. **Hypothyroidism** occurs in 50% of neck radiotherapy patients at 1 to 20 years after treatment. The risk of coronary artery disease is also increased, especially for patients irradiated when <30 years old. The risk of infertility and **secondary MDS/leukemia** is low with standard ABVD chemotherapy but higher in patients who receive dose-intensive regimens.

Special Topics

Nodular lymphocyte-predominant HL is a distinct subtype of HL and is best characterized as an indolent B cell lymphoma with a good prognosis. For patients with stage I disease, IFRT alone should be considered, and clinical trials exploring single-agent rituximab have shown promising results. For advanced-stage presentation (uncommon), treatment with systemic chemotherapy used in indolent B cell NHL should be considered (e.g., R-CHOP; see below).

NON-HODGKIN LYMPHOMA

Introduction

The most common "prototype" indolent (follicular; FL) and aggressive (DLBCL) NHL are presented in this chapter, with additional clinical situations and subtypes briefly reviewed under Special Topics.

Pathophysiology

NHL is defined by the growth and/or survival of a clonal population of lymphocytes, which are B cells in both FL and DLBCL. The genetic hallmark of FL is the translocation of chromosomes 14 and 18, t(14;18)(q32;q21), involving the BCL-2 gene and the immunoglobulin heavy-chain locus. This translocation results in the dysregulation and increased expression of BCL2, an antiapoptotic survival factor for B cells. DLBCL has genetic and molecular heterogeneity revealed by gene expression profiling, which suggests a number of molecular subtypes of DLBCL exist. One common (~40%) change in DLBCL involves abnormalities of the BCL-6 gene on chromosome 3q27, which typically results in overexpression. BCL-6 is a transcription factor that regulates genes involved in apoptosis, the cell cycle, and lymphocyte development. The pathological determination of NHL subtype is based on morphology, immunophenotype, and genetic and molecular analysis.

Presentation

The most common presentation of NHL is **painless enlarged lymph nodes** similar to those in HL; however, NHL hematogenously spreads to multiple noncontiguous lymph node groups. In FL lymph nodes typically enlarge slowly over months to years (and may wax and wane), while in DLBCL lymph nodes enlarge over weeks to months. Systemic B symptoms are observed in about one third of DLBCL and one fifth of FL patients. Extranodal involvement is more common in DLBCL (~40%) and may involve the bone marrow, skin, GI tract, testes, salivary glands, liver, spleen, breast, adrenals, bone, sinuses, and CNS. The majority of FL patients present with involvement of the liver, spleen, or bone marrow at diagnosis.

Management

Workup

Staging and Lab Tests. The routine staging and laboratory testing for NHL is very similar to that for HL (Table 30-3). Routine lab tests include LDH, CBC with differential, and chemistries. A precise determination of the subtype of NHL (Table 30-2) by a hematopathologist examining adequate biopsy material is essential to define prognosis and guide treatment.

Prognosis

The prognosis of NHL is determined by multiple factors but starts with defining the subtype of NHL. In general, indolent NHLs are not considered curable, while aggressive NHL patients have a significant chance for long-term disease-free survival after initial therapy. The **international prognostic index (IPI)** was developed to help predict complete remission and long-term survival in aggressive NHL such as DLBCL at a time when CHOP-like chemotherapy was standard treatment. Subsequently, the IPI factors were used to develop a revised IPI to provide prognostic information with current front-line treatment approaches that combine the anti-CD20 monoclonal antibody rituximab with CHOP chemotherapy (Table 30-6). The follicular lymphoma IPI (FLIPI) was developed to define overall prognosis (Table 30-7) in FL, and results have shown that this index is useful in patients treated with current chemotherapy. Additional laboratory parameters, gene expression profiling, and molecular analyses have been correlated with prognosis but are not routinely used in clinical practice.

Treatment

Indolent Non-Hodgkin Lymphoma. In general, advanced-stage indolent NHLs are not considered curable with current standard therapeutic approaches. Clinical data with long follow-up has shown that a considerable percentage of these FL patients may initially be safely observed without intervention, and in fact, a substantial number of patients (15% to 20%) never require therapy. Indications for treatment include bulky lymphadenopathy, B symptoms, threatened end-organ damage, cytopenias, and eligibility for a clinical trial. The "watchful waiting" approach does not alter overall survival but requires a reliable patient, and this paradigm may change in the future as more effective therapies are developed.

- **Treatment of early-stage indolent NHL.** A minority of FL patients present with early stage (I/II) disease and have a good prognosis when treated with IFRT or IFRT plus chemotherapy (e.g., R-CHOP; Table 30-8), with a 10-year progression-free survival rate of 50% to 70%.
- **Treatment of advanced-stage indolent NHL.** When FL patients have an indication for therapy, standard treatment includes **rituximab plus chemotherapy** (e.g., CHOP, CVP, FND, fludarabine), with a 3-year progression-free survival rate of 50% to 77%. There is no clear superiority of one combination regimen; however, R-CHOP is a reasonable choice, as nonrandomized trials have shown high remission rates with

TABLE 30-6 INTERNATIONAL PROGNOSTIC INDEX (IPI) FOR NHL

Risk Factors

1. Age >60 yr
2. LDH >normal
3. ECOG PS 2–4
4. Stage III or IV
5. ≥2 extranodal sites

Standard IPI Score	Risk	CR (%)	OS at 5 yr (%)
0–1	Low	87	73
2	Low-intermediate	67	51
3	High-intermediate	55	43
4–5	High	44	26

Revised IPI Score	Risk	PFS at 4 yr (%)	OS at 4 yr (%)
0	Very good	94	94
1–2	Good	80	79
3–5	Poor	53	55

CR, complete remission; ECOG, Eastern Cooperative Oncology Group; LDH, lactate dehydrogenase; OS, overall survival; PFS, progression-free survival; PS, performance status.

Data from: A predictive model for aggressive non-Hodgkin's lymphoma. The International Non-Hodgkin's Lymphoma Prognostic Factors Project. *N Engl J Med.* 1993;329(14):987–994, and Sehn LH, Berry B, Chhanabhai M, et al. The revised International Prognostic Index (R-IPI) is a better predictor of outcome than the standard IPI for patients with diffuse large B-cell lymphoma treated with R-CHOP. *Blood.* 2007;109(5):1857–1861.

TABLE 30-7 FOLLICULAR LYMPHOMA INTERNATIONAL PROGNOSTIC INDEX (FLIPI)

FLIPI Factors

1. Age >60 yr
2. Stage III or IV
3. >4 nodal areas
4. LDH >normal
5. Hemoglobin <12 g/dl

Risk	Factors	5-yr OS (%)	10-yr OS (%)	Patients (%)
Low	0–1	91	71	36
Intermediate	2	78	51	37
High	≥3	53	36	27

OS, overall survival.

From Solal-Celigny P, Roy P, Colombat P, et al. Follicular lymphoma international prognostic index. *Blood.* 2004;104(5):1258–1265, with permission.

TABLE 30-8	COMMONLY USED CHEMOTHERAPY REGIMENS IN NON-HODGKIN LYMPHOMA
R	Rituximab (commonly combined with chemotherapy regimens, e.g., R-CHOP)
CHOP	Cyclophosphamide, doxorubicin, vincristine, prednisone
CVP	Cyclophosphamide, vincristine, prednisone
ESHAP	Etoposide, methylprednisolone, high-dose Ara-C, cisplatin
DHAP	Dexamethasone, high-dose Ara-C, cisplatin
ICE	Ifosfamide, carboplatin, etoposide
EPOCH	Etoposide, vincristine, doxorubicin, cyclophosphamide, prednisone
FND	Fludarabine, mitoxantrone, dexamethasone
FR	Fludarabine-rituximab

Ara-C, cytosine arabinoside.

a long median progression-free survival (>5 years). In elderly patients, single-agent rituximab is also an alternative approach. The use of maintenance rituximab (e.g., q3months × 2 years) following rituximab-containing combination regimens has shown improved progression-free survival but not overall survival. Current clinical trials are comparing front-line rituximab-chemotherapy combinations, evaluating radioimmunotherapy in the front-line setting, as well as evaluating the optimal dose, schedule, and duration of maintenance rituximab.

- **Treatment of relapsed indolent NHL.** The treatment of relapsed FL depends on the time frame of relapse and prior therapy. Patients who initially receive R-chemotherapy and relapse <1 year from initial therapy are typically considered for aggressive salvage approaches. Alternative treatment regimens include other R-chemotherapy combinations, radioimmunoconjugates that combine monoclonal antibodies and a radioactive isotope (e.g., tositumomab-^{131}I, ibritumomab-^{90}Y), autologous or allogeneic SCT (see Chap. 31), and investigational agents. New agents being evaluated include immune-based strategies such as idiotype vaccines, which vaccinate patients against their own lymphoma clone following treatment.

Aggressive Non-Hodgkin Lymphoma

- **Treatment of early-stage aggressive NHL.** Only a minority (<20%) of DLBCL patients present with early stage (I/II) disease, and these patients have a good prognosis, with 10-year survival estimates of 70% to 90%. Current treatment approaches include combined modality therapy with three cycles of R-CHOP plus IFRT or six cycles of R-CHOP chemotherapy. Patients with bulky stage II DLBCL have a worse prognosis and are typically treated as advanced stage disease.
- **Treatment of advanced-stage aggressive NHL.** In contrast to indolent NHL, advanced-stage DLBCL is initially treated with curative intent using rituximab plus anthracycline-containing combination chemotherapy (e.g., R-CHOP × 6–8 cycles). Patients with CNS relapse risk factors (testicular, breast, ovarian, bone marrow, or epidural involvement) should receive CNS prophylaxis with intrathecal chemotherapy or high-dose methotrexate (which crosses the blood-brain barrier). Similarly to cHL, clinical trials evaluating use of high-dose chemotherapy and autologous SCT in first complete remission have not demonstrated any survival benefit, and this approach is reserved for patients who relapse. Current clinical trials are evaluating

R-CHOP followed by autologous SCT in high-risk patients, and alternative doses/schedules of CHOP-like chemotherapy (e.g., dose-adjusted EPOCH-R).

- **Treatment of relapsed aggressive NHL.** DLBCL patients who relapse after obtaining a complete remission may also be treated with curative intent. Standard treatment including salvage chemotherapy (e.g., ESHAP or ICE) followed by SCT in appropriate candidates results in long-term disease-free survival in ~30% to 40%.

Follow-up

Similarly to HL, follow-up for DLBCL during the first 2 years after obtaining a remission includes H&P, CBC, LDH, and complete metabolic panel at 3-month intervals, with imaging typically repeated at 1 and 2 years and as clinically indicated. After 2 years, follow-up intervals may be lengthened, and after 5 to 10 years without relapse, patients may be followed by their primary care physician. For indolent NHL, follow-up is typically every 3 to 4 months, with imaging repeated annually and as clinically indicated.

Special Topics

- **Transformation to aggressive lymphoma.** Indolent NHL patients have a 1% to 3%/year risk of transforming into aggressive NHL (most commonly DLBCL), which commonly manifests as rapid enlargement of a single lymph node group, sudden rise in LDH, decline in performance status, hypercalcemia, or new extranodal involvement. Transformed NHL occurs regardless of treatment approach for the indolent NHL, it has a poor prognosis, and the optimal therapy is unclear. Therefore, these patients are encouraged to enroll in a clinical trial. If a trial is not available, they are typically treated similarly to patients with high-risk, relapsed DLBCL.
- **Marginal-zone lymphoma.** MALT marginal-zone lymphomas commonly present with localized disease (approximately two-thirds) involving the GI tract, thyroid, orbit/conjunctiva, lung, breast, or salivary glands. Gastric MALT lymphomas are associated with *H. pylori*, and complete responses are seen after antibiotic therapy aimed at eradicating the infection. At other sites, early-stage disease has an excellent prognosis with IFRT alone. Advanced-stage MALT lymphomas are treated with chemotherapy, similarly to FL. Splenic marginal-zone lymphoma also has an excellent prognosis, and first-line therapy involves splenectomy or single-agent rituximab, both of which may result in a high rate of complete remissions and long-term disease-free survival. Nodal and extranodal marginal-zone lymphomas are treated in a similar fashion to FL.
- **Mantle cell lymphoma.** Mantle cell lymphoma is an aggressive NHL characterized by t(11;14), a translocation that results in the overproduction of **cyclin D1**, which is identified by immunostains or molecular analysis as a key factor for diagnosis. Cure rates of mantle cell NHL are low with standard aggressive NHL therapy, and in appropriate candidates, aggressive chemotherapy regimens are warranted, preferably as part of a clinical trial. Typical approaches off-study include rituximab plus hyper-CVAD (hyperfractionated cyclophosphamide, vincristine, adriamycin, dexamethasone) alternating with high-dose methotrexate and cytosine arabinoside (Ara-C).
- **Burkitt lymphoma.** Burkitt lymphoma/leukemia is a highly aggressive NHL that may be endemic (e.g., equatorial Africa), associated with immunodeficiency (HIV), or sporadic (most common in the United States). The sporadic form is characterized by overexpression of the *c-myc* proto-oncogene, usually via the t(8;14) translocation. This NHL is rapidly life-threatening without therapy, has a poor prognosis, commonly involves the bone marrow and CNS, and is treated with aggressive combination chemotherapy (e.g., hyper-CVAD regimen) with CNS prophylaxis.
- **Lymphoblastic lymphoma.** Lymphoblastic lymphoma is another highly aggressive NHL, which is combined with acute lymphoblastic leukemia (ALL) in the WHO

classification. This disease is treated identically to ALL, with intensive chemotherapy, and also requires CNS prophylaxis (see Chap. 29). Prognosis is good for early-stage disease and intermediate for advanced-stage disease, with ~80% and ~50% chance of long-term disease-free survival, respectively.

- **Primary CNS lymphoma.** This entity is an aggressive NHL that presents with isolated CNS disease and, if untreated, has a rapidly fatal natural history. Compared to systemic DLBCL, its prognosis is worse, and treatment approaches include radiation therapy and/or chemotherapy that penetrates into the CNS (e.g., high-dose methotrexate).
- **AIDS-associated lymphoma.** See Chapter 32.
- **Cutaneous T cell lymphoma/mycosis fungoides.** Cutaneous T cell lymphomas typically present as erythematous plaques or exfoliation of skin but may progress to involve lymph nodes. They are treated with topical medications (steroids, retinoids, chemotherapy), local radiation, PUVA therapy, oral methotrexate and retinoids, interferon, and, at advanced stages, combination chemotherapy.
- **Anaplastic large-cell lymphoma.** This aggressive NHL typically involves both nodal and extranodal sites (e.g., skin, lung, bone, soft tissues) and is characterized by overexpression of anaplastic lymphoma kinase (ALK)-1, usually via a t(2;5) translocation. The presence of ALK-1 confers a much more favorable prognosis, compared with ALK-1-negative cases. Standard treatment is anthracycline-containing combination chemotherapy similar to DLBCL (e.g., CHOP), with good results (~70% long-term disease-free survival).

KEY POINTS TO REMEMBER

- To evaluate for suspected lymphoma, a generous incisional/excisional biopsy is critical to provide a WHO diagnosis and thereby inform prognosis and therapy.
- Lymphoma patients should have a definite diagnosis and complete staging workup prior to initiation of treatment.
- HL generally spreads in a contiguous fashion along lymph node chains and has a good chance for long-term disease-free survival with standard therapy.
- Indolent NHLs such as follicular lymphoma are usually incurable, but they have a long natural history and respond to chemotherapy.
- Aggressive NHLs such as DLBCL have a substantial chance for cure with chemotherapy; however, they have a high chance of being life-threatening if they do not respond to initial treatment.

REFERENCES AND SUGGESTED READINGS

Abramson JS, Shipp MA. Advances in the biology and therapy of diffuse large B-cell lymphoma: moving toward a molecularly targeted approach. *Blood.* 2005;106(4):1164–1174.

Armitage JO, Bierman PJ, Bociek RG, et al. Lymphoma 2006: classification and treatment. *Oncology (Williston Park).* 2006;20(3):231–239.

Bartlett NL. Therapies for relapsed Hodgkin lymphoma: transplant and non-transplant approaches including immunotherapy. *Hematology (Am Soc Hematol Educ Program).* 2005:245–251.

Canellos GP, Anderson JR, Propert KJ, et al. Chemotherapy of advanced Hodgkin's disease with MOPP, ABVD, or MOPP alternating with ABVD. *N Engl J Med.* 1992;327(21):1478–1484.

Cheson BD. Monoclonal antibody therapy for B-cell malignancies. *Semin Oncol.* 2006;33(2; Suppl 5):S2–S14.

Coiffier B, Lepage E, Briere J, et al. CHOP chemotherapy plus rituximab compared with CHOP alone in elderly patients with diffuse large-B-cell lymphoma. *N Engl J Med.* 2002;346(4):235–242.

DeVita VT, Hellman S, Rosenberg SA. *Cancer: Principles and Practice of Oncology.* 7th ed. Philadelphia: Lippincott Williams & Wilkins; 2005.

Diehl V, Franklin J, Pfreundschuh M, et al. Standard and increased-dose BEACOPP chemotherapy compared with COPP-ABVD for advanced Hodgkin's disease. *N Engl J Med.* 2003;348(24):2386–2395.

Hasenclever D, Diehl V. A prognostic score for advanced Hodgkin's disease. International Prognostic Factors Project on Advanced Hodgkin's Disease. *N Engl J Med.* 1998;339 (21):1506–1514.

International Non-Hodgkin's Lymphoma Prognostic Factors Project. A predictive model for aggressive non-Hodgkin's lymphoma. The International Non-Hodgkin's Lymphoma Prognostic Factors Project. *N Engl J Med.* 1993;329(14):987–994.

Jaffe ES, Harris NL, Stein H, et al. Pathology and genetics of tumours of haematopoietic and lymphoid tissues. In: *World Health Organization Classification of Tumours.* Lyon, France: IARC Press; 2001.

Lister TA, Crowther D, Sutcliffe SB, et al. Report of a committee convened to discuss the evaluation and staging of patients with Hodgkin's disease: Cotswolds meeting. *J Clin Oncol.* 1989;7(11):1630–1636.

Miller TP, Dahlberg S, Cassady JR, et al. Chemotherapy alone compared with chemotherapy plus radiotherapy for localized intermediate- and high-grade non-Hodgkin's lymphoma. *N Engl J Med.* 1998;339(1):21–26.

National Comprehensive Cancer Network, Inc. The NCCN Practice Guidelines in Non-Hodgkin Lymphoma, and Hodgkin Disease/Lymphoma. Clinical Practice Guidelines in Oncology. Version 2.2007, Version 1.2007. Available at: http://www.nccn.org. Accessed August 1, 2007. (To view the most recent and complete version of the guideline, go to www.nccn.org.)

Non-Hodgkin's Lymphoma Classification Project. A clinical evaluation of the International Lymphoma Study Group classification of non-Hodgkin's lymphoma. The Non-Hodgkin's Lymphoma Classification Project. *Blood.* 1997;89(11):3909–3918.

Philip T, Guglielmi C, Hagenbeek A, et al. Autologous bone marrow transplantation as compared with salvage chemotherapy in relapses of chemotherapy-sensitive non-Hodgkin's lymphoma. *N Engl J Med.* 1995;333(23):1540–1545.

Sehn LH, Berry B, Chhanabhai M, et al. The revised International Prognostic Index (R-IPI) is a better predictor of outcome than the standard IPI for patients with diffuse large B-cell lymphoma treated with R-CHOP. *Blood.* 2007;109(5):1857–1861.

Solal-Celigny P, Roy P, Colombat P, et al. Follicular lymphoma international prognostic index. *Blood.* 2004;104(5):1258–1265.

Winter JN, Gascoyne RD, Van Besien K. Low-grade lymphoma. *Hematology (Am Soc Hematol Educ Program).* 2004:203–220.

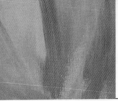

Introduction to Hematopoietic Stem Cell Transplantation

31

Pablo Ramirez

INTRODUCTION

Adult hematopoietic stem cells (HSCs) have two main characteristics: they are able to make identical copies of themselves for long periods of time (known as long-term self-renewal), and they can give rise to mature cells with specialized functions. Primitive stem cells create intermediate cells called precursor cells. Under specific signals these cells divide and become differentiated cells that finally mature to specialized blood cells.

The first therapeutic uses of HSCs began in the 1950s in patients with hematological malignancies, initially from allogeneic donors and later from autologous donors. The development of techniques that identified human tissue antigens, the discovery of the importance of histocompatibility, and studies showing improved outcomes when donor and recipient leukocyte antigens matched allowed transplants to gain more importance as a curative procedure.

Sources of Hematopoietic Stem Cells

HSC transplant is a general term referring to the reconstitution of a patient's hematopoietic system by the administration of stored HSCs. The most common source of HSCs in adults is **peripheral blood,** accounting for ~67% of transplants. **Bone marrow** is a source of HSCs in 30% of adult transplants. Cells are harvested directly from the bone marrow, usually from the iliac crests, under general anesthesia. **Umbilical cord blood** HSCs are currently used in 3% of transplants in adults, and the results are comparable to those achieved with adult unrelated donors.

Types of Hematopoietic Stem Cell Transplants

HSC transplants are divided into **allogeneic** and **autologous** transplants, depending on the relationship between the recipient and the donor.

Allogeneic transplant, where the donor is different from the recipient, can be classified as **sibling-derived** or **matched unrelated donor.** The two main sources of matched unrelated donor transplants are **adult unrelated donors** and **umbilical cord blood.** In addition to the effect of the preparative high-dose chemotherapy, the antitumoral effect of allogeneic transplants is mediated by the **graft-versus-tumor effect** (GvT), which consists in the immune destruction of residual tumor cells by the donor's immune system. In general, sibling transplants suffer fewer problems with rejection and **graft-versus-host disease** (GvHD) than matched unrelated donor transplants, and thus, recipients of the latter usually need more intensive immunosuppressive therapy in the posttransplant period (see Complications Related to Transplant, below).

Autologous transplant refers to the infusion of a patient's own HSCs to reconstitute all of the hematopoietic lineages. This approach is used to allow very high doses of chemotherapy to be administered. Infusion of autologous HSCs rescues a patient's bone marrow function from the effects of the myeloablative doses of chemotherapy.

Transplant Immunology

The major determinants of **histocompatibility** between donor and recipient, and thus risk for GvHD, are encoded by the **human leukocyte antigen** (HLA) **system** on chromosome 6. These proteins normally function in antigen presentation in adaptive immunity. The HLA class I antigens are called A, B, and C and are found on all nucleated cells. Class II proteins, called DR, DQ, and DP, are found only on dendritic cells, B lymphocytes, and macrophages. Traditionally, at the time of HSC matching of a potential donor, A, B and DR proteins are typed phenotypically by allele. If the donor and the recipient share the same alleles at these loci, then they are considered completely matched. Fortunately, the HLA locus can be considered a haplotype, so that all of the genes on one chromosome are inherited together (HLA A, B, and DR). This means that the region can effectively be thought of as one gene passed by Mendelian inheritance, owing to the low incidence of meiotic recombination between the loci at this site. Thus, for any given patient, the probability is one in four that a sibling will share the same two haplotypes and make a complete match. Currently, in unrelated transplants, the replacement of serological tissue typing for a DNA-based tissue typing has allowed more precise HLA matching between donor and recipient, improvement in overall survival, reduction in incidence of GvHD, and improvement in engraftment rate.

Other antigens called **minor histocompatibility antigens** (MHCs) are peptides also presented by HLA proteins but that elicit weaker responses compared to major antigens. These antigens are related to both GvHD and GvT effect. MHCs expressed only on the recipient HSCs will cause a GvT effect. MHCs expressed on both epithelial cells and HSCs will cause both GvHD and GvT.

THE TRANSPLANT PROCEDURE

Mobilization and Collection of Hematopoietic Stem Cells

In order to collect the necessary number of HSCs from the donor and to ensure rapid engraftment in the recipient's bone marrow, autologous and allogeneic HSCs are most commonly collected by leukapheresis from the peripheral blood after pretreatment with drugs that mobilize the HSCs from the bone marrow endosteal and vascular niches (**mobilization**). The most extensively studied mobilizing agent is granulocyte colony-stimulating factor (G-CSF). For G-CSF, the peak mobilization occurs after 4 to 6 days of daily treatment. During the harvest procedure, called **leukapheresis**, leukocytes are separated and removed from the other components of the blood by a cell-separator machine. The cells are then processed and stored for infusion into the patient.

Preparative Regimens

In **allogeneic transplants**, the traditional preparative regimens are **ablative regimens**, consisting of very high doses of chemotherapy drug combinations intended primarily to eliminate the tumor cells and secondarily to suppress the donor immune system. Due to the high toxicity associated with this approach, and in order to extend transplants to older patients or patients with comorbidities, **reduced intensity** and **nonmyeloablative regimens** have been developed. The basic principle is to give drugs that are immunosuppressive to allow the GvT effect.

In the **autologous** setting, the objective is to give high-dose chemotherapy to eliminate the tumor cells and then rescue the patient from aplasia with his or her own previously harvested and stored HSCs. In this case there is no GvT effect, and the disease control is exclusively due to the high-dose chemotherapy.

Among the most commonly used drugs are cyclophosphamide, busulfan, fludarabine, melphalan, etoposide, and antithymocyte globulin. **Total-body irradiation**-based regimens combine high-dose chemotherapy with irradiation to the whole body.

After the conditioning regimen is administered, patients will become profoundly pancytopenic (absolute neutrophil count, <100; platelet count, <10,000 cells/µL) for a period of between 12 and 24 days, depending on the source of HSCs (autologous or allogeneic) and preparative regimen used (ablative or nonablative).

Homing and Engraftment

After infusion, HSCs migrate to specific sites in the bone marrow called niches, where they reside and undergo self-renewal and differentiation. The process of migration and adhesion is called **homing**. The interaction between HSC and their niches will result ultimately in **engraftment** and long-term durable repopulation. The processes of both homing and engraftment require several adhesion molecules. The most important correspond to axes SDF-1/CXCR4, VLA-4/ VCAM-1, and CD44/hyaluronic acid.

Ten to fourteen days after the HSC infusion, there is evidence of marrow expansion, and by 10 to 21 days, neutrophils can be detected in the peripheral blood. Factors affecting time to recovery include the use of G-CSF during mobilization and harvest, degree of pretreatment chemotherapy, use of peripheral blood HSCs instead of bone marrow HSCs, and presence of infections. By days 18 to 21, natural killer cells are expected and will provide antiviral responses. Platelet recovery is more prolonged. Patients will require blood and platelet support during this time. Monocytes typically are the first cells to recover, and their presence often heralds initial neutrophil and platelet recovery.

SUPPORTIVE CARE

The posttransplant period is a critical time for patients who have undergone transplant. They become profoundly pancytopenic. During this time, there is significant potential morbidity and mortality from infectious agents, drug toxicity, and bleeding complications. Intensive care in a dedicated unit experienced in HSC transplant is required to support patients and provide optimal outcome.

Blood Products

All cytomegalovirus (CMV)-seronegative patients should receive CMV-negative blood and platelet products both prior to and during the transplant period. Blood products should also be irradiated or leukodepleted to avoid T cell responses against host tissue (i.e., GvHD caused by the transfusion). Platelet products derived from a single donor are preferred to reduce alloantigen exposure.

Growth Factors

For both allogeneic and autologous transplants, **hematopoietic growth factors** have shown small reductions in the risk of documented infections, but with no effect on infection or treatment-related mortality. Specifically, in patients undergoing allogeneic HSC transplantation for myeloid leukemias, no long-term risk or benefit of using G-CSF after transplantation has been demonstrated. G-CSF shortens the posttranplantation neutropenic period by 4 to 5 days, without substantially affecting the hospitalization period or treatment-related mortality at days +30 and +100. Probabilities of acute and chronic GvHD, leukemia-free survival, and overall survival are similar whether or not G-CSF is given.

Recombinant human keratinocyte growth factor (Palifermin) is a monoclonal antibody approved by the FDA in December 2004 to decrease the incidence and duration of severe oral mucositis in patients with hematologic malignancies who are receiving myelotoxic therapy requiring HSC support. The mechanism of action involves induction of epithelial proliferation and differentiation. Clinical data show a decrease in frequency of severe mucositis, less narcotic use, and a decreased incidence of total parenteral nutrition use.

COMPLICATIONS RELATED TO TRANSPLANT

Graft-versus-Host Disease

GvHD corresponds to an immune response of the donor T cells against the recipient. It is the main cause of morbidity and mortality after allogeneic HSC transplants. The exact cause and pathogenesis are still not completely understood but are believed to be caused by a reaction of donor T cells against the receptor HLA class I antigens. This inflammatory response is augmented by intestinal damage caused by the preparative regimens, which cause leakage of bacterial lipopolyssacharides into the bloodstream, increasing and maintaining the cytokine storm and tissue damage.

GvHD has been divided into two phases, according to the timing of the symptoms. **Acute GvHD** occurs within 100 days after the transplant, and **chronic GvHD** occurs 100 days or more after the transplant, although the correlation between the two forms of GvHD is not very well understood. Moreover, not all cases of chronic GvHD are preceded by acute GvHD, although acute GvHD is the most important risk factor for chronic GvHD.

Acute GvHD is graded as stages 0 to IV (most severe) according to the intensity of the symptoms. The usual organs compromised are the skin, mucous membranes, gastrointestinal tract, and liver. The risk factors for acute GvHD include HLA disparity, matched unrelated donors, older patients, gender-mismatched HLA, donors previously sensitized by transfusion or pregnancy, and CMV-positive donors.

The most effective measure to prevent GvHD is an accurate HLA matching between donor and receptor. Other measures include posttransplant immunosuppressive drugs (methotrexate, cyclosporine, tacrolimus), immunosuppressive antibodies (anti-interleukin 2 and anti-tumor necrosis factor), and in vivo and ex vivo T cell depletion.

Once GvHD is established, the first-line treatment remains corticosteroids. Second-line treatments include high-dose corticosteroids, antithymocyte globulin, monoclonal antibodies against interleukin 2 receptor and tumor necrosis factor, mycophenolate mofetil, and cellular therapy.

Chronic GvHD develops in >50% of long-term survivors after HSC transplantation and affects both quality of life and survival. Manifestations resemble autoimmune diseases, suggesting T cell immune deregulation, and include dermal, hepatic, ocular, oral, pulmonary, gastrointestinal, and neuromuscular manifestations.

In contrast to acute GvHD, little is known about the causes and pathobiology of chronic GvHD. Presumably, MHCs would be both responsible for and targets of this disease. It is also believed that chronic T cell stimulation (as occurs in acute GvHD) could deregulate T cells, predisposing to chronic GvHD.

The most important risk factor for chronic GvHD is previous acute GvHD. Thirty percent of patients with grade 0 acute GvHD, versus 90% of grade IV acute GvHD patients, will develop chronic GvHD. Among patients with no or grade I acute GvHD, recipient age >20 years, use of non-T cell-depleted bone marrow, and alloimmune female donors for male recipients predict a greater risk of chronic GvHD.

Prevention of chronic GvHD includes drugs such as cyclosporine, methotrexate, tacrolimus, corticosteroids, in vivo and ex vivo T cell depletion, and monoclonal and polyclonal antibodies. Treatment of chronic GvHD includes immunosuppressive drugs such as corticosteroids and tacrolimus. Also under research is the use of thalidomide, pentostatin, mycophenolate mofetil, and extracorporeal photopheresis.

Sinusoidal Obstruction Syndrome (Veno-occlusive Disease)

Sinusoidal obstruction syndrome (SOS) is a feared complication with a high mortality rate that can occur after either allogeneic or autologous transplant. The incidence ranges from 0% to 50%, depending on the preparative regimen. Almost 50% of patients receiving total-body irradiation or cyclophosphamide will develop SOS. Experimental studies have shown that the main damage occurs in the hepatic sinusoid.

The gold standard diagnostic test is a hepatic biopsy. However, because a biopsy is high risk in these patients, the major features accepted for diagnosis are jaundice, rising conjugated bilirubin, tender hepatomegaly, and ascites with fluid retention 10 to 20 days after the start of preparative regimen. There are no other specific lab tests to confirm this complication.

There is no effective therapy for SOS. In 50% to 80% of patients, there is a gradual spontaneous resolution of the symptoms and signs in a 3-week period after onset of disease.

Mucositis

Mucositis is extremely common during the neutropenic period and corresponds to the painful desquamation of the gastrointestinal epithelium. Almost 100% of patients will develop some grade of mucositis after the conditioning regimen, usually starting 3 to 5 days after the preparative regimen and lasting for 7 to 14 days.

The only demonstrated preventive treatment currently available is Palifermin (keratinocyte growth factor), which is able to reduce the frequency of severe mucositis significantly, from 60% to 20%. Others measures after mucositis is established include bland rinses, topical anesthetics, mucosal coating agents, and topical and systemic analgesics.

Infections

Patients undergoing HSC transplantation are at very high risk of infection due to the disease itself, previous chemotherapies, the preparative regimen, mucosal barrier breakdown, GvHD, and immunosuppressive drugs.

There are three periods of host defense recovery after HSC transplantation, and particular infections pose a threat in each period. The **early period**, the first 6 weeks posttransplant, is marked by **severe neutropenia** and mucosal barrier damage. As such, the patient is at risk of infection with skin and gastrointestinal organisms. Gram-negative bacilli, *Escherichia coli*, *Pseudomonas*, *Klebsiella*, and other enterics may cause local infection or sepsis. Enterococci or *viridans* streptococci may also cause bacteremia. Catheter-related bloodstream infection can be caused by staphylococci, particularly *Staphylococcus epidermidis*. Fungi, including *Candida* species and *Aspergillus*, may cause disseminated disease. Viral reactivation with herpes simplex virus (HSV) is common, as is varicella zoster virus (VZV), causing shingles. Human herpesvirus 6 commonly reactivates and is implicated in graft failure. BK virus is associated with encephalitis, hepatitis, and cystitis. Adenovirus and rotavirus may cause enteritis. Respiratory pathogens include adenovirus, influenza, parainfluenza, and respiratory syncytial virus.

Special consideration is given to nosocomial transmission of pathogens, including drug-resistant organisms. Thus, vigilance for methicillin-resistant *Staphylococcus aureus* is necessary, and broad coverage with vancomycin may be appropriate in the setting of neutropenic fevers without a known focus. Vancomycin-resistant enterococcus is commonly isolated from the stool but is often nonpathogenic; however, it requires treatment if isolated from the blood. *Clostridium difficile* causing colitis and diarrhea is problematic, as many patients receive broad antibiotics at some point during transplant. Contact isolation and strict adherence to routine hand washing are necessary to prevent outbreaks of nosocomial pathogens.

The **midrecovery** period, from 2 to 3 months posttransplant, is characterized by intense cellular and humoral immunodeficiency, the appearance of GvHD, and increased risk of CMV reactivation.

The **late recovery** period is characterized by a T **cell-mediated immunodeficiency.** Several studies have demonstrated that although innate immunity recovers within several weeks, B cell and CD8 T cell counts take several months to normalize, and CD4 T cells can take several years or, indeed, may never recover in the presence of chronic GvHD.

Among the most common infections in the later stages after transplantation is recurrent encapsulated bacterial infection, CMV reactivation, which can cause interstitial pneumonia and retinal compromise, and VZV reactivation. Patients are also at risk of *Pneumocystis jiroveci* (formerly *P. carinii*) and *Aspergillus* sp. pneumonia.

Prevention of Infections

Strict adherence to hand-washing procedures and isolation precautions (visitor screening, HEPA filtered air, no fresh flowers) is mandatory in the care of the HSC transplant patient. Avoidance of unwashed fruits, vegetables, and raw food is recommended but its impact on infection prevention is not known. Also, good oral and body hygiene is recommended. Gut decontamination with antibiotics is no longer recommended.

Routine prophylaxis includes trimethoprim-sulfamethoxazole against *Pneumocystis*, acyclovir against HSV and VZV, and fluconazole or itraconazole against candidemia. Vaccination with inactivated vaccines can proceed >12 months posttransplant, and patients will require a 23-valent pneumococcal vaccine as well as yearly influenza vaccinations (resuming 6 months posttransplant). Recent data show that a heat-inactivated varicella vaccine may be effective in this population in preventing VZV reactivation. Complete guidelines for preventing opportunistic infections among hematopoietic stem cell transplant recipients can be found at http://www.cdc.gov/mmwr/preview/mmwrhtml/rr4910a1.htm.

General Principles of Treatment of Infections

Workup should be directed at the most likely organisms based on time after HSC transplant. Under the minimal suspicion of infection, rapid labs and imaging, such as blood and urine cultures, CMV or aspergillus serologies, chest x-ray, and sinus or chest CTs, should be done. Treatment often requires broad-spectrum antibiotics and antifungals, which should be started as soon as possible and normally without knowing the causative agent. Acyclovir is used for HSV and VZV at therapeutic doses. For CMV, ganciclovir or foscarnet is required. Human herpesvirus 6 is responsive to ganciclovir or foscarnet. *Candida albicans* and *tropicalis* are sensitive to fluconazole but disseminated infection may require caspofungin, voriconazole, or amphotericin. Other *Candida* species, such as *Candida glabrata* and *Candida krusei*, respond to itraconazole, voriconazole, caspofungin, or amphotericin. For aspergillosis, amphotericin is the standard; however, voriconazole and caspofungin are very effective, with fewer side effects. If IV amphotericin is required, lipid formulations may be used to reduce renal toxicity.

HEMATOPOIETIC STEM CELL TRANSPLANT PROGNOSIS

Despite significant advances in the knowledge of the biology and results of HSC transplantation, infections and other treatment-related complications are still a limiting factor in improving outcomes. Many complications are emergent and require admission to an ICU. Respiratory failure due to infections is common and may require mechanical ventilation. In addition, GvHD, infections and medication toxicities may contribute to multiple-organ dysfunction syndrome. The mortality rate is high in these situations, and overall prognosis should be discussed with the patient and family members promptly. Long-term survivors are at risk of complications such as chronic GvHD and secondary malignancies and should be closely followed. Factors such as age, comorbidities, and indication for and type of transplantation all contribute to the overall prognosis in each individual patient.

- Adult HSCs can be used to restore a patient's own hematopoiesis and immunity after ablative chemotherapy.
- The source of HSCs can be the patient (autologous) or a donor (allogeneic).
- If an infection is suspected in a neutropenic or immunosuppressed patient, broad-spectrum antibiotics must be started urgently.
- The most important causes of morbidity and mortality after the transplant are bacterial and viral infections (both autologous and allogeneic transplants) and acute and chronic GvHD (allogeneic transplants).

REFERENCES AND SUGGESTED READINGS

Bacigalupo A. Management of acute graft-versus-host disease. *Br J Haematol.* 2007;137: 87–98.

Copelan EA. Hematopoietic stem-cell transplantation. *N Engl J Med.* 2006;354: 1813–1826.

Geddes M, Storek J. Immune reconstitution following hematopoietic stem-cell transplantation. *Best Pract Res Clin Haematol.* 2007;20:329–348.

Holler E. Risk assessment in haematopoietic stem cell transplantation: prevention and treatment. *Best Pract Res Clin Haematol.* 2007;20:281–294.

Schlomchik WD, Lee SJ, Couriel D, et al. Transplantation's greatest challenges: advances in chronic graft-versus-host disease. *Biol Blood Marrow Transplant.* 2007;13:2–10.

Thomas ED, Blume KG, Forman SJ, et al. *Thomas' Hematopoietic Cell Transplantation.* 3rd ed. Cambridge, MA: Blackwell; 2004.

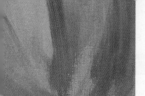

Human Immunodeficiency Virus-Related Malignancies

32

Giridharan Ramsingh and Nina Asrani

INTRODUCTION

Patients infected with human immunodeficiency virus (HIV) are at significantly increased risk of developing a malignancy compared with the general population. The possible mechanisms and pathways responsible for development of cancer include tumorigenic effects of coinfection with other viruses, HIV infection-induced immune dysregulation causing chronic immune stimulation, cytokine activation with resultant immunosuppression, and confounding epidemiological risk factors for malignancies. HIV is not an oncogenic virus by itself. AIDS-defining malignancies include Kaposi sarcoma (KS), primary central nervous system lymphoma (PCNSL), non-Hodgkin lymphoma (NHL), and invasive cervical cancer. In addition, patients with HIV infection are also at increased risk of developing certain non-AIDS defining malignancies. Introduction of highly active antiretroviral therapy (HAART) has resulted in a significant change in the epidemiological and clinical profile of cancers in HIV-infected patients by decreasing the mortality associated with opportunistic infections and by improving the longevity of the patients. Although a significant decrease has been reported in certain AIDS-defining malignancies such as KS in the developed world, as patients live longer with chronic HIV infection, malignancy is becoming an important cause of morbidity and mortality. Immune reconstitution following HAART and advances in chemotherapy and supportive care have resulted in improved outcomes of cancer compared to the pre-HAART era.

KAPOSI SARCOMA

Epidemiology

KS is the most common HIV-related malignancy. Though the incidence of KS has decreased significantly since HAART, it continues to be a problem of epidemic proportion in the parts of the world where HIV remains untreated. KS-associated herpes virus, human herpes virus 8 (HHV-8), infection is found in all forms of KS. HHV-8 infection is transmitted by sexual contact, but it is also found in the saliva of infected patients. Though patients on HAART have a less severe disease at presentation, the natural course of disease does not change with prior HAART.

Pathophysiology

KS lesions are histologically characterized by neoangiogenesis and proliferating spindle-shaped cells admixed with an inflammatory infiltrate of lymphocytes, plasma cells, and macrophages. The malignant spindle-shaped cells are thought to be derived from lymphatic endothelial cells. The HHV-8 virus expresses proteins that are homologous to interleukin 6, chemokines of the macrophage inflammatory protein family, and antiapoptotic molecules of the bcl-2 family.

Clinical Presentation

The clinical presentation of KS varies from minimal to fulminant disease. AIDS-related KS is generally an aggressive cancer resulting in serious morbidity and mortality. Although no organ is spared from involvement with KS, the most commonly involved sites are skin, mucous membranes, lymph nodes, gastrointestinal tract, and lungs. The cutaneous lesions are typically multifocal, plaquelike or papular, and pinkish to violaceous in color, although they may evolve into nodules and ultimately ulcerate. Lymph node involvement can cause lymphedema. Internal disease can present with vague symptoms and can occur in the absence of mucocutaneous manifestations. Gastrointestinal involvement can cause abdominal pain or bleeding.

Management

Diagnosis is established by biopsy of lesions; bronchoscopy or esophagoduodenoscopy may be necessary for internal involvement. Serology for anti-HHV-8 antibodies is not central to the diagnosis. It is important to note that KS is not considered a curable malignancy. The treatment decisions are based on the presence and extent of symptomatic and extracutaneous manifestations. Optimization of HAART therapy is the first line of therapy. Local therapy is used for bulky lesions or for cosmesis. Therapeutic options for local treatment include topical alitretinoin, intralesional chemotherapy with vinblastine, radiation therapy, laser therapy, and cryotherapy. Individuals with more advanced or progressive disease are treated with systemic chemotherapy. First-line chemotherapeutic drugs are liposomal anthracyclines such as doxorubicin and daunorubicin. Paclitaxel is a second-line agent. High-dose interferon-alpha therapy can be used for patients following immune reconstitution, but it is associated with significant side effects. Drugs inducing antiangiogenesis are being investigated.

Prognosis

The AIDS Clinical Trials Group classifies patients with AIDS-related KS into good- and poor-risk groups based on tumor burden, CD4 counts, and the presence of systemic illness. However, in the post-HAART era, the CD4 count is less important. Advanced age and associated AIDS-defining illnesses also affect the outcome of patients with KS.

HUMAN IMMUNODEFICIENCY VIRUS-RELATED LYMPHOMAS

Epidemiology

HIV-associated lymphomas constitute the second most common type of malignancy encountered in patients with HIV infection. Introduction of HAART has not changed the overall incidence of HIV-associated lymphomas significantly; however, if HAART therapy is available and accessible in the community, the incidence of the NHL subtypes associated with severe immunosuppression is decreased. Systemic NHL is the most common type, although the greatest increase in risk over the general population seems to be with PCNSL.

Pathophysiology

Various pathogenic mechanisms are attributed to development of lymphoma in HIV, including HIV-induced immunosuppression, chronic antigenic stimulation, genetic abnormalities, cytokine dysregulation, dendritic cell impairment, and viral infections associated with Epstein-Barr virus (EBV) and HHV-8.

Non-Hodgkin Lymphoma

Classification and Clinical Presentation

HIV-related NHLs are a heterogeneous group of tumors. More than 95% of the tumors are derived from B cells. Notable differences between HIV-related lymphoma and NHL in the general population include propensity for advanced disease, presence of B symptoms, extranodal disease including bone marrow involvement, leptomeningeal disease, and disease in unusual locations.

- **Diffuse large B cell lymphoma** (DLBCL) is the most common HIV-related lymphoma. It is divided into centroblastic and immunoblastic types. The immunoblastic type is more characteristic of HIV infection and is more frequently associated with EBV infection (90%) compared to the centroblastic type (30%). Amplification of bcl-6, a proto-oncogene product, is usually associated with centroblastic and not immunoblastic DLBCL.
- **Burkitt lymphoma** accounts for 30% of HIV-related lymphoma. It is associated with c-myc oncogene activation. Only 30% to 50% of HIV-related Burkitt lymphoma are associated with EBV infection, suggesting other pathogenic mechanisms in the oncogenesis.
- **PCNSL** represents a distinct extranodal presentation of DLBCL in HIV infection. It is usually of the immunoblastic type and is associated with severe immunosuppression (CD4 count, <50) and universal EBV infection. Its involvement is usually confined to the craniospinal axis, without any systemic involvement. Its prognosis is extremely poor.
- **Primary effusion lymphoma** represents <5% of HIV-related lymphomas. It is associated with HHV-8 infection and frequent coinfection with EBV. It is an aggressive tumor and morphologically varies from the immunoblastic to the anaplastic type. It is of B cell origin but does not express B cell antigens.
- **Plasmablastic lymphoma** is a subtype that typically involves the oral cavity and jaw. It is highly associated with EBV infection and lacks HHV-8 infection. The tumor consists of large plasmablast cells with the morphological features of immunoblasts but the immunophenotypic features of plasma cells.

Workup

Since many other HIV-associated diseases, including various infections, can mimic the clinical and imaging features of lymphoma, biopsy is typically needed for diagnosis. The **staging workup** includes CT of the chest, abdomen, and pelvis and bone marrow evaluation. Because CNS involvement is common, MRI of the brain and lumbar puncture for cerebrospinal fluid (CSF) analysis should be considered for all patients with HIV-related lymphoma.

The **workup of a brain mass** requires special consideration. CNS imaging cannot reliably differentiate between CNS lymphoma and toxoplasmosis. A solitary lesion is more likely to be lymphoma. Antitoxoplasma antibody titers (IgG and IgM) should be obtained. If the serology is positive, the patient can be treated with empiric antibiotic therapy followed by repeat imaging in 10 days to look for regression. If the lesions worsen, brain biopsy is necessary to rule out lymphoma. CSF EBV DNA is 80% sensitive and 10 % specific for PCNSL and, hence, could substitute for a diagnostic biopsy.

Treatment

With the use of HAART and anticipated immune restoration, standard-dose chemotherapy is the standard of care in patients with HIV-related NHL. The regimens that have been studied include standard CHOP (cyclophosphamide, vincristine, doxorubicin, and prednisone) and dose-adjusted EPOCH (etoposide, prednisone, doxorubicin, cyclophosphamide, and vincristine). Whether HAART needs to be given concurrently with chemotherapy remains unanswered. If HAART is used with chemotherapy, zidovudine should be avoided due to an increased risk of myelosuppression. Also, caution should be exercised with didanosine, stavudine, and zalcitabine, which may potentiate vincristine-induced neuropathy. The role of rituximab in AIDS-related lymphoma remains unclear. Prophylactic intrathecal methotrexate may be delivered at the time of initial CSF analysis to reduce the risk of leptomeningeal disease, particularly in patients with Burkitt lymphoma, Burkitt-like lymphoma histology, bone marrow, paranasal or paraspinal involvement, or EBV virus coinfection. PCNSL is treated with high-dose methotrexate chemotherapy and/or whole-brain irradiation. Select patients with relapsed or refractory lymphoma can be considered for high-dose chemotherapy with stem cell support.

Prognosis
Poor prognostic factors include low CD4 counts (<100), elevated lactate dehydrogenase, poor performance status, presence of extranodal disease, prior-AIDS defining illness, advanced stage, and aggressive histology of lymphoma.

Hodgkin Lymphoma
Clinical features of HIV-associated Hodgkin lymphoma include a high frequency of B symptoms, advanced-stage disease, a higher incidence of bone marrow involvement, and universal EBV coinfection. Histological subtypes most often seen are mixed cellularity and lymphocyte depleted. Although chemotherapy outcomes are improving in the post-HAART era, the prognosis is significantly worse than that for HIV-negative patients. Timing of HAART therapy again remains inconclusive. Chemotherapy regimens that have been studied include ABVD (doxorubicin, bleomycin, vinblastine, and dacarbazine), BEACOPP (bleomycin, etoposide, doxorubicin, cyclophosphamide, vincristine, procarbazine, and prednisone), and the Stanford V regimen (doxorubicin, vinblastine, meclorethamine, etoposide, vincristine, bleomycin, prednisone, and involved field radiation for initial bulky disease).

CERVICAL CANCER

HIV infection is a strong risk factor for cervical cancer independent of the usual demographic and behavioral risk factors for cervical cancer. HIV-positive women have significantly increased rates of cervical intraepithelial neoplasia compared to HIV-negative individuals, and the incidence of cervical intraepithelial neoplasia increases with the severity of immunosuppression. However, there has been no convincing evidence to show increased invasive cervical neoplasm in HIV-infected individuals compared to HIV-negative women. HIV-positive patients are more likely to be infected with the oncogenic human papilloma virus (HPV) strains 16, 18, and 31 and, also, with multiple strains compared to HIV-negative individuals. HPV infection is more persistent in HIV-positive patients and correlates with the severity of immunosuppression. The Centers for Disease Control recommends two Pap smears at a 6-month interval for any woman newly diagnosed with HIV. If both are negative, a Pap smear should be repeated annually. HIV-positive patients with cervical cancer have more intractable disease and have a higher relapse rate compared to the HIV-negative group. Restoring immune function with HAART may improve the treatment outcome.

OTHER CANCERS

In large database studies of linked HIV and cancer registries, several other cancers have been shown to be increased in incidence compared to that in the general population: invasive anal carcinoma (an HPV-associated illness), multiple myeloma, leukemia, lung cancer, and malignancies of the oral cavity, lip, esophagus, stomach, liver, pancreas, larynx, heart, vulva, vagina, kidney, and soft tissues. Multiple myeloma in HIV-infected individuals occurs at a younger age and has a more aggressive clinical picture. The most common epithelial neoplasms seen in the general population—breast cancer, colon cancer, and prostate cancer—do not appear to occur more frequently in HIV-infected patients. In contrast to the adult malignancies, the clinical pathology and optimal therapy of AIDS-related malignancies in children are unclear.

KEY POINTS TO REMEMBER

- Patients with HIV infection are at increased risk of several malignancies including KS, NHL, and cervical cancer.
- KS is caused by HHV-8 virus coinfection in patients with HIV.
- The use of HAART results in a dramatic improvement in KS but less so in other malignancies.
- NHLs in HIV-positive individuals have certain unique features including advanced disease with higher incidence of CNS involvement at presentation.
- CNS lymphoma should be differentiated from CNS toxoplasmosis.
- HIV patients should be actively screened for cervical cancer and treated early.

REFERENCES AND SUGGESTED READINGS

Abeloff MD. *Clinical Oncology.* 3rd ed. New York: Churchill Livingstone; 2004.

Antman K, Chang Y. Kaposi's sarcoma. *N Engl J Med.* 2000;342:1027–1038.

Cheung MC, Pantonowitz L, Dezube BJ. AIDS-related malignancies: emerging challenges in the era of highly active antiretroviral therapy. *Oncologist.* 2005;10:412–426.

Ferenczy A, Coutlee F, Franco E, et al. Human papillomavirus and HIV coinfection and the risk of neoplasia in the lower genital tract: a review of recent developments. *Can Med Assoc J.* 2003;169(5):431–434.

Krown SE, Testa MA, Huang J. AIDS-related Kaposi's sarcoma: prospective validation of the AIDS Clinical Trials Group staging classification. AIDS Clinical Trials Group Oncology Committee. *J Clin Oncol.* 1997;15:3085.

Lim ST, Levine A. Recent advances in acquired immunodeficiency syndrome (AIDS)-related lymphoma. *CA Cancer J Clin.* 2005;55;229–241.

Mandell GL. *Principles and Practice of Infectious Diseases.* 6th ed. New York: Churchill Livingstone; 2004.

Pagano JS. Viruses and lymphomas. *N Engl J Med.* 2002;347:78–79.

Stebbing J, Sanitt A, Nelson M, et al. A prognostic index for AIDS-associated Kaposi's sarcoma in the era of highly active antiretroviral therapy. *Lancet.* 2006;367:1495–1502.

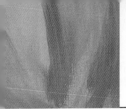

Cancer of Unknown Primary Site

33

Lukas D. Wartman

INTRODUCTION

Definition

Cancer of unknown primary site (CUPS) is defined as a biopsy-proven malignancy for which the site of origin is not defined by a thorough history and physical, imaging studies, chemistries (including tumor markers), and detailed pathologic evaluation. This is a heterogeneous group of patients and the median survival is 6 to 9 months, with little response to therapy. There are **subgroups,** however, with treatment-responsive disease, who may be able to achieve long-term disease-free survival. The workup of the patient with an unknown primary tumor is focused on identifying these patients with treatable disease. An exhaustive search for the primary tumor after these treatable cases have been excluded adds little to the overall management of the patient, as the primary tumor site is located in <30% of patients before death and is often not even found at autopsy.

Epidemiology

CUPS accounts for ~5% of all initial cancer diagnoses. It is generally a disease of the middle-aged, with the median age at diagnosis about 60. Equal numbers of men and women are affected. As noted earlier, the **median survival is poor**—6 to 9 months—regardless of treatment.

Classification

Light microscopy is the first step in the pathologic classification of these malignancies. There are **four major classifications:** moderately to well-differentiated adenocarcinoma (~60% of cases), poorly differentiated carcinoma/adenocarcinoma (~30%), poorly differentiated neoplasm (~5%), and squamous cell carcinoma (~5%).

- **Immunohistochemistry** is widely available and is often useful in classifying these tumors. Staining for the cytokeratins, CK7 and CK20, is the most common first step in trying to identify an occult adenocarcinoma. CK7-positive tumors include lung, urothelial, ovary, endometrium, and breast. CK20-positive tumors include gastrointestinal, urothelial, and Merkell cell carcinomas. Common leukocyte antigen (CD45) can distinguish lymphoma from carcinoma. *Neuroendocrine tumors* often stain positive for neuron-specific enolase, chromogranin, and synaptophysin. Prostate-specific antigen (PSA) staining is suggestive of *prostate cancer*, and estrogen receptor/progesterone receptor (ER/PR) and HER-2/neu staining is suggestive of *breast cancer*. Thyroglobulin is a marker of *thyroid cancer* and thyroid transcription factor (TTF-1) is a marker of *lung adenocarcinoma* and *thyroid tumors*. Alpha-fetoprotein (AFP) and beta-human chorionic gonadotropin (β-hCG) are markers for *germ cell cancers*. *Melanoma* often stains positive for vimentin, HMB-45, and S-100. *Sarcoma* may stain positive for vimentin, desmin, and von Willebrand antigen. Finally, CA125 is a marker of *ovarian cancer*, and the CDX2 transcription factor is a marker of *gastrointestinal tumors*.

- **Electron microscopy** is not widely available and is expensive, but it may contribute to the diagnosis in rare cases. For example, secretory granules are seen in neuroendocrine tumors, Weibel-Palade bodies in angiosarcomas, and premelanosomes in melanomas.
- **Cytogenetics** may also be useful. Isochromosome 12p and 12q⁻ are seen in germ cell tumors. The t(11;22) translocation is seen in Ewing sarcoma and primitive neuroectodermal tumor. The t(8;14) translocation is seen in some lymphoid malignancies, most commonly Burkitt lymphoma.

CLINICAL PRESENTATION

Patients typically present with symptoms of widely metastatic disease and often have multiple symptoms. Pain is the most common presenting symptom and is present in 60% of patients. Other symptoms include weight loss, anorexia, fatigue, new mass, lymphadenopathy, CNS abnormalities, and bone pain or fracture. Common **sites of metastasis** include lymph nodes, bone, liver, lung, brain, and skin. Cervical adenopathy can be a manifestation of primary lung, breast, or head and neck cancer, as well as lymphoma. A midline mass in the mediastinum or retroperitoneum is worrisome for an extragonadal tumor. One must remember that CUPS can metastasize to any site and that the pattern of metastasis, while sometimes suggestive of an underlying primary tumor, does not confirm the diagnosis.

MANAGEMENT

Workup

The workup of an occult primary tumor includes evaluation for the most common malignancies: breast, colon, prostate, and lung. Lung and pancreatic cancer are the primary tumors most likely to present as an unknown primary metastasis. Evaluation includes adequate **biopsy specimen** of the metastatic tumor with appropriate immunohistochemical pathologic studies, thorough **history and physical exam** (especially of head, neck, breast, pelvis, and rectum), **chest x-ray**, chemistries and blood counts, occult blood testing of stool, and consideration of CT imaging of the abdomen and pelvis. Tumor markers such as CEA, CA19-9, and CA125 are nonspecific and are generally not helpful in establishing a diagnosis; exceptions include checking serum AFP and β-hCG when a germ cell tumor is considered, as well as PSA screening in men if prostate cancer is considered. In addition, the workup of CUPS includes a **mammogram** in women with an occult adenocarcinoma. Additional imaging studies such as testicular ultrasound or breast MRI depend on the site of the metastasis and features on pathology. Endoscopy is generally indicated only in the presence of suggestive signs or symptoms.

The use of **fluorodeoxyglucose (FDG)-PET scans**, now routinely done in conjunction with a noncontrast CT study to provide better anatomic localization, are often performed in cases of CUPS. Small studies suggest that PET/CT may be more sensitive than traditional imaging studies in locating a primary tumor, but larger follow-up studies have yet to be reported. For now, clinical judgment governs the use of PET/CT in the workup of CUPS, and clinicians should consider this imaging test if the results would significantly change further management.

Poorly Differentiated Neoplasm

Poorly differentiated neoplasms account for ~5% of CUPS. Further pathologic studies are very important in this group, as treatment may differ radically depending on the results. Many of these tumors can be characterized as atypical lymphomas, neuroendocrine tumors, or germ cell tumors by careful pathologic testing. If a specific diagnosis cannot be made, then poorly differentiated neoplasms are treated the same as poorly differentiated adenocarcinomas. If a male patient <50 years old presents with a poorly differentiated neoplasm (especially with mediastinal or retroperitoneal mass), particular attention should focus on making the diagnosis of an atypical germ cell tumor, and presumptive treatment with a cisplatin-based chemotherapy regimen is standard because of the high response rate in this group.

Poorly Differentiated Carcinoma or Adenocarcinoma

Poorly differentiated carcinoma or **adenocarcinoma** accounts for ~30% of CUPS. Two thirds of these patients will have poorly differentiated carcinoma, and one third will have adenocarcinoma. In comparison to patients with moderately or well-differentiated adenocarcinoma, these patients tend to be younger, to have more rapidly progressive symptoms, and to have involvement of lymph nodes. Overall, this subset of patients has a better response to chemotherapy as well.

Treatment

Treatment regimens used include carboplatin- or cisplatin- and paclitaxel-based regimens. These have been found to prolong survival in some studies. The decision to treat must be individualized and based on performance status and the patient's desire to proceed.

Prognosis

The median survival of patients with poorly differentiated carcinoma is 13 months. For patients with poorly differentiated adenocarcinoma, the median survival is 8 months. Certain clinical features, such as young age, nonsmoking status, single metastatic site, neuroendocrine features, and lymph node location, have been associated with a more favorable prognosis.

Low-Grade Neuroendocrine Tumor

These tumors have features typical of carcinoid and islet cell tumors and usually involve liver or bone. They may be associated with syndromes such as Zollinger-Ellison and carcinoid. In some patients, a primary site is found in the small intestine, rectum, pancreas, or bronchus. These tumors are generally indolent and may progress slowly over many years. Patients are treated as they would be for metastatic carcinoid or islet cell malignancies.

Extragonadal Germ Cell Tumor

Extragonadal germ cell tumors present in patients <50 years old with midline tumors, short duration of symptoms, good response to chemotherapy or radiation, and elevation of tumor markers (AFP and β-hCG). Poorly differentiated carcinoma in young men with mediastinal or retroperitoneal tumors should be treated as germ cell tumors with platinum-based regimens. Approximately 30% to 40% of these patients may be cured.

Gestational Choriocarcinoma

Gestational choriocarcinoma should be suspected in young women with poorly differentiated carcinoma and pulmonary nodules. A recent history of pregnancy, spontaneous abortion, or missed menses may be elicited. β-hCG is often elevated in these patients. Most patients are cured with chemotherapy.

Well-Differentiated or Moderately Differentiated Adenocarcinoma

Well-differentiated or **moderately differentiated adenocarcinoma** is the most frequent type of CUPS, accounting for 60% of cases. The patients are typically elderly, with multiple sites of metastasis. The primary tumor will become apparent in 15% to 20% of patients. At autopsy, the most common primary malignancies found include lung and pancreas, which account for 40% of cases. Immunohistochemistry is of limited value in this group of patients, although identification of **ER/PR status** or **PSA** is valuable for treatment and prognosis.

Prognosis

The median survival is 3 to 4 months with this diagnosis.

Workup

Evaluation of patients should include thorough history and physical, chemistries, urinalysis, and chest x-ray. Women should have a **breast exam and mammogram,** and men should have a **prostate exam and PSA** check. CT imaging of the abdomen may provide a diagnosis in 10% to 35% of patients and may identify additional sites of metastasis.

Treatment

Approximately 10% of patients fit into subsets with a favorable response to chemotherapy, which is discussed later. The remainder of patients do not fit into these groups and are mainly treated for **palliation** of symptoms. Multiple chemotherapy regimens have been evaluated in these patients, with little evidence of improvement in survival. Features such as lymph node location, female gender, and poor differentiation predict a better response to chemotherapy. Liver and bone involvement predict a poor response. Recent trials have suggested that taxane-based chemotherapy regimens may improve survival, and newer agents, such as gemcitabine and topotecan, are being evaluated. However, randomized controlled trials are lacking. Patients with a good performance status should be considered for regimens such as these and for clinical trials.

- **Women with peritoneal carcinomatosis.** Women may present with peritoneal carcinomatosis suggestive of **ovarian cancer,** and histologic features, such as psammoma bodies and papillary structure, may be found. Patients often have elevated CA-125 levels, and metastases outside the peritoneal cavity are rare. These women should be treated as for stage III ovarian cancer (see Chap. 27), with surgical cytoreduction and chemotherapy with paclitaxel and platinum. Approximately 15% to 25% of patients will have long-term survival with this regimen.
- **Women with axillary lymph node adenocarcinoma. Breast cancer** should be suspected in this group of patients. Breast exam and mammography should be performed, as well as staining for ER/PR. Breast MRI can now also be used if prior studies are unrevealing. In this group of patients with negative exams and imaging, breast adenocarcinoma is found in 40% to 80% of mastectomy specimens. Patients should be evaluated for other metastatic disease, and if evaluation is negative, they should be treated for stage IIB breast cancer. Primary therapy consists of modified radical mastectomy versus lymph node dissection and breast irradiation. Patients should receive adjuvant treatment based on their age, lymph node status, ER/PR status, and her-2/neu status. If patients are found to have additional metastatic disease, they should be treated according to guidelines for stage IV breast cancer (see Chap. 18).
- **Men with elevated PSA and/or osteoblastic bone metastases.** Patients with these features or with PSA staining of their tumors should undergo hormonal treatment

for **prostate cancer** even if the clinical features are atypical, as many will have significant palliation.

- **Patients with a single metastatic lesion.** On occasion, only one site of metastasis is found even with complete evaluation. The possibility of a primary cancer of an unusual site, such as apocrine cancer presenting as a skin lesion, should be considered. Treatment should include local therapy with surgical resection or radiation or a combination of the two modalities. Many patients can have prolonged survival with this type of treatment. The role of systemic treatment is not yet defined in these patients but may be considered for patients with good performance status and poor differentiation, especially in the context of clinical trials.

Squamous Cell Carcinoma

Squamous cell carcinoma accounts for 5% of cases of CUPS. Most of the patients are elderly and have a significant history of alcohol and/or tobacco abuse. Most of these tumors arise in the lung or head and neck. Additional sites include the esophagus, cervix, anus, rectum, and bladder. For patients who do not fit into the specific subsets that follow, the prognosis is poor. These patients likely have occult lung cancer and should be evaluated with CT and bronchoscopy. Chemotherapy regimens used for non-small-cell lung cancer should be considered. If features are atypical for lung cancer, patients should be carefully evaluated for other sites, as adenocarcinoma may undergo squamous differentiation. Immunohistochemistry may be helpful in these patients.

Squamous Cell Carcinoma Involving High Cervical Lymph Nodes

Primary head and neck cancer should be suspected in patients with squamous cell carcinoma involving high cervical lymph nodes. CT evaluation of the head and neck may better define the disease and identify a primary site. Careful endoscopic evaluation should also be performed in these patients. These studies usually result in location of the primary cancer, but as many as 15% may not be identified. These patients should be treated for locally advanced head and neck cancer. In patients treated with local therapy alone, long-term survival has been seen in 30% to 40% of patients. The role of chemotherapy is undefined, but recent trials with concurrent chemotherapy and radiation are promising, and this approach should be considered in appropriate patients.

Squamous Cell Carcinoma Involving Low Cervical or Supraclavicular Lymph Nodes

Patients with squamous cell carcinoma involving low cervical or supraclavicular lymph nodes presentation should be evaluated for lung cancer with CT and bronchoscopy. The prognosis is not as favorable for this subgroup as for patients with high cervical lymph nodes, but 10% to 15% may have long-term survival. These patients do not typically respond well to systemic therapy; therefore, local treatment with radiation therapy should be offered.

Squamous Cell Carcinoma Involving Inguinal Lymph Nodes

In most patients with inguinal lymph node involvement, careful exam of the perineum will reveal a primary site. All patients should undergo sigmoidoscopy, and female patients should undergo pelvic examination. If no primary site is identified with these studies, patients should undergo inguinal lymph node dissection with radiation therapy if extensive disease is identified. The role of systemic chemotherapy is not defined, but given the role of combined-modality therapy in cervical and anal cancers, platinum-based regimens should be considered.

KEY POINTS TO REMEMBER

- CUPS accounts for 2% to 5% of cancers and includes numerous clinical presentations and histologies.
- There are four main light microscopy classifications for these tumors, and further studies, such as immunohistochemistry, should be used in poorly differentiated tumors.
- A number of patient subsets have been identified who have a more favorable prognosis and better response to treatment.
- In most patients, the search for the primary cancer should be brief and based on the site and histology of the metastasis.
- Overall, the median survival is poor regardless of treatment.

REFERENCES AND SUGGESTED READINGS

Chorost MI, McKinley B, Tschoi M, et al. The management of the unknown primary. *J Am Coll Surg.* 2001;193:666–677.

DeVita VT, Rosenberg SA, Hellman S, eds. *Cancer: Principles and Practice of Oncology.* 7th ed. Philadelphia: Lippincott Williams & Wilkins; 2005:2213–2234.

Hainsworth JD, Greco FA. Management of patients with cancer of unknown primary site. *Oncology.* 2000;14:563–574.

Hainsworth JD, Greco FA. Treatment of patients with cancer of unknown primary site. *N Engl J Med.* 1993;329:257–263.

National Comprehensive Cancer Network. NCCN Clinical Practice Guidelines in Oncology: Occult Primary. v2.2007. Available at: www.nccn.org. Accessed July 2007.

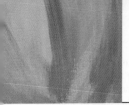

Supportive Care in Oncology

34

Brian A. Van Tine

INTRODUCTION

Supportive care addresses the physical, mental, and spiritual needs of the cancer patient. Physical symptoms can arise from the cancer itself, the side effects of therapy, medications, or comorbid medical conditions. This chapter focuses on symptom control as an important element of oncology practice, including pain management, nausea and vomiting, mucositis, diarrhea, anorexia, and dyspnea. It also addresses the emotional issues of depression, anxiety, and delirium, and presents an approach to addressing spiritual needs of the cancer patient.

PHYSICAL SYMPTOM MANAGEMENT

Pain Management

Background
Pain is a prevalent complaint in cancer patients, occurring in 50% to 70% of all patients with cancer. More than one half of cancer patients experience moderate to severe pain, and 50% to 80% of cancer patients are not satisfied with their pain relief. The undertreatment of cancer pain can be attributed to multiple barriers, including physician, patient, and societal factors. It must be remembered that each person's pain is different and must be treated as such.

Definition
Pain is always subjective. The International Association for the Study of Pain defines pain as "an unpleasant sensory and emotional experience associated with actual or potential tissue damage, or described in terms of such damage. Each individual learns the application of the word through experiences related to injury early in life." Acute pain may be associated with physical signs, including tachycardia, hypertension, hyperventilation, facial grimacing, and verbalizations. However, patients with chronic pain may not exhibit any of these overt physical signs and may not "appear in pain." It is important to remember that pain is *always* subjective, and the patient's self-reporting is a key element to an accurate pain assessment.

Pain Assessment
- The first step in the management of pain depends on a comprehensive pain assessment gathered through history, physical exam, and review of laboratory and radiology studies. Important pain characteristics to elicit from the patient should be descriptions of the pain with regard to **onset, duration, intensity, quality,** and **exacerbating or relieving factors**. The physician can use each of these characteristics to identify potential etiologies and institute the appropriate pain management plan.

- Simple tools can reliably aid in the measurement of pain. The most common clinical assessment tools are verbal rating scales and visual analogue scales. A verbal rating scale uses words to describe pain such as none, mild, moderate, severe, or excruciating. A visual analogue scale uses a line with or without verbal clues or numbers and asks patients to place their pain rating on this scale. The specific scale used to measure pain is less important than the consistent use of a scale over time. For illiterate or pediatric patients, a visual analogue scale can be used with pictures to describe the levels of pain for a better pain assessment tool. Examples of pain scales can be found at http://www.nci.nih.gov/cancerinfo/understanding-cancer-pain/.

Management
Analgesic Ladder

- The World Health Organization (WHO) recommends the use of an analgesic ladder in the approach to the selection of opioids to treat cancer pain. Analgesic selection should be guided by the severity of cancer pain. Patients with mild to moderate pain are usually started on acetaminophen or nonsteroidal anti-inflammatory drugs (NSAIDs). Patients with moderate to severe pain, or those who had insufficient relief after a trial of acetaminophen or NSAIDs, are treated with an opioid used for moderate pain, such as codeine, hydrocodone, dihydrocodeine, and oxycodone. This opioid may be combined with acetaminophen or an NSAID or an alternative adjuvant drug (tricyclic antidepressant, anticonvulsant, or topical anesthetic). Many of the drugs used for moderate to severe cancer pain are available in the United States as a combination of the opioid and acetaminophen or aspirin (ASA). The drug can be titrated until the maximum safe dose of acetaminophen (4 g/day) or ASA is reached.
- Patients with severe pain, including those who fail to reach adequate pain relief with drugs from the second step on the WHO ladder, should receive an opioid that is useful in the treatment of severe cancer pain. The drugs useful in the treatment of severe cancer pain include morphine, hydromorphone, fentanyl, oxycodone, and methadone. These opioids may also be combined with acetaminophen or an NSAID or an adjuvant drug when needed. Patients can experience a variation of analgesia and side effects between the different opioids. A clinician may need to rotate among the various opioids to identify the drugs that have the correct balance between pain control and side effects. These drugs should be titrated to analgesic effect or intolerable side effects. There is no maximum dose limitation on the opioid medication itself.

Acute and Chronic Pain

- In the treatment of cancer pain, it is important to distinguish between acute and chronic pain, as the goals of treatment are slightly different. Acute pain is a linear event; the pain starts, and, with relief of the offending event, the pain stops. Chronic pain is cyclical in nature, repeating itself over time. For acute pain, the goal of treatment is pain relief. To accomplish pain relief, the drugs administered should have a rapid onset of action, with the desired duration of action (e.g., 2 to 4 hours). These drugs are given as needed. Common side effects, such as sedation, are usually acceptable and well tolerated by the patient. An example of an acute pain scenario is the patient who falls and suffers a hip fracture at the site of a previous bone metastasis. The patient is treated with short-acting IV narcotics until surgery can be performed to stabilize the fracture.
- Chronic pain management has a different focus. The overall goal is pain prevention and the avoidance of undesirable side effects, such as sedation. The analgesic regimen should include long-acting narcotics administered on a regular schedule and should be individualized for the patient based on side effects. Patients with chronic

pain also need to have the understanding of how to manage acute exacerbations with short-acting, rapid-onset analgesics, most commonly referred to as breakthrough pain relief. Many cancer patients have chronic pain. Chronic pain is ineffectively managed when the clinician focuses on acute control of the pain in this setting.

- Opioid therapy can provide effective pain relief to the majority of patients with cancer pain. Opioids can be classified as pure agonists or agonist antagonists, based on their interactions with opioid receptors in the body. The drugs that are included in the agonist-antagonist subclass include butorphanol (Stadol), nalbuphine (Nubain), pentazocine (Talwin), and buprenorphine (Buprenex). Drugs in this subclass have a ceiling effect for analgesia and may reverse the effects of pure agonists. For these reasons, use of the mixed agonist-antagonist subclass is not recommended in the treatment of cancer pain.

Treatment

- When managing chronic pain, it is important to remember that there are wide variations in dose requirements. This variation is not based on the size or age of the patient or the amount of disease present. The analgesic dose required to keep a patient out of pain cannot be predicted, but rather, must be determined by educated trial and error. The following are guidelines for opioid use in chronic pain patients.
- Start with one drug at the lowest effective dose. Titrate the drug to pain relief or intolerable side effects. If the patient is unable to tolerate one narcotic due to undesirable side effects, switch to an alternative agent.
- Use around-the-clock dosing schedules to avoid peaks and valleys in serum analgesic levels.
- Sustained or long-acting release preparations of narcotics are very useful in this population. When converting between modes of administration or drugs, calculate the equianalgesic dosages to avoid undermedicating a patient. See Table 34-1.
- Breakthrough pain medications should be the same or a similar drug used for long-acting pain relief. The minimum effective breakthrough pain medication dose should be equivalent to 12.5% of the patient's total daily narcotic requirements, or 25% of a single BID dose.
- Keep the regimen as simple as possible. Avoid mixing a variety of analgesic regimens.
- Always start a bowel regimen when placing a patient on narcotics, as constipation is a side effect of all narcotics.
- Educate the patient and family about dosing and side effects. Discuss and reassure the patient and family about addiction, tolerance, and physical dependence.

TABLE 34-1	EQUIVALENT OPIOID DOSES	
	PO (mg)	SC/IV (mg)
Morphine	30	10
Hydromorphone	7.5	1.5
Methadone	20	10
Codeine	180	NA
Oxycodone	20	NA
Fentanyl	NA	0.67

NA, not available.

- **Morphine** is the drug of choice for moderate to severe cancer pain. It has a wide range of doses available and flexible methods of delivery. Morphine is available as sustained-release, immediate-release, liquid/sublingual, and parenteral preparations. The sustained-release tablets may be given per rectum or sublingually in patients unable to swallow. **Oxycodone** is available orally as immediate- and sustained-release preparations. **Fentanyl** is available in the parenteral route, as well as the fentanyl (Duragesic) patch for patients unable to swallow or who cannot tolerate morphine or oxycodone. The patches are applied to the chest wall or back and changed every 48 to 72 hours. The onset of action in these long-acting preparations is 12 hours. When starting a patient on long-acting agents, the clinician needs to provide the patient with immediate-relief preparations for use in the interim, until the long-acting narcotic can achieve adequate serum levels for analgesia.
- Meperidine (Demerol) should be avoided in the treatment of chronic pain. Meperidine has the very short half-life of 2 to 3 hours. This is ineffective in the management of chronic pain. Meperidine has a toxic metabolite, normeperidine, which is a weaker analgesic but a potent CNS stimulant. Normeperidine has a half-life of ≥ 25 to 30 hours in the setting of renal failure. This can rapidly lead to accumulation of the drug when used for more than 48 to 72 hours. CNS toxicity can include irritability, tremors, myoclonus, agitation, and seizures. When CNS toxicity occurs, it is important to stop the drug. Naloxone (Narcan) should not be administered, as the effects of normeperidine are not reversed with naloxone and can precipitate worsening CNS toxicity.
- Propoxyphene (Darvon-N) is another narcotic agent that is ineffective in the treatment of chronic pain. Despite its widespread use, the drug has no more analgesic properties than ASA (650 mg). Propoxyphene has the long half-life of 6 to 12 hours. It also has a toxic metabolite, norpropoxyphene, with a half-life of 30 to 36 hours. Norpropoxyphene has been associated with pulmonary edema, cardiotoxicity, and cardiac arrest.
- IM injections should be avoided for the management of cancer pain. The use of IM injections is painful, and absorption is unreliable. The onset of action can be 30 to 60 minutes, and this is not acceptable in the acute pain setting. IV or transmucosal (sublingual or rectal) routes are much more efficacious at getting rapid onset of action in the acute pain setting.
- The perception that the administration of opioid analgesics for chronic pain management causes addiction is prevalent and is a barrier to adequate pain control. Confusion about the differences among addiction, tolerance, and physical dependence is in part responsible. **Addiction** is a pattern of drug abuse characterized by drug craving and overwhelming behaviors to obtain the drug. **Tolerance** is a state in which escalating doses of opioids are needed to achieve pain control as the drug effectiveness reduces over time. Tolerance occurs with all of the side effects of narcotics, with the exception of constipation. It is important to educate patients and family members that tolerance to many of the common side effects, such as itching or sedation, will develop, and that the drug should not be abruptly discontinued. **Physical dependence** is the onset of signs and symptoms of withdrawal with abrupt discontinuation of the opioid. Abrupt withdrawal may result in tachycardia, hypertension, diaphoresis, nausea, vomiting, abdominal pain, psychosis, and hallucinations. This is not the same as addiction. Physical dependence and addiction are not synonymous. When stopping chronic opioid medications, the dose should be reduced in increments of 20% every 2 to 3 days to avoid the risk of withdrawal symptoms. Finally, it should be remembered that patients experiencing inadequately controlled pain may engage in what appears to be drug-seeking behavior, which is easy to confuse with addiction.

- **Adjuvant analgesics** can be important in the treatment of cancer pain. Adjuvant analgesics include antidepressants, anticonvulsants, corticosteroids, and local anesthetics. Within the antidepressants, tricyclics are the most effective as an adjunctive therapy for neuropathic pain. Common side effects from the tricyclics include orthostatic hypotension, sedation, urinary retention, confusion, and sexual dysfunction. Doses of the tricyclic antidepressants should be started low and titrated for analgesia. Anticonvulsants are also helpful adjunctive therapies in the treatment of neuropathic pain syndromes. These drugs include carbamazepine (Tegretol), phenytoin (Dilantin), gabapentin (Neurontin), and pregabalin (Lyrica). The usual initiating dose of gabapentin is 100 mg TID titrated up to a maximum of 3600 mg per day. Side effects of these drugs can be self-limiting, including sedation, confusion, and dizziness.
- Corticosteroids can be useful in the management of bone metastases, nerve compression, elevated intracranial pressure, and obstruction of a hollow viscus. Local anesthetics, such as nerve blocks, lidocaine patches, and eutectic mixture of local anesthetics (EMLA) cream, can aid in the treatment of cancer pain. In extreme cases, IV administration of anesthetics can be used in conjunction with IV or intraspinal narcotics to allow the clinician to administer lower doses of narcotics and spare the patient the complications of sedation seen with high doses of narcotics.
- Bisphosphonates (pamidronate, zoledronic acid) and calcitonin have been used to treat pain from bony metastases. Clinical trials have failed to demonstrate clear evidence for the ability of bisphosphonates to deliver an analgesic benefit over placebo. Calcitonin provides no benefit in metastatic bone pain over placebo, but some studies suggest that it may reduce the intensity and frequency of neuropathic pain.

Constipation

Causes
Differential Diagnosis. Most constipation in cancer comes from opioid pain management, but the differential diagnosis of constipation is broad. Before assuming that all constipation is pain medicine related in the cancer patient, one must remember to consider bowel obstruction, spinal cord compression, hypercalcemia, hypokalemia, diabetes mellitus, hypothyroidism, timing of chemotherapy, uremia, etc., as these must be treated differently. Other possible considerations are different classes of drugs, such as: antacids, anticholinergics, antidepressants, calcium channel blockers, cholestyramine, clonidine, diuretics, levodopa, NSAIDs, psychotropics, and sympathomimetics.

Presentation
During opioid treatment, constipation should be expected. Prophylactic measures should always be initiated with the start of opioid therapy. Constipation occurs with all opioids, and pharmacologic tolerance rarely develops. Symptoms from constipation may become so severe that patients may decide to discontinue pain medications. This is preventable with the use of an aggressive laxative regimen.

Management
- Dietary interventions are almost never sufficient to prevent constipation. Combinations of agents are often necessary. Clinicians should also avoid the use of bulk-forming agents in the absence of a motility agent, especially in debilitated or anorectic patients. When using these agents, it should be remembered that stool softeners and bulking agents do little to relieve constipation but may make stools more comfortable to pass. Their sole use will only lead to constipation with soft stools, and another agent is necessary for adequate treatment. Also, it should be remembered that the onset of abdominal pain or nausea in a patient taking opioids may be due to unrecognized constipation.

TABLE 34-2	LAXATIVES
Stimulant laxatives	
Senna	2 tablets bid, titrated to effect (up to 8/day)
Bisacodyl (Dulcolax)	5 to 15 mg PO or 10 mg PR qhs
Osmotic laxatives	
Lactulose	20 g/30 mL PO every 4 to 6 hours, titrated to effect (or every 2 hours in severe constipation)
Sorbitol	30 mL PO every 4 to 6 hours, titrated to effect
Milk of magnesia	15 to 30 mL per day or twice daily
Magnesium citrate	300-mL bottle per day, bid, scheduled or prn
Detergent laxatives	
Docusate sodium or calcium	100 mg PO per day or twice daily
Phosphosoda enema	prn

- Laxatives can be classified into three categories: stimulant, osmotic, and detergent agents (Table 34-2). **Stimulant laxatives** irritate the bowel, leading to increased peristaltic activity. **Osmotic laxatives** draw water into the bowel lumen and increase the moisture content of the stool. In addition, they add to overall stool volume. **Detergent laxatives** facilitate the dissolution of fat in water and increase the water content of stool. Laxatives can be titrated to a maximal therapeutic dose. Clinicians should try to simplify the bowel regimen, as this will improve patient compliance. Combinations of stimulant and detergent laxatives such as docusate/senna (Senokot-S) are ideal for preventing opioid-induced constipation.
- Prokinetic agents such as metoclopramide (Reglan) can increase peristaltic activity and facilitate stool movement. This agent can be used in combination with other laxative agents. Lubricant stimulants and large-volume enemas can also be used but are not recommended for daily use and prophylaxis of opioid-related constipation. The use of these agents is effective while titrating other laxatives to ensure that the patient is having regular bowel movements.
- Often patients present with constipation from narcotics of the order of days to weeks in duration. It is important to identify this immediately and treat it aggressively. One can use enemas or suppositories per rectum, or oral regimens such as lactulose, 20 g every 2 hours, until the bowels move. Patients should be instructed to inform their physician if they do not have a bowel movement within any 48-hour time period while they are on narcotics to avoid potentially life-threatening complications.

Diarrhea

Introduction

Diarrhea can be defined as stools that are looser than normal and that may be increased in number over baseline. The definition is based on the frequency, volume, and consistency of stools.

Causes

Differential Diagnosis. Potential causes of diarrhea in the cancer patient can include infections, malabsorption, gastrointestinal bleeding, medications, chemotherapy (particularly 5-FU), radiation to the abdomen or pelvis, and overflow incontinence. It is important to remember that herbals such as ginkgo biloba, ginseng, and licorice may cause diarrhea.

Natural History. In cancer patients, getting up to go to the bathroom multiple times day and night can be exhausting. If persistent, diarrhea can lead to dehydration and electrolyte abnormalities that can lead to the need for a hospital admission.

Management

Treatment. Patients should be instructed on the establishment of normal bowel habits. Any change from the normal baseline should be reported to the physician to avoid severe dehydration or electrolyte imbalances. Patients should be counseled on the avoidance of foods containing lactose or other gas-forming foods that can increase abdominal cramping and pain. Another general approach to diarrhea is to increase the bulk of the stools with the addition of psyllium, bran, or pectin. However, sometimes bulk-forming agents can worsen abdominal cramping and bloating.

For the medical management of transient or mild diarrhea, the use of attapulgite (Kaopectate) or bismuth salts (Pepto-Bismol) can be useful. Care should be taken to rule out infection by checking *Clostridium difficile* toxin before using antiperistaltic medications in the setting of recent antibiotic use. Potential infectious workup may include checking for fecal leukocytes, ova, and parasites and stool culture. For more persistent and severe diarrhea, agents that slow down peristalsis are more useful, including the following:

- Loperamide (Imodium), 2 to 4 mg PO every 6 hours (maximum, 8 tablets/day)
- Diphenoxylate/atropine (Lomotil), 2.5 to 5 mg PO every 6 hours (maximum, 8 tablets/day)
- Tincture of opium, 0.7 mL PO every 4 hours and titrated as needed (Belladonna can be added as an antispasmodic agent.)
- Octreotide (Dandostatin LAR Depot), 10 to 20 mg IM every 4 weeks.

For persistent, severe secretory diarrhea, the patient should be admitted for parenteral fluid support and the initiation of octreotide.

- Octreotide (Sandostatin), 50 to 500 µg SC/IV every 8 to 12 hours. Begin at 50 µg SC/IV, then titrated up 100 µg per dose every 48 hours to a maximum of 500 µg SC every 8 hours, with titration based on response; may also be given as a continuous IV infusion, 10 to 80 µg/hour.

Nausea and Vomiting

Introduction

Background. Nausea and vomiting are commonly associated with advanced malignancies as a direct result of the disease or as side effects of chemotherapy or other medications. There are multiple potential causes of nausea and vomiting in the cancer patient. Different etiologies for nausea and vomiting may require different interventions for control of the symptoms.

Classification. The three most common forms of chemotherapy-associated nausea are **acute**, which begins within 1 to 2 hours of chemotherapy; **delayed**, which occurs 24 hours to 5 days after chemotherapy; and **anticipatory**, which is a conditioned response from prior occurrences of chemotherapy.

Causes

A thorough assessment of nausea and vomiting is important to gain an understanding of potential etiologies and allow for an appropriate choice of antiemetics. A common mnemonic for potential etiologies is the "11 M's of emesis": metastases, meningeal irritation, movement, mental (anxiety), medications, mucosal irritation, mechanical obstruction, motility, metabolic, microbes, and myocardial (ischemia, congestive heart failure). Identification of the source of nausea and vomiting dictates treatment.

Management

Treatment. For prevention of chemotherapy-associated acute nausea, the three classes of drugs with the highest efficacy are corticosteroids (dexamethasone), 5-HT$_3$ receptor antagonists (dolasetron, granisetron, ondansetron, palonosetron), and the neurokinin-1 (NK1) receptor antagonist aprepitant (Emend). Treatment recommendations for acute nausea and vomiting are dependent of the emetogenic potential of the chemotherapy. For low-emetogenic therapies, dexamethasone or metoclopramide (a dopamine antagonist) is used. For moderately emetogenic therapies, a 5-HT$_3$ is combined with dexamethasone. For highly emetogenic chemotherapies, such as platinum-based regimens, aprepitant is combined with a 5-HT$_3$ and dexamethasone. For delayed nausea, either single-agent dexamethasone or dexamethasone plus metoclopramide is recommended. If the combination treatment does not work, aprepitant should be considered. Anticipatory emesis is a conditioned response from prior cycles of chemotherapy. Patients benefit from benzodiazepines and behavioral therapy (hypnosis, desensitization, relaxation, etc.). The best way to prevent anticipatory emesis is good control of acute and delayed emesis in prior cycles of chemotherapy.

Nausea and vomiting from a bowel obstruction can be a challenge to treat, especially when surgery is not an option. Octreotide has been shown to effectively inhibit the secretion of fluid into the intestinal lumen and decrease bloating and abdominal pain, as well as nausea and vomiting. It may be started by continuous infusion or intermittent SC injection at a dose of 100 μg every 8 to 12 hours and titrated every 24 to 48 hours for effect.

Dopamine antagonists are one of the most frequently used antiemetics. These medications have the potential to cause sedation and extrapyramidal symptoms. Medication options include the following.

- Haloperidol (Haldol), PO, IV, SC
- Prochlorperazine (Compazine), PO, PR, IV
- Droperidol (Inapsine), IV
- Promethazine (Phenergan), PO
- Perphenazine (Trilafon), PO, IV
- Trimethobenzamide (Tigan), PO, PR
- Metoclopramide (Reglan), PO, IV

Histamine antagonists may also cause sedation and can have a beneficial effect in some patients. The antihistamines also have the added benefit of anticholinergic properties, which can also be beneficial in patients with dual etiologies of nausea. These drugs include the following.

- Diphenhydramine (Benadryl), PO, IV
- Meclizine (Antivert), PO
- Hydroxyzine (Atarax), PO, IV

Scopolamine is an anticholinergic agent that is useful in treating nausea induced by the vestibular apparatus. It can also be used adjunctively with other antiemetics in empiric therapy. Scopolamine can be given as an IV or SC scheduled or continuous infusion but is also conveniently available as a transdermal patch.

Serotonin antagonists have been effective in the treatment of chemotherapy-associated nausea and vomiting. They are also useful for refractory nausea but are typically tried when other medications have failed. The medications available are as follows.

- Ondansetron (Zofran), PO, IV
- Granisetron (Kytril), PO, IV
- Dolasetron (Anzemet), PO, IV
- Palonosetron (Alopi), IV

The NK1 receptor antagonist aprepitant has become first-line therapy on day 1 for highly emetogenic chemotherapies.

- Aprepitant (Emend) PO

The use of dronabinol (Marinol) and benzodiazepines is beneficial in some patients, but the mechanism of action remains unclear. Benzodiazepines (i.e., lorazepam [Ativan] at a 1-mg dose) often are useful in conjunction with other classes of antiemetics and may have a synergistic effect.

Mucositis

Introduction
Mucositis refers to painful inflammation and ulceration of the oral mucosa. Mucositis can result from chemotherapy or radiation therapy.

Causes
Chemotherapeutic agents that are associated commonly with mucositis include melphalan, methotrexate, etoposide, and vinblastine. Radiation to the head and neck may also cause mucositis. Patient factors that can contribute to worsening symptoms include poor-fitting oral prostheses, periodontal disease, and overall poor oral hygiene. Patients should undergo repair of ill-fitting prostheses, tooth extraction, and repair of periodontal disease before the initiation of chemotherapy. In the event that repair cannot be done before chemotherapy, the physician should make a referral to an oral surgeon once the patient's peripheral blood counts have returned to baseline.

Management
  Diagnosis. A mucositis grading system established by the National Cancer Institute allows the physician to assess mucositis severity in terms of both pain and the patient's ability to continue to eat or drink, graded on a scale from 0 to 4. A score of 0 is given when there is no evidence of mucositis. When a patient develops nonpainful erythema or ulcers, but is able to eat or drink, a score of 1 is given. A score of 2 is given when there are mildly to moderately painful erythema or ulcers, but the patient is still able to eat or drink without difficulty. This may require intermittent analgesia. Severe erythema, painful ulcers that cause interference with eating and drinking requiring constant analgesia, scores a 3. Finally, a score of 4 is given when the severity of symptoms requires parenteral analgesia and/or nutritional support.
  Treatment. A standardized approach to the prevention and treatment of mucositis is essential to quality care in the oncology patient. The prophylactic measures usually used include mouth rinses with sodium chloride, sodium bicarbonate, or chlorhexidine (Peridex). Regimens commonly used for the treatment of mucositis and the associated pain include a local anesthetic such as lidocaine, magnesium-based antacids (Maalox, Mylanta), diphenhydramine (Benadryl), and an antifungal such as nystatin (Mycostatin) or Mycelex. These agents are used either alone or at equal concentrations in a mouthwash. The patient can use the mouthwash up to five times per day for relief. In the treatment of severe mucositis, narcotics may need to be used in addition to the agents mentioned earlier.
  Recently, palifermin (Kepivance), keratinocyte growth factor-1, has been studied for the prevention of mucositis. At this time, it is only approved for use in leukemia and lymphoma patients who are undergoing stem cell transplant.

Anorexia and Cachexia

Introduction
  Background. Anorexia and cachexia frequently occur with advanced malignancies and are characterized by a loss of muscle mass and adipose tissue. The increased catabolism

of cancer and the anorexia that accompanies it result in increased muscle protein break-down and lipolysis.

Etiology. The specific etiologies of these symptoms are not well understood. Anorexia and cachexia are significant causes of distress to the patient and family members. These symptoms typically represent progression of disease and are not reversible with parenteral or enteral nutrition. The clinician should always assess for other potential etiologies underlying the loss of appetite and weight such as dysphagia, odynophagia, infections, and side effects of medications. Some medications may improve appetite and allow the patient to gain weight, although none of these therapies improves survival.

Management

There are several approaches to the general management of anorexia and cachexia. Patients should be offered their favorite foods and nutritional supplements if the patients enjoy them. Any dietary restrictions should be eliminated. Portion sizes can be reduced, and food should be made to look appetizing. Foods that have potent odors should be avoided.

There is a variety of pharmacologic approaches for improving appetite. Corticosteroids have an appetite-stimulating effect, as well as effects on the patient's mood and energy level. Dexamethasone (Decadron) at doses of ≤4 mg/day is recommended. Dexamethasone is preferred because of the relative lack of mineralocorticoid effects, but any steroid will be efficacious. Steroids are considered only for short-term treatment, as they lose their efficacy over days to weeks. If longer treatment is anticipated, megestrol (Megace) has also been shown to improve appetite in cancer patients. There is a large variation in the effective dose of megestrol between individual patients. One should begin with 200 mg PO every 6 to 8 hours and titrate up to 400 to 800 mg/day or Megace ES, 650 mg PO daily. The cannabinoids, such as dronabinol (Marinol), also have been shown to promote weight gain in cancer patients.

It should be understood that clinical studies have demonstrated no impact on overall survival or improvement in quality of life when anorexia and cachexia are pharmacologically managed. Thus, treatment of anorexia and weight loss is done primarily because anorexia is distressing to the patients and their families.

Dyspnea

Introduction

Dyspnea can be one of the most frightening symptoms to patients and family members. Some patients with severe tachypnea will not complain of dyspnea, while others who are not tachypneic report severe dyspnea. For the majority of patients, relief of dyspnea can be achieved with simple interventions.

Presentation

Clinical Presentation. Respiratory rate, O_2 saturation, and blood gas levels often do not correlate with the patient's subjective report. The clinician must accept the patient's self-report and try to identify and/or correct the underlying etiology of the symptom.

Evaluation. In patients with known advanced disease, the burden of investigating the etiology of the dyspnea must be weighed against the limited potential benefit from therapeutic interventions.

Management

There are three widely used medical approaches for symptomatic breathlessness: supplemental O_2, opioids, and anxiolytics. A therapeutic trial of supplemental O_2 may be beneficial; it has been suggested that there is a placebo effect in nonhypoxemic patients. In addition, the cool air moving across the patient's face from the supplemental O_2 can also have a calming effect and help to relieve the feelings of air hunger. Studies have reported that stimulation of the trigeminal nerve with oxygen can cause a central inhibitory effect and relieve dyspnea. A fan in the room can also help achieve this effect.

Opioids can provide relief in dyspnea without any measurable effect on respiratory rate or blood gas measurements. The precise mechanism by which opioids exert this effect is not known. In an opioid-naïve patient, doses lower than those used to achieve analgesia may be effective. Doses of hydrocodone, 5 mg PO every 4 hours, or codeine, 30 mg PO every 2 hours, can be beneficial in these patients. Other opioids can be useful and administered IV for urgent situations or when the PO route is not available. Patients can be maintained on a fixed schedule of opioid IV every 4 to 6 hours. An additional dose of a short-acting opioid, equivalent to 25% to 50% of the amount of baseline opioid taken every 4 hours can be used hourly for intermittent periods of worsening dyspnea. Sublingual morphine can also be helpful in the terminal dyspneic patient.

Dyspnea may cause severe anxiety. Some patients with dyspnea may need more effective treatment for their anxiety. Benzodiazepines can be used in addition to opioids and other nondrug therapies to reduce dyspnea. The clinician should begin with low doses and titrate for desired effects. Sublingual lorazepam has been shown to be quite effective if there is no IV access.

Anemia

Causes
Anemia in cancer patients may be due to the effects of their underlying malignancy (particularly when there is bone marrow involvement) and/or treatment. The basic mechanisms involved are decreased erythropoiesis, impaired iron metabolism, and decreased survival time for RBCs. In addition, erythropoietin production may be impaired.

Management
Current treatment approaches are aimed at treating the underlying malignancy and boosting red cell mass. Transfusions offer only transient effects and have side effects such as transfusion reactions, iron overload, volume overload, and cardiac congestion. It is recommended that transfusions be administered only to those patients who are suffering from symptoms of anemia with hemoglobin <8 g/dL. Recombinant erythropoietin has been shown to reduce transfusion requirements and improve outcomes in terms of quality of life and response to treatment. For treatment of chemotherapy-associated anemia, epoetin should be dosed at 150 units/kg three times a week or 40,000 units per week. Alternatively, darbepoetin can be given at 2.25 μg/kg per week. If there is no response within 4 weeks, the dose should be increased by 25%. Recent studies of erythropoiesis-stimulating agents (ESAs) in non-chemotherapy-associated anemia have suggested worse outcomes in this setting; the current FDA recommendation is that utilizing erythropoiesis-stimulating agents to treat anemia in cancer patients who are not receiving chemotherapy provides no benefit and may be harmful.

EMOTIONAL SYMPTOM MANAGEMENT

Depression
Depression occurs in approximately half of cancer patients, though it is often underdiagnosed and undertreated. Specific problems facing these patients include pain, medication side effects, and changes in functional status.

Presentation
Typical features of major depression may also be present, such as depressed mood for at least 2 weeks, feelings of guilt or worthlessness, inability to concentrate, decreased energy,

preoccupation with death or suicide, anhedonia, and changes in eating or sleeping habits. In the cancer patient, one must be aware that drugs such as prednisone, dexamethasone, procarbazine, vincristine, and vinblastine can cause depression like symptoms. Loss of appetite, fatigue, or insomnia may be secondary to chemotherapy, the cancer itself, or pain, making it difficult to diagnose depression. Excessive guilt, low self-esteem, the wish to die, and hopelessness are most diagnostic of depression in the cancer patient. One must be careful to screen for suicidal ideation, as the incidence of suicide is higher in both men and women with cancer.

Management
Depression should be screened for and treated in all cancer patients. In addition to counseling by oncologic psychologists, medications can by useful in the treatment of depression. Antidepressants may require up to 6 weeks before symptoms are alleviated. The selective serotonin reuptake inhibitors (e.g., citalopram, 20 to 80 mg PO daily), bupropion SR (200 to 400 mg PO daily), and mirtazapine (usual dosage range, 30 to 45 mg PO daily; mirtazapine has sedating effects but may aid those with insomnia) are all reasonable first-line agents. Tricyclic antidepressants have the ability to treat depression and potentiate the effects of opioids on neuropathic pain. Imipramine, amitriptyline, and doxepin are started at 25 mg PO at bedtime, then titrated up 25 to 50 mg every 24 to 48 hours until the desired effect is achieved.

The psychostimulants methylphenidate, dextroamphetamine, and modafinil are an alternative for depressed patients with cancer (e.g., methylphenidate, 5 mg PO at 9:00 a.m. and noon daily). They begin to work within a short period of time, provide relief from the sedating effects of opioids, and give the patient improved energy. Tolerance can develop to stimulants, and dosages may have to be adjusted over time.

Anxiety

Presentation
The diagnosis and recognition of anxiety can be challenging. Patients often complain of physical and somatic manifestations of anxiety. The patient's subjective level of distress from fear, isolation, estrangement, or other common stressors is often the impetus for treatment.

Management
Anxiety is usually treated with benzodiazepines, neuroleptics, antihistamines, or nonpharmacologic psychotherapies. Benzodiazepines are first-line therapy for the treatment of anxiety disorders.

- Lorazepam, 0.5 to 2.0 mg PO, IV, or IM, every 3 to 6 hours
- Alprazolam, 0.25 to 1.0 mg PO, every 6 to 8 hours
- Diazepam, 2.5 to 10 mg PO, PR, IM, or IV every 3 to 6 hours
- Clonazepam, 1 to 2 mg PO, every 8 to 12 hours

Other anxiolytics include the following.

- Haloperidol (0.5 mg to 5 mg PO, IV, or SC every 2 to 12 hours), if there is concern about respiratory depression
- Thioridazine (10 to 25 mg PO tid), if insomnia and agitation are also present
- Hydroxyzine (25 to 50 mg every 4 to 6 hours PO, IV, or SC), which has mild anxiolytic, sedative, and analgesic properties
- Buspirone (10 mg PO tid), a nonbenzodiazepine anxiolytic that is useful in patients with chronic anxiety or anxiety related to adjustment disorders

Nonpharmacologic interventions for anxiety and distress include supportive psychotherapy and behavioral interventions used alone or in combination, relaxation, guided imagery, and hypnosis.

Delirium

Causes
Delirium is common in advanced cancer and is strongly associated with mortality. The differential diagnosis for delirium in the cancer patient includes dehydration, hypo- and hypernatremia, hypocalcemia, uremia, liver failure, drugs (opiates, radiation, chemotherapeutics, benzodiazepines, tricyclic antidepressants, etc.), brain metastases, paraneoplastic syndrome, and infection.

Management
Diagnosis. One must identify the underlying cause so that supportive therapies can be given. Many scales exist for the diagnosis of delirium, including the Mini Mental Status Exam and Memorial Delirium Assessment Scale, and these should be used to both diagnose and follow delirium.

Treatment. If supportive techniques do not work, treatment with neuroleptics or sedative medications can be tried.

- Haloperidol (Haldol), 0.5 to 1 mg every 1 to 2 hours PO, IV, or SC is the first drug of choice for treatment of delirium and is usually effective for agitation, paranoia, and fear.
- Zyprexa, 5 to 10 mg PO, sublingually, is another possible first-line agent, as it can be given under the tongue.
- Lorazepam, 0.5 to 1.0 mg PO or IV, plus haloperidol (but not lorazepam alone) can be tried next.
- Chlorpromazine can be used if no response to antipsychotics is observed within 24 to 48 hours, as it is much more sedating.

Insomnia

Introduction
Insomnia is often a result of pain, medications, anxiety, or a mood disorder. Poor sleep can be distressing in the cancer patient, as it can make pain, anxiety, and delirium worse. Proper sleep hygiene and adequate management of pain and other symptoms are beneficial.

Management
Benzodiazepines (e.g., lorazepam, 0.5 to 2 mg PO qhs) or antidepressants with sedating effects (e.g., trazodone, 50 mg PO qhs, or amitriptyline, 25 to 50 mg PO qhs) may be used in conjunction with the nonpharmacologic measures. Newer agents such as Ambien/Ambien CR (5 to 10 mg/6.25 to 12.5 mg PO qpm), Lunesta (2 to 3 mg PO qpm), and Rozerem (8 mg PO qpm) can be tried. One should be careful when treating insomnia in terminally ill patients, as these can be hypnotic drugs. For some patients, improved cognition may be achieved by discontinuing the medications without an effect on insomnia.

ADDRESSING SPIRITUAL CARE

When a person has a malignancy, suffering occurs at many levels. Religion or spiritual belief can be a source of great strength or considerable pain to a patient. Some find new faith during a cancer experience, while others find great turmoil. Spiritual care for the oncology patient can be either uncomfortable for the physician or, if the physician is overzealous, uncomfortable for the patient. Many doctors and nurses are appropriately uneasy when it comes to talking about religion because they fear they might be imposing their religious beliefs on others. The role of the physician is to advocate and try to connect a patient with chaplains, the patient's own religious community, or nonreligious groups that might help to provide solace.

The role of the oncologic chaplain can greatly aid in the spiritual journey of a patient, both as an inpatient and as an outpatient. Chaplains can help identify patients in spiritual distress and address the religious or spiritual issues raised by their illness. Those who have never had strong religious beliefs may not feel an urge to turn to religion, but as trained listeners, chaplains can help patients identify core beliefs, recognize coping skills, and, potentially, help patients to find sources of strength within or beyond themselves.

Chaplains also help families identify spiritual resources to enhance their coping with the level of distress during a loved one's illness. Often, chaplains are privy to information that may not be provided to the medical professional. This can, with permission, be shared for the benefit of the patient and improvement of care. Therefore, it is appropriate to involve chaplaincy in a patient's care. It is not necessary to ask whether a patient would like a chaplain, as the patient may feel undue pressure based on distorted understandings of a professional chaplain's role. A trained chaplain showing up at the bedside can lead to positive outcomes, even if the patient is enabled to say, "No, thank you" to spiritual care. Chaplains work to help people in crisis find a measure of control in the midst of what can feel like chaos.

KEY POINTS TO REMEMBER

- Pain is a common complaint in cancer patients, and is often inadequately controlled.
- The WHO recommends the use of an analgesic ladder based on pain severity in the approach to the selection of opioids to treat cancer pain.
- When starting narcotics to manage chronic pain, start with one drug at the lowest effective dose and titrate the drug to pain relief. Sustained-release preparations are extremely useful in the management of chronic pain.
- Breakthrough medications should be offered to all patients on chronic analgesics for acute situations. The minimum effective dose should be equivalent to 25% of the twice daily narcotic dose.
- Constipation should always be expected during opioid therapy, and prophylactic laxatives and/or stool softeners should be started with the initiation of narcotic medications.
- Nausea and vomiting are commonly associated with advanced malignancies for a variety of reasons. Effective medications are now available to decrease the morbidity associated with these symptoms.
- Diarrhea can be debilitating to an oncology patient. Patient education and management with antidiarrheal agents are most often effective in preventing patients from requiring hospitalizations for severe dehydration or electrolyte imbalances.
- Anorexia and cachexia are frequent symptoms of advanced malignancies. Some drugs, such as dexamethasone and megestrol, can assist in improving appetite, but more often, education of the patient and family members is most beneficial.
- O_2, opioids, and anxiolytics can be useful in the relief of dyspnea in the terminal patient.
- Anemia should be treated with transfusion only if the patient is symptomatic from anemia, with a hemoglobin of <8 g/dL.
- Depression is underdiagnosed and undertreated. First-line therapy is with selective serotonin reuptake inhibitors (SSRIs). Patients benefit from working with an oncologic psychologist for therapy.
- Anxiety should be addressed and treated with benzodiazepines as a first-line therapy. Chronic anxiety issues can be treated with long-acting benzodiazepines or buspirone.
- An underlying cause of delirium should be sought. Delirium may be treated with neuroleptics.
- Often chaplains are privy to information that may not be provided to the medical professional. This can, with permission, be shared for the benefit of the patient and overall improvement of patient care.

REFERENCES AND SUGGESTED READINGS

Berger J. Identifying spiritual landscapes among oncology patients. *Chaplaincy Today.* 1998;4(2):15–21.

Bonica JJ, Ventafridda V, Twycross RG. Cancer pain. In: Bonica JJ, ed. *The Management of Pain.* 2nd ed. Philadelphia: Lea & Febiger; 1990:400–460.

Levy MH. Drug therapy: pharmacologic treatment of cancer pain. *N Engl J Med.* 1996;335:1124–1132.

Ludwig H, Zojer N. Supportive care. *Ann Oncol.* 2007;18(Suppl 1):i37–i44.

National Comprehensive Cancer Network. Cancer pain treatment guidelines for patients. Version II, August 2005. Cancer pain. In: National Comprehensive Cancer Network Practice Guidelines in Oncology, 2005:1. Available at: http://www.nccn.org. Accessed June 2007.

National Comprehensive Cancer Network. Nausea and vomiting treatment guidelines for patients with cancer. Version III, June 2005. In: National Comprehensive Cancer Network Practice Guidelines in Oncology. Available at: http://www.nccn.org. Accessed June 2007.

Pharo GH, Zhou L. Pharmacologic management of cancer pain. *J Am Osteopath Assoc.* 2005;105(11; Suppl 5):S21–S28.

Rogakos J, Boyer S. Psychiatric disorders. In: Lin TL, Rypkema SW, eds. *The Washington Manual of Ambulatory Therapeutics.* Philadelphia: Lippincott Williams & Wilkins; 2002.

Schultz MZ. Oncology and palliative care. In: Lin TL, Rypkema SW, eds. *The Washington Manual of Ambulatory Therapeutics.* Philadelphia: Lippincott Williams & Wilkins; 2002:344–358.

Oncologic Emergencies

35

Lukas D. Wartman

INTRODUCTION

True oncologic emergencies are relatively infrequent. However, physicians who treat cancer patients are often called on to rule out an oncologic emergency. To diagnose and appropriately treat an oncologic emergency, physicians must have a working knowledge of the distinct presentation, appropriate diagnostic testing, and management of a wide array of complications that are often unique to cancer patients. These complications primarily result from pressure or obstruction by space-occupying lesions, metabolic abnormalities, or cytopenias.

MALIGNANT PERICARDIAL EFFUSION AND TAMPONADE

Introduction

Malignancy is a frequent cause of pericardial disease including pericardial effusion, cardiac tamponade, and constrictive pericarditis. Autopsy studies have reported that between 10% and 20% of patients with cancer will have malignant pericardial disease at the time of death. However, many of these cases were not clinically significant. Malignant pericardial disease is generally a manifestation of an advanced malignancy. The most common malignancies associated with pericardial involvement are lung cancer, breast cancer, and lymphoma.

Causes

Pathophysiology

Breast and lung tumors generally spread locally to cause pericardial disease. Lymphomas involving the mediastinum can involve the pericardium, whereas leukemias can infiltrate the myocardium, resulting in a pericardial effusion. Tumors in the pericardial space can cause bleeding and create a more rapidly accumulating effusion than in an exudative or transudative process. Patients with acute promyelocytic leukemia treated with all-trans retinoic acid can develop a treatment-related pericardial effusion.

Differential Diagnosis

The differential diagnosis of pericardial disease in a patient with malignancy also includes nonmalignant causes, such as radiation-induced effusion, hypothyroidism, autoimmune disorders, infection, uremia, and idiopathic pericardial disease.

Other pathologic entities may present with similar symptoms in the cancer patient. Cardiotoxicity leading to **congestive heart failure** can result from chemotherapy (such as anthracyclines, mitoxantrone, ifosfamide, and cyclophosphamide) or biologics (such as the monoclonal antibody trastuzumab). 5-Flurouracil (5-FU), a commonly used antimetabolite, is associated with acute cardiotoxicity that can lead to cardiac arrhythmia, myocardial ischemia, and, rarely, cardiogenic shock. Radiation therapy can also cause cardiomyopathy in the absence of pericardial disease (especially in the setting of mediastinal radiation for non-Hodgkin or Hodgkin lymphoma and left breast radiation for breast cancer). One must always consider other causes of cardiovascular emergencies in the cancer patient, such as coronary artery disease, heart failure, and infectious endocarditis.

Clinical Presentation

Patients with small, slowly expanding effusions may present with subtle nonspecific complaints such as weakness, fatigue, and dyspnea. If a large effusion accumulates rapidly, patients can develop cardiac tamponade and hemodynamic collapse. On evaluation, patients with tamponade exhibit signs of hypotension, tachycardia, jugular venous distention, and dulled heart tones. Another sign indicative of tamponade is pulsus paradoxus, or a >10 mm Hg decrease in systolic blood pressure with inspiration.

Management

Diagnosis

Patients with suspected pericardial disease should have an immediate chest radiograph and electrocardiogram (ECG). On chest x-ray, in the presence of a large effusion, the cardiac silhouette is enlarged in a globular, symmetric fashion. Chest x-ray may also reveal signs of pulmonary congestion and/or pleural effusions. ECG commonly shows sinus tachycardia and may reveal reduced voltage or, with very large effusions, electrical alternans. Transthoracic echocardiography is the diagnostic test of choice and should be ordered emergently whenever the diagnosis of tamponade is suspected. It will diagnose the effusion and indicate the degree of hemodynamic compromise. Early signs of tamponade on echo include right atrial and ventricular collapse.

Treatment

With severe hemodynamic compromise, emergent **pericardiocentesis** by a percutaneous, subxiphoid approach should be performed. Giving a **rapid IV fluid bolus and inotropics** can be temporizing measures to support the patient until echocardiographic guidance is available, as this method is much safer than a "blind" approach. A pericardial drain or a pericardial window may be necessary. To prevent recurrence, sclerosing agents such as thiotepa are available but are often less effective and have more risks than placing a **surgical pericardial window.** A surgical pericardial window is generally the definitive treatment for a clinically significant pericardial effusion. Radiation therapy can be used to manage pericardial effusions secondary to radiosensitive tumors such as leukemia and lymphoma. Small asymptomatic effusions may be observed without therapy.

SUPERIOR VENA CAVA SYNDROME

Introduction

Superior vena cava syndrome (SVCS) is the result of **obstruction of the SVC,** by either external compression or internal thrombosis.

Presentation

Patients typically present with swelling of the neck, face, and upper extremities. Jugular venous distention, cyanosis, and facial plethora may also be present. Shortness of breath, dizziness, and, rarely, obtundation from cerebral edema are possible if the onset is rapid. Very rarely, the process causes laryngeal edema and compromise of the upper airway. Vocal cord paralysis and Horner syndrome are also possible if neural structures are invaded.

With slowly progressive obstruction, collateral flow has time to develop, and symptoms related to vascular obstruction may be subtle.

Causes

Lung cancer (non-small-cell lung cancer followed by small-cell lung cancer) and lymphoma are the most common causes (~85%), although SVCS has been reported in breast cancer and other malignancies of the chest as well. These less common malignancies of the chest include germ cell tumors, thymoma, and mesothelioma. **Thrombosis of the SVC** in patients with central venous catheters is an increasingly common cause of SVCS. Other nonmalignant causes of SVCS include granulomatous infections, goiter, aortic aneurysms, and fibrosing mediastinitis.

Management

Diagnosis

CT scan of the chest with IV contrast is the diagnostic test of choice. CT findings are notable for reduced or absent opacification of central venous structures with prominent collateral venous circulation. **Chest radiography** may show a widened superior mediastinum and pleural effusions. There is no advantage of MRI over CT. A diagnosis of the mass should be attempted before treatment is begun if the tissue type of tumor is unknown. Sputum cytology, biopsy of lymph nodes, bronchoscopy, thoracentesis (if a pleural effusion is present), mediastinoscopy, or thoracotomy can be diagnostic. The workup generally progresses first through less invasive diagnostic testing (e.g., sputum cytology) before more invasive tests are performed (e.g., mediastinoscopy).

Treatment

Supportive measures including a low-salt diet, head elevation, and oxygen can be temporizing. Diuretics and corticosteroids (e.g., dexamethasone, 4 mg IV every 6 hours) have traditionally been used for treatment at presentation, although corticosteroids are likely only helpful in SVCS caused by lymphoma, and diuretics have not been shown to be helpful at all. If compression is not life-threatening, then a tissue diagnosis should be made before beginning treatment. **Radiation therapy** is useful for non-small-cell lung carcinoma and other metastatic solid tumors. Chemotherapy is more useful in small-cell lung cancer and lymphoma owing to their exquisite chemosensitivity, but small trials suggest that chemotherapy may be as effective as radiation therapy in treating SVCS secondary to non-small-cell lung cancer, which is relatively chemoinsensitive. SVCS resulting from catheter-related thrombus is treated by anticoagulation and, in limited cases, fibrinolysis. For emergent cases in which a prompt response is needed, experienced centers can perform angioplasty and stent placement. These approaches have largely replaced open surgical intervention, which is now generally done only when the surgical resection of the tumor is of benefit.

Prognosis

Multiple studies suggest that patients with SVCS do not have worsened survival compared to similarly staged patients with the same underlying malignancy and no history of SVCS.

ACUTE TUMOR LYSIS SYNDROME

Introduction

Acute tumor lysis syndrome (ATLS) represents a myriad of metabolic and electrolyte abnormalities that results from the release of intracellular products by rapidly dividing tumor cells prior to therapy or from the **lysis** of sensitive tumor cells **during therapy**. ATLS usually occurs in the setting of therapy of rapidly growing, hematologic malignancies,

TABLE 35-1   RISK FACTORS FOR TUMOR LYSIS SYNDROME

Patients at risk for acute tumor lysis syndrome

Tumor type
  High-grade non-Hodgkin lymphoma (example: Burkitt lymphoma)
  Acute leukemia (AML or ALL)
  Rapidly-growing solid tumors (small cell lung cancer)

Extent of disease
  Bulky tumors
  Elevated lactate dehydrogenase
  Elevated WBC count

Underlying renal dysfunction/oliguria

Elevated pre-treatment uric acid

Adapted from DeVita VT, Rosenberg SA, Hellman S, eds. *Cancer: Principles and Practice of Oncology.* 7th ed. Philadelphia: Lippincott, Williams & Wilkins; 2005:2292–2294.

classically acute lymphoblastic leukemia and high-grade non-Hodgkin lymphoma (e.g., Burkitt lymphoma). Rarely, ATLS has been described after the treatment of solid tumors such as breast cancer. The size of the tumor, rate of tumor growth, and sensitivity of the tumor cells to chemotherapy determine the risk of development of ATLS (Table 35-1).

Presentation

ATLS is characterized by the following electrolyte derangements: hyperuricemia, hyperkalemia, hyperphosphatemia, and hypocalcemia. These electrolyte abnormalities place patients at risk for cardiac arrhythmias and seizures. Acute renal failure and uremia can develop from precipitation of uric acid and calcium phosphate crystals in the renal tubules (Table 35-2).

TABLE 35-2   CAIRO-BISHOP DEFINITION OF ACUTE TUMOR LYSIS SYNDROME

Laboratory tumor lysis syndrome
  Uric acid >8 mg/dL or 25% increase from baseline
  Potassium >6 mEq/L or 25% increase from baseline
  Phosphorus >4.49 mg/dL or 25% increase from baseline
  Calcium <7 mg/dL or 25% decrease from baseline

Clinical tumor lysis syndrome
  Creatinine >1.5 times the upper limit of normal (adjusted for age)
  Cardiac arrhythmia or sudden death
  Seizure

Adapted from Cairo MS, Bishop M. Tumour lysis syndrome: new therapeutic strategies and classification. *Br J Haematol.* 2004;127:3–11.

Management

The best management of ATLS includes identifying patients at risk for ATLS and taking preventive measures.

- **IV hydration** should occur 24 to 48 hours before initiation of chemotherapy (3 liters/m^2/day) and during therapy. Consider using IV furosemide (Lasix) to improve urine flow rate if it is <100 mL/m^2/day. Electrolytes including phosphorus, calcium, and magnesium; uric acid; blood urea nitrogen; and creatinine should be measured three times a day in patients at risk for ATLS.
- **Hyperkalemia** should be treated with standard therapy: glucose and insulin (acutely), sodium-potassium exchange resins (Kayexalate), and IV calcium if ECG changes are noted.
- **Hyperuricemia** can be controlled with allopurinol (maximum 800 mg/day PO or 600 mg/day IV in adults) and/or rasburicase. Uric acid is relatively insoluble and can precipitate in renal tubules, causing acute renal failure. Allopurinol decreases the production of uric acid by inhibiting the enzyme, xanthine oxidase, which converts xanthine and hypoxanthine to uric acid. Allopurinol must be dose-reduced in patients with renal failure. Also, allopurinol inhibits the degradation of 6-mercaptopurine and azathioprine so these drugs must be dose-reduced if the patient is taking allopurinol. Allopurinol does not decrease the amount of uric acid already present. **Thus, one must initiate allopurinol before chemotherapy in patients with pre-existing hyperuricemia or in those at high risk for ATLS.**
- Rasburicase is a recombinant form of the enzyme, urate oxidase, which is derived from yeast and not found in humans. Urate oxidase breaks down uric acid to form allantoin. Allantoin is much more soluble in the urine than uric acid and can thus be renally excreted. Rasburicase is contraindicated in patients with glucose-6-phosphate dehydrogenase deficiency, as it can cause hemolysis. Other side effects of rasburicase include methemoglobinemia, bronchospasm, and anaphylaxis. The dosing of rasburicase is still not defined, but many institutions use 0.2 mg/kg for one dose and repeat doses only if hyperuricemia is still present. Rasburicase has not yet been rigorously tested in randomized, controlled trials in adults; however, case reports and pediatric data have demonstrated its efficacy. Rasburicase is now generally the standard of care for pediatric and adult patients with ATLS, while allopurinol remains the standard prophylactic therapy.
- Alkalinization of the urine to increase uric acid excretion can also be considered in the treatment of hyperuricemia. However, there is no clear evidence that it improves outcomes.
- **IV calcium should not be administered for hypocalcemia unless the patient is symptomatic.** Symptoms of hypocalcemia include muscular (cramps, spasms, and tetany), cardiac (arrhythmias and hypotension), and neurologic (confusion or seizures) abnormalities. A positive Chvostek or Trousseau sign is indicative of symptomatic hypocalemia. With a high serum phosphate level, IV calcium repletion may result in metastatic calcification and renal failure.
- In the setting of **hyperphosphatemia,** mild cases may be managed with PO antacids (phosphate binders), but **dialysis** may be necessary in patients with poor renal function or metabolic abnormalities not corrected by conservative measures.

HYPERCALCEMIA OF MALIGNANCY

Introduction

Hypercalcemia is the most common paraneoplastic syndrome, seen in 10% to 20% of patients with cancer. Malignancies of the lung, breast, head/neck, and kidney, as well as multiple myeloma, are most often associated with hypercalcemia.

Causes

Most commonly, a tumor causes hypercalcemia by producing ectopic parathormone-related protein (PTHrP), which stimulates osteoclasts to cause bone resorption as well as causing renal tubular calcium retention. Less commonly, tumor in bone can have a direct osteolytic activity through local cytokines. Rarely, lymphomas can produce ectopic activated vitamin D to cause hypercalcemia.

Presentation

Presentation is often nonspecific. Common symptoms include fatigue, anorexia, constipation, polydipsia, polyuria, nausea, vomiting, lethargy, and apathy. Nephrolithiasis is possible. In severe cases, mental status alterations, seizures, and coma can be seen. Hypercalcemia can cause renal parenchymal damage and nephrogenic diabetes insipidus. Hypercalcemia produces a brisk diuresis, and patients are often severely volume depleted. Most clinicians will remember the symptoms of hypercalcemia from the mnemonic: "stones, bones, abdominal groans, and psychic moans."

Management

Workup

Management includes obtaining an ionized calcium level (or an albumin level to correct for the hypoalbuminemia that is frequently seen in cancer patients). Serum intact parathormone (PTH) levels should be checked to rule out primary hyperparathyroidism. Intact PTH levels are suppressed in the hypercalcemia of malignancy. There is generally no need to check a PTHrP, as the diagnosis of malignant hypercalcemia is often made by history alone. Other causes of hypercalcemia such as thiazide diuretics, granulomatous disease, and vitamin D intoxication can also be ruled out by history alone. A serum phosphate level must be checked, as hypercalcemia often leads to clinically significant hypophosphatemia.

Treatment

- The acute treatment of hypercalcemia **begins with IV fluids** (4 to 8 liters). Normal saline is started at 200 to 500 mL/hour and decreased after the volume deficit is corrected. At least 3 to 4 liters should be given in the first 24 hours, and a positive fluid balance of at least 2 liters should be achieved. Further saline diuresis (100 to 200 mL/hour) will aid in calcium excretion. Serum electrolytes, including potassium, phosphate and magnesium, should be measured every 6 to 12 hours and corrected accordingly. Oral phosphate repletion is standard if the serum phosphate level is low and the patient has normal renal function. With IV phosphate repletion, there is the risk of calcium phosphate precipitation and renal failure. Its use should be reserved for serious cases of hypophosphatemia managed by experienced physicians. Furosemide can lead to greater calcium loss through the urine; however, its use is **contraindicated** until the patient is euvolemic and it is generally not necessary.
- Other than IV fluids, the mainstay of the treatment of hypercalcemia is a **bisphosphonate**. Two bisphosphonates are FDA approved for the treatment of hypercalcemia of malignancy: pamidronate (Aredia; 60 to 90 mg IV over 2 hours) and zoledronic acid (Zometa; 4 mg IV over 15 minutes). Bisphosphonates work by inhibiting bone resorption by osteoclasts. Side effects include flulike symptoms and fever, as well as renal failure (rarely). These drugs must be used with extreme caution in patients with underlying renal insufficiency and generally avoided in patients with significant renal impairment (creatinine clearance, <30 mL/min). Also, the dose of bisphosphonates will often need to be reduced in patients with renal insufficiency. Rarely, patients treated with bisphosphonates develop osteonecrosis of the jaw. The onset of action of the bisphosphonates is at between 2 and 4 days, with the peak effect generally between day 4 and day 7.

- **Glucocorticoids** (e.g., prednisone at an initial dose of 0.5 to 1 mg/kg/day) may be effective in hypercalcemia due to some hematologic malignancies and myeloma. Results may take up to 10 days and side effects of steroid treatment are common. In addition, dialysis is effective if other treatments fail. Other drugs that are rarely used (now mostly in hypercalcemia refractory to bisphosphonates) include calcitonin, gallium nitrate, and plicamycin (mithramycin). Of course, the definitive treatment of hypercalcemia is successful treatment of the underlying malignancy.

SYNDROME OF INAPPROPRIATE ANTIDIURESIS AND HYPONATREMIA

Introduction

The syndrome of inappropriate antidiuresis (SIAD) was formerly known as the syndrome of inappropriate secretion of andiurectic hormone (SIADH). It is now recognized that antidiuretic hormone (ADH)/vasopressin levels are commonly suppressed in patients with the syndrome, but affected patients have their homeostatic set-point for sodium set at a lower level than normal. SIAD is seen most commonly in small-cell lung cancer but can also be seen in many other malignancies including tumors of the upper gastrointestinal and genitourinary tract.

Causes

In addition to SIAD directly related to the malignancy, drugs can also cause the inappropriate release of vasopressin or attenuate its action. Common drugs that can cause SIAD include morphine, vincristine sulfate, and cyclophosphamide. Pulmonary and central nervous system disease can also cause SIAD that is not related to an underlying malignancy.

Presentation

Patients with SIAD and hyponatremia may present with complaints of anorexia and nausea. With rapid and severe decline in serum sodium concentrations, they may also present with confusion, coma, and seizures. Look for decreased serum osmolality (<270 mOsm/L) and urine that is not maximally dilute (>100 mOsm/L). In addition to the previously mentioned findings, the diagnosis of SIAD requires the absence of a hypervolemic state (manifest by ascites, edema) and absence of volume contraction, along with normal thyroid, renal, and adrenal function.

Management

Acute management includes IV normal saline or, in more severe cases, 3% sodium chloride (which should typically *only* be given with the assistance of someone skilled in its use, such as a nephrologist). Allow only 1 to 2 mEq/L/hour of correction for the first 3 to 4 hours and ≤ 0.5 mEq/L/hour thereafter to avoid *demyelination* syndromes (use even lower rates of correction for patients with chronic hyponatremia or hyponatremia of unknown duration—generally 0.5 to 1 mEq/L/hour). To avoid potentially catastrophic demyelination, the overall rate of correction is limited to 8 to 10 mEq/L/day. Furosemide may add to free water loss when given with saline. Demeclocycline is an antibiotic that lowers urine osmolality and can be useful in long-term therapy, but renal toxicity limits its use.

Finally, **vasopressin-receptor antagonists** are a new option for the treatment of SIAD. The first to be FDA approved was conivaptan (Vaprisol), an IV formulation that blocks both the V_{1A} and the V_2 vasopressin receptors. Newer drugs that are currently being tested include tolvaptan and lixivaptan. Both are selective V_2 antagonists (and thus have less potential for causing hypotension) and are available in oral formulations. The role of the new vasopressin-receptor antagonists in the management of SIAD will be defined over the next several years.

NEUTROPENIC FEVER

Introduction
Background
Neutropenic fever is one of the most common complications of chemotherapy. Risk of infection is slightly increased with granulocyte counts <1000/μL, markedly increased with granulocytes <500/μL, and highest with granulocyte counts <100/μL. Eighty percent of infections in the neutropenic patient originate from the patient's own flora. As many neutropenic patients also have long-term vascular access in place, these are common sources as well. Likely microbes include both gram-positive (*Staphylococcus, Streptococcus*) and gram-negative aerobes (*Escherichia coli, Klebsiella pneumonia, Pseudomonas aeruginosa*).

Definition
Neutropenic fever is defined as a single **temperature >38.3°C** (or a temperature >38.0°C for >1 hour) in patients with an **absolute neutrophil count <500/μL** (or <1000/μL that is expected to decrease to <500/μL).

Presentation
Signs of infection, such as exudate, erythema, and warmth, may not be evident because of the reduced numbers of neutrophils. Pneumonias may only be evident by rales, and an infiltrate on chest x-ray may be lacking. Physical exam should focus on the skin, ocular fundus, sinuses, CNS, pelvis, and perirectal area.

Management
Workup
Management includes searching for a **source of infection** by obtaining two sets of blood cultures, with one set from any indwelling intravascular catheter. Sputum and urine cultures are indicated, and chest x-ray should also be obtained. If diarrhea is present, a workup for infectious etiologies is indicated including stool culture and *Clostridium difficile* antigen testing. Lumbar puncture is not indicated unless clinical signs of meningitis are present, as neutropenia does not predispose to meningitis. In addition, lumbar puncture in the setting of thrombocytopenia can be dangerous.

Treatment
    Antimicrobial Therapy. Antimicrobial therapy should not await the results of diagnostic tests, as patients can die of gram-negative sepsis in a matter of hours after their first fever, despite appearing well at initial presentation.

Empiric Antimicrobial Therapy in Neutropenic Fever
- Initial therapy is antipseudomonal beta-lactam ± aminoglycoside. A single agent such as cefepime (2 g IV every 8 hours in patients with normal renal function) may be used, depending on local sensitivities.
- If the patient is still febrile after 3 days of treatment: add vancomycin (1 g IV every 12 hours in normal renal function or adjusted based on trough levels).
- If the patient is still febrile after 5 to 7 days, antifungal coverage should be added. Caspofungin, voriconazole, and posaconazole are reasonable choices, depending on the clinical circumstances. Treatment with amphotericin B is usually limited to refractory infections or critically ill patients who have not responded to the above agents.

The above are only general guidelines. If the patient is penicillin allergic, consider substituting a fourth-generation fluoroquinolone. If contraindications to aminoglycosides are present, substitute a fluoroquinolone or aztreonam. One should consider using vancomycin as initial therapy in addition to the previously mentioned antibiotics if the patient is hypotensive, has severe mucositis, is colonized with methicillin-resistant *Staphylococcus aureus*, or has signs of obvious catheter infection. Antibacterial choice may vary depending on organisms and resistance patterns at particular hospitals or communities. Always consider other causes of fever in the febrile neutropenic, such as thrombosis. The role of colony-stimulating factors in neutropenic fever is controversial, but administration should be considered in critically ill patients. Antimicrobials should be continued until the neutrophil count rises above $500/\text{mm}^3$ for 2 days and the patient has been afebrile without evidence of infection for the same duration. Other precautions, such as visitor screening, hand washing, and proper isolation measures, should be maintained during this period.

EPIDURAL SPINAL CORD COMPRESSION

Introduction

Epidural spinal cord compression (ESCC), occurring in 5% of cancer patients, is one of the most common oncologic emergencies. The dural sac is compressed by tumor in the epidural space at the level of the spinal cord or cauda equine; neurologic deficits may result. *If ESCC is caught early, when pain is the only symptom, the patient can be spared significant disability.*

Causes

Any malignancy can produce epidural compression, with lung, breast, and prostate cancers being the most common, followed by lymphoma, myeloma, and sarcoma. The thoracic spine is the most common location, followed by the lumbosacral and then the cervical spine. Osteolytic lesions of the vertebral column cause most cases. Compression occurs either by direct extension from metastases in the vertebral bone or by tumor growth through the intervertebral foramina. On occasion, tumor can metastasize directly to the epidural space.

Presentation

Back pain is the first symptom in 90% of patients. The pain localizes in the back, near the midline, and is frequently accompanied by referred or radicular pain. The pain, unlike the pain of a herniated disc, may be exacerbated by recumbency and improved by the upright position. Many patients are unaware that back pain is related to their underlying malignancy and do not seek treatment. Weakness and sensory impairment may follow from hours to months after the onset of pain. Regardless of the spinal compression site, weakness tends to begin in the proximal legs. The weakness can progress to **paraplegia** and can occasionally develop abruptly without prior clinical signs. At presentation, about 80% of patients complain of weakness, usually affecting gait. About 50% of patients have sensory complaints at presentation. These complaints range from paresthesias to loss of sensation. Autonomic dysfunction, including impotence and bowel/bladder dysfunction, occurs late and is generally not the sole presenting symptom.

Management

Diagnosis

Whole-spine MRI is the diagnostic test of choice for ESCC. **The entire spine should be imaged because of the high incidence of asymptomatic multilevel disease.** CT myelography is necessary for patients with contraindications for MRI. In published studies, CT myelography is as accurate as MRI, but MRI is noninvasive, safer, and better tolerated. One must also consider other causes of spinal cord dysfunction, such as myelopathy, intramedullary metastases, hematoma, and abscess. Lumbar puncture to search for additional causes should not be performed until spinal cord compression is excluded.

Treatment

Dexamethasone is the indicated medical treatment of nearly all patients with ESCC. Treatment should begin immediately after the diagnosis is suspected and not be delayed until the results of imaging studies are available. The dose is controversial, but a common regimen is a 10-mg IV bolus followed by 4 mg IV every 6 hours (although this regimen is not supported by published evidence). Next, all patients should have an immediate neurosurgical consultation. Patchell and colleagues (2005) published a pivotal randomized study showing that initial operative treatment benefits a subgroup of patients with ESCC. The general indications for surgery include spinal instability with bony compression, neurologic progression during or after radiation therapy, unknown primary site with surgical decompression and biopsy, and a single site of cord compression. The exclusion criteria of the published study were patients with paraplegia for >48 hours prior to study entry, multiple compressive lesions, pre-existing neurologic conditions including brain metastases, and radiosensitive tumors (lymphoma, leukemia, multiple myeloma, and germ cell tumors). Radiation therapy is also indicated in nearly all patients with ESCC, either in lieu of surgery or after surgery. The most common regimen is 10 uninterrupted fractions of 3 Gy each.

OTHER NEUROLOGIC EMERGENCIES

- **Increased intracerebral pressure and cerebral herniation** (from brain metastases, hemorrhage, venous sinus thrombosis, meningitis, head trauma, infarction, or abscess). Again, immediate consultation with neurosurgery is often essential. The patient should be stabilized, and maneuvers to lower intracranial pressures such as hyperventilation and IV mannitol and/or dexamethasone should be attempted. A head CT scan can aid in determining whether surgery is indicated.
- **Status epilepticus** (from brain metastases, metabolic derangement, or neurotoxicity of cancer therapy). Ensuring an airway should be the first and foremost concern. Laboratory studies such as glucose, electrolytes, Ca, Mg, serum and urine toxicology screens, serum alcohol level, CBC, urinalysis, and any pertinent medication levels must be obtained. IV benzodiazepines, phenytoin, and barbiturates are used in the treatment of status epilepticus. If the patient does not have IV access, benzodiazepines are also available in rectal, IM, or intranasal formulations.
- **Intracerebral hemorrhage** (from metastatic tumor, thrombocytopenia, or leukostasis). Headache, vomiting, and mental status changes are symptoms of significantly increased intracranial pressure and hemorrhage. Workup should include imaging with a STAT noncontrast head CT scan and possibly a lumbar puncture (if CT is nondiagnostic). Therapy largely focuses on maintenance of adequate blood pressure, supportive care, correction of coagulopathy and thrombocytopenia, and surgical consultation when appropriate.

PATHOLOGIC FRACTURES

Definition

Pathologic fractures are defined as fractures occurring in diseased bone.

Causes

Breast, prostate, kidney, and lung are the most common carcinomas to metastasize to bone and potentially cause fracture. The majority of patients have multiple metastatic lesions.

Presentation

Symptoms include new-onset bone pain in patients with a history of a primary carcinoma.

Management

In the management of the pathologic fracture, consider life expectancy, as most fractures are best treated surgically with internal fixation. IV narcotics and fracture immobilization are used to control pain and bleeding. Consultation with orthopedics is necessary. Hip and femur fractures will require traction, whereas casts or splints may be used for distal fractures. Radiographs of the region in at least two planes are needed. A bone scan may be obtained to locate occult lesions. Radiographs of involved bones may identify other areas of impending fracture. Both the pathologic fracture and impending fractures could thus be repaired during one surgery. Bisphosphonates have an expanding role in the prevention of further pathologic fracture, and treatment with pamidronate or zoledronic acid should be considered in patients with pathologic fracture. Consultation with radiation oncology is indicated to determine whether the patient could benefit from radiation therapy as well.

KEY POINTS TO REMEMBER

- The amount of disability after treatment of spinal cord compression is directly related to both the pre-event level of function and the swiftness of diagnosis. When it is suspected, use MRI liberally to diagnose ESCC, and image the entire spine.
- Give steroids for suspected spinal cord compression before awaiting the results of imaging studies.
- Antimicrobial therapy for neutropenic fever must start immediately with broad-spectrum agents before any test results are back.
- The initial treatment of both hypercalcemia and tumor lysis syndrome includes IV fluids.

REFERENCES AND SUGGESTED READINGS

Brigden ML. Hematologic and oncological emergencies: doing the most good in the least time. *Postgrad Med.* 2001;109(3):143–163.

Cairo M, Bishop M. Tumour lysis syndrome: new therapeutic strategies and classification. *Br J Haematol.* 2004;127:3–11.

De Vita VT, Rosenberg SA, Hellman S, eds. *Cancer: Principles and Practice of Oncology.* 7th ed. Philadelphia: Lippincott, Williams & Wilkins; 2005:2292–2294.

Ellison DH, Berl T. The syndrome of inappropriate antidiuresis. *N Engl J Med.* 2007;356:2064–2072.

Hughes WT, Armstrong D, Bodey GP, et al. 2002 Guidelines for the use of antimicrobial agents in neutropenic patients with cancer. *Clin Infect Dis.* 2002;34:730–751.

Patchell RA, Tibbs PA, Regine WF, et al. Direct decompressive surgical resection in the treatment of spinal cord compression caused by metastatic cancer: a randomized trial. *Lancet.* 2005;366:643–648.

Retter AS. Pericardial disease in the oncology patient. *Heart Dis.* 2002;4:387–391.

Sood AR, Burry LD, Cheng KF. Clarifying the role of rasburicase in tumor lysis syndrome. *Pharmacotherapy.* 2007;27(1):111–121.

Stewart AF. Hypercalcemia associated with cancer. *N Engl J Med.* 2005;352:373–379.

Wilson LD, Detterbeck FC, Yahalom J. Superior vena cava syndrome with malignant causes. *N Engl J Med.* 2007;356:1862–1869.

Index

Page numbers followed by *f* refer to figures; page numbers followed by *t* refer to tables.